Pregnancy For Dumm

Important Phone Numbers and Addresses

Your GP:

Name ______________________

Phone number ______________________

Address ______________________

Your midwife or consultant:

Name ______________________

Phone number ______________________

Address ______________________

Hospital or birthing centre:

Name ______________________

Phone number ______________________

Address ______________________

Labour ward:

Phone number ______________________

Things to Remember to Take to the Hospital

- ❑ Your partner or birthing partner (!)
- ❑ A dressing gown, nightgown, slippers, and socks
- ❑ Toiletries
- ❑ Sturdy underwear (that you don't mind soiling with blood), nursing bras, and breast pads
- ❑ A change of clothes to wear home, including comfortable, roomy shoes
- ❑ Baby clothes
- ❑ Infant car seat (your partner can bring this item on the day of discharge)
- ❑ Sanitary pads (if you don't want to use the archaic ones that most hospitals provide)
- ❑ A camera (don't forget the film!)
- ❑ A hot water bottle (for pain relief)
- ❑ Telephone numbers of family and friends you may want to call
- ❑ Radio/cassette/CD player, if you want
- ❑ Change for telephones, parking, or vending machines

Item 7042-0.

For more information about John Wiley & Sons, call (+44) 1243 779777.

For Dummies: Bestselling Book Series for Beginners

Pregnancy For Dummies®

Cheat Sheet

A Typical Schedule for Antenatal Visits and Tests

Your abdomen, blood pressure, and urine will usually be examined at every appointment – if an appointment has no additional information next to it, that's what you can expect. Other routine tests, which are needed at particular stages, are listed. Extra tests may be needed if any abnormalities are found.

Weeks	*Schedule and Tests*
5–8	GP visit for referral for antenatal care; delivery, weight, and height tests
11–14	Hospital booking appointment – screening tests for foetal abnormalities, ultrasound, and blood tests
16	Discuss results of tests to date
18–20	Ultrasound to check for foetal anatomy and abnormalities
25*	Routine appointment
28	Tests for anaemia and Rhesus antibodies if Rhesus negative, first Anti-D treatment
31*	Routine appointment
34	Second Anti-D treatment if Rhesus negative
36	Check if baby is cephalic (head down) and discuss birth options if not
38	Routine appointment
40*	Routine appointment
41	Options for membrane sweep and/or induction

** indicates visit in first pregnancies only*

Commonly Used Medical Abbreviations

Abbreviation	*What It Stands For*
Ceph	Cephalic (baby's head facing down into your pelvis)
CRL	Crown-Rump Length
CTG	Cardiotocograph (a tracing of your baby's heart and your contractions)
CVS	Chorionic Villus Sampling
EDD	Estimated Date of Delivery or Estimated Due Date
FBC	Full Blood Count (to test for anaemia infection and clotting problems)
FHHR	Foetal Heart Heard Regular
FMF	Foetal Movement Felt
G-P-	Gravida-Para- (gravida is the number of pregnancies, para the number of births)
GTT	Glucose Tolerance Test (to check for diabetes)
IUGR	Intrauterine Growth Restriction or Retardation
LMP	Last Menstrual Period
NAD	No Abnormality Detected (often used when urine is checked)
N/E	Not Engaged (the widest part of your baby's head has not moved into your pelvis)
OP	Occipito-posterior (baby's head facing backwards, with its spine lying along yours)

Your Baby's Growth

Weeks Pregnant (measured from LMP)	*Average Weight*	*Average Length*	*Weeks Pregnant (measured from LMP)*	*Average Weight*	*Average Length*
8	0.035 oz (1 g)	1.5 in (3.81 cm)	26	2 lb (0.91 kg)	12.5 in (31.75 cm)
10	0.175 oz (5 g)	2.4 in (6.10 cm)	28	2 lb 12 oz (1.25 kg)	13.7 in (34.80 cm)
12	0.7 oz (20 g)	3.5 in (8.89 cm)	30	3 lb 10 oz (1.65 kg)	14.8 in (37.60 cm)
14	2.1 oz (60 g)	4.1 in (10.41 cm)	32	4 lb 6 oz (2.00 kg)	15.6 in (39.62 cm)
16	4.2 oz (0.12 kg)	6.25 in (15.88 cm)	34	5 lb 3 oz (2.35 kg)	16.4 in (41.66 cm)
18	8.0 oz (0.23 kg)	7.8 in (19.81 cm)	36	6 lb (2.72 kg)	17.5 in (44.45 cm)
20	12.0 oz (0.34 kg)	9.75 in (24.77 cm)	38	6 lb 12 oz (3.10 kg)	18.7 in (47.50 cm)
22	1 lb (0.45 kg)	11.0 in (27.94 cm)	40	7 lb 8 oz (3.40 kg)	19.5 in (49.53 cm)
24	1 lb 8 oz (0.68 kg)	11.7 in (29.72 cm)			

lb = pounds   cm = centimetres   oz = ounces   g = grams   in = inches   kg = kilograms

Pregnancy FOR DUMMIES®

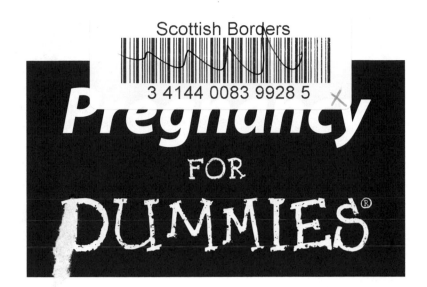

Pregnancy FOR DUMMIES®

by Dr Sarah Jarvis, GP, Joanne Stone, MD,
Keith Eddleman, MD, and Mary Duenwald

JOHN WILEY & SONS, LTD

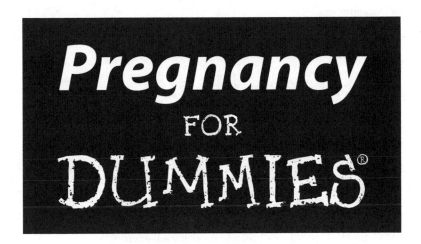

Pregnancy For Dummies®
Published by
John Wiley & Sons, Ltd
The Atrium
Southern Gate
Chichester West Sussex

E-mail (for orders and customer service enquires): cs-books@wiley.co.uk

Visit our Home Page on www.wileyeurope.com

Wiley also publishes its books in a variety of electronic formats. Some content that appears in print may not be available in electronic books.

A catalogue record for this book is available from the British Library.

ISBN 978-07645-7042-1 (PB)

Printed and bound in Great Britain by TJ International, Padstow, Cornwall

10 9 8 7 6

WILEY

About the Authors

Joanne Stone, MD, is a full-time faculty member in the internationally renowned Division of Maternal-Fetal Medicine at The Mount Sinai Medical Center in New York City. She is the director of the Perinatal Ultrasound Unit and also cares for patients with problem pregnancies. She has lectured throughout the USA, is widely published in medical journals, and has been interviewed frequently for television and magazines on topics related to pregnancy, with a special emphasis on the management of multifoetal pregnancies. She was a co-star in the critically acclaimed series *Pregnancy For Dummies* on the Discovery Health Channel. Away from the hospital she loves to spend time with her husband, George, and her two little girls, Chloe and Sabrina.

Keith Eddleman, MD, works with Joanne at Mount Sinai. He is also a full-time faculty member and is the Director of the Division of Maternal-Fetal Medicine. He teaches medical students, residents, and fellows; lectures throughout the world; and appears often on television to discuss issues concerning the care of pregnant women. His areas of special expertise are ultrasound and reproductive genetics. He was also a co-star on the critically-acclaimed series *Pregnancy For Dummies* on the Discovery Health Channel. His free time, when he has any, is split between spending time with his family at their apartment in Manhattan or at their country house in upstate New York.

Mary Duenwald is a writer and editor who has for many years specialised in medicine and science journalism. She has written for *The New York Times*, *Discover*, *Smithsonian*, and *Departures*. She has been executive editor of *Harper's Bazaar*, *Women's Sports & Fitness*, and *The Sciences* magazines and a senior editor for *Vogue*. She is currently a contributing editor for *GQ*. She is also the mother of 14-year-old twins, Nick and Claire Murray.

Dr Sarah Jarvis is a GP and GP trainer in inner city London. She is a Fellow of, and the Women's Health spokesperson for, the Royal College of General Practitioners (RCGP). She was a founder member, and later chair, of the Women's Taskforce at the RCGP. She was also the medical advisor/presenter of the television series, *The Maternity Guide*, on Channel Health. She is also a medical writer and broadcaster, and appears regularly on Radio Five Live, GMTV, and ITN lunchtime news, as well as being the Radio 2 doctor. She writes regularly for a variety of magazines, including *Good Housekeeping*, *Women's Health*, *Pregnancy*, and *Baby and You*. Her great passion (as far as work is concerned) is patient education, and she has written over 500 patient information leaflets, as well as two previous books, *A Younger Woman's Diagnose-It-Yourself Guide to Health* and *Diabetes For Dummies*. Her other great passion is her family, and she loves spending time with her husband, Simon, their two children, Seth and Matilda, and their dog, Dascha.

Dedication

Joanne, Keith, and Mary:

To George, Chloe, Sabrina, Regina, Philip, Frank, Melba, Jack, Nick, and Claire for all their love and support.

Sarah:

To Seth and Matilda, who remind me daily that pregnancy was worth it.

Authors' Acknowledgements

Writing this book was truly a labour of love. We would like to thank everyone who played a part in the 'birth' of this book, and specifically the following:

Kathy Cox, Traci Cumbay, Chad Sievers, Tami Booth, Jennifer Ehrlich, Christy Beck, Elizabeth Kuball, Paula Lowell, and the other folks at Wiley, who conceived this idea and walked us through the whole process. Sophia Seidner, Carolyn Krupp, and the folks at International Management Group for connecting us with Wiley. Dr Jill Fishbane-Mayer for establishing the initial connection. Drs Jeffrey Penman, Lynn Friedman, Mary D'Alton, Richard Berkowitz, and Ramona Slupik for excellent comments and suggestions. Dr Ian Holzman for nurturing us through the newborn chapter. Kathryn Born for taking our scrap art and turning it into terrific illustrations. And to all our patients over the years whose inquisitive minds and need for accurate information inspired us to write this book.

— Joanne, Keith, and Mary

I would like to thank my husband, Simon, who is the best father in the world – and the source of more than his fair share of pregnancy-related anecdotes; my children, who have been remarkably patient as I laboured through the writing of not just one, but two *For Dummies* books; my mother-in-law, Lotte, who has been a fount of common sense as well as invaluable medical input; and my father Derek, who reminds me what bravery is all about. I would also like to acknowledge the enduring support of all my colleagues at the Richford Gate Medical Practice, and of Mr Silesh Kumar, who nurtured me through the sections on maternal-foetal medicine.

— Sarah

Publisher's Acknowledgements

We're proud of this book; please send us your comments through our Dummies online registration form located at www.dummies.com/register/.

Some of the people who helped bring this book to market include the following:

Acquisitions, Editorial, and Media Development

Project Editor: Daniel Mersey

Executive Editor: Jason Dunne

Executive Project Editor: Amie Tibble

Assistant Editor: Samantha Clapp

Copy Editor: Martin Key

Technical Reviewer: Jane Bashford

Special Help: Zoë Wykes

Cover Photos: © Getty Images/ Jack Hollingsworth

Cartoons: Ed McLachlan

Composition

Project Coordinator: Erin Smith

Layout and Graphics: Carl Byers, Amanda Carter, Andrea Dahl, Lauren Goddard, Joyce Haughey, Clint Lahnen, Barry Offringa, Jacque Roth, Heather Ryan

Proofreaders: Laura Albert, Carl Pierce, Brian H. Walls, TECHBOOKS Production Services

Indexer: TECHBOOKS Production Services

Publishing and Editorial for Consumer Dummies

Diane Graves Steele, Vice President and Publisher, Consumer Dummies

Joyce Pepple, Acquisitions Director, Consumer Dummies

Kristin A Cocks, Product Development Director, Consumer Dummies

Michael Spring, Vice President and Publisher, Travel

Brice Gosnell, Associate Publisher, Travel

Kelly Regan, Editorial Director, Travel

Publishing for Technology Dummies

Andy Cummings, Vice President and Publisher, Dummies Technology/General User

Composition Services

Gerry Fahey, Vice President of Production Services

Debbie Stailey, Director of Composition Services

Contents at a Glance

Table of Contents

Introduction

Our goal, in writing *Pregnancy For Dummies*, has been to write a scientifically correct, comprehensive guide to what is one of the most memorable experiences in anyone's life – pregnancy. We have dozens of years of experience caring for pregnant women from all walks of life and, equally relevant, many of us have been pregnant, allowing us to look at this life-changing event from both sides of the coin.

About This Book

We want this book to be practical, as well as theoretically accurate – and there's nothing like personal experience to make you realise that intellect and human nature are sometimes mutually exclusive! For example, if Sarah had been asked to talk on her radio show about the scare relating to second-hand cot mattresses and cot death in 1994, she would have dismissed it as unscientific scaremongering – as it was, she sat on a postnatal ward with her one-day-old first baby, refusing to take her son home until her husband had bought a new cot mattress! In this book, we don't just roll out the party-line answer, or the safe answer; instead, we base our response on medical research. Sometimes, no solid evidence exists to indicate whether something is safe or unsafe, and when this is the case, we tell you.

Too often, our patients come to us incredibly worried about something they've read in another book (or a newspaper) that's either outdated, lacks any real scientific basis, or is exaggerated way out of proportion. Our experience of medical scare stories in the media is that they will often give only one side of the story, in order to make more dramatic headlines. For example, a headline that shouts 'Caffeine linked to miscarriage' will sell more papers than 'Women who drink large quantities of coffee may have a higher chance of miscarriage; however, there's a significant chance that this relationship is a link, rather than a causal association, and moderate intake is unlikely to be a factor'.

We don't aim to ignore these scares – our own experience has shown us that intelligent women (and men) need informing, not patronising. So, we put facts and figures into perspective and provide you with enough information to come to a really informed decision for yourself. Pregnancy should be a joy, not a worry. A big part of our philosophy in writing this book is to reassure pregnant women (and their partners) whenever medically possible, rather than to add to the unnecessary worries they already have.

Our experience has shown us that prospective parents also want to know about the real medical aspects of pregnancy. When is the baby's heart formed? When are fingers developed? What blood tests should be done, and why? What options are available for detecting various problems? In addressing these topics, we have attempted to write a book that is essentially a medical text on obstetrics for the layperson.

We trust that you will use this book as a companion to regular medical care. Perhaps some of the information in it will lead you to ask your practitioner questions that you may not otherwise have thought to ask. Because there isn't always just one answer, or even a right answer, to every question, you may find that your practitioner holds a different point of view than we do in some areas. This difference of opinion is only natural, and in fact, we even occasionally disagree with each other. The bottom line is that this book provides a lot of factual information, but do not consider it 'gospel'. Remember also that many topics we discuss apply to pregnancy in general, but your particular situation may have unique aspects to it that warrant different or extra consideration.

Conventions Used in This Book

Understanding a few conventions that we used while writing this book can help you when reading this book.

We try to be respectful of the fact that although traditional husband-wife couples still account for the majority of expectant parents, babies are born into many different circumstances.

We also realise that doctors aren't the only health professionals who help women through pregnancy. (See Chapter 2 for specific descriptions of the many kinds of professionals who can play a major role in helping women through pregnancy and childbirth.) That is why, in many cases, we refer to your pregnancy professional as your 'practitioner'. In some cases, we do specify 'doctor', but usually only when we describe a situation that clearly calls for the services of an obstetrician (or sometimes your GP).

What You're Not to Read

Any text preceded by a Technical Stuff icon contains information for the very curious and offers deeper, usually scientific or (of course) technical explanations of topics. These nuggets of information may be of interest to you, or they may not, but rest assured that you may safely skip them and still find everything you need to know about pregnancy.

Foolish Assumptions

As we wrote this book, we made some assumptions about you and what your needs may be:

- You may be a woman who is considering pregnancy, planning to have a baby, or already pregnant.
- You may be the partner of the mother-to-be.
- You may know and love someone who is, or plans to be, pregnant.
- You want to find out more about pregnancy but have no interest in becoming an expert on the topic.

If you fit any of these criteria, then *Pregnancy For Dummies* gives you the information you're looking for!

How This Book Is Organised

The parts and chapters of this book represent a logical flow of information about the pregnancy process. However, you don't have to read it in order. You can pick up this book, thumb through it and read what stands out, look up specific topics in the table of contents or index, or read it cover to cover. Check out the following sections for a more detailed overview.

Part I: The Game Plan

Of course, some women get pregnant 'accidentally'. In fact, the UK has one of the highest rates of unplanned pregnancy in Europe. But for many women these days, pregnancy is a conscious choice. Planning ahead is a good idea – even seeing your GP before you conceive. Even if it's already too late to plan that far ahead, this part of the book fills you in on what's happening to your body during the first days and weeks of pregnancy. In this part, you can also find out what happens at an antenatal visit, as well as your legal entitlements. And you can find out the general scope of what your life will be like for the next 40 weeks.

Part II: Pregnancy: A Drama in Three Acts

Like all good narratives, pregnancy has a beginning, a middle, and an end – called *trimesters*. Because pregnancy is about nine months' long, the trimesters are divided into (approximately) three periods of 13 weeks – 0–12, 13–26 and 27–40. The way you feel and the kind of care you need vary with each stage. In this part, you get an idea of how each trimester unfolds.

Part III: The Big Event: Labour, Delivery, and Recovery

After you've put in your nine months, it's time for the flurry of activity that results in the birth of your baby. At this point, a lot is going on in a short time. Your experience depends heavily on what kind of delivery you have and how long it takes. This part covers the basic scenario of labour, delivery, and recovery – plus many possible variations on the theme.

Part IV: Special Concerns

This part is where to look for information about all kinds of special concerns that you may have as new parents – from practical challenges like how to introduce older siblings to the new baby to health problems that sometimes arise during pregnancy.

In an ideal world we would not need a section about problems that come up during pregnancy because every woman's experience would be perfectly trouble-free. On the other hand, many of the difficulties that sometimes arise need not develop into full-blown problems if they are properly taken care of. For this reason, we offer information about how to deal with anything that can come up. This part is the one to consult if you think you're having any kind of difficulty, from the serious to the mundane.

Part V: The Part of Tens

The 'Part of Tens' is standard in all *For Dummies* books. Before we began writing the book, we weren't sure how to make this part of our book useful. But in the end, we were very glad to have a place where we could put many aspects of pregnancy in a nutshell. Here you find out more about how the baby grows and how you can view him or her on ultrasound. We also dispel some common myths and give you some good reasons to relax and enjoy your pregnancy.

Appendix

In most pregnancy books, the father of the baby is, sadly, overlooked. We think that's a shame. Dads are, of course, welcome to read any part of the book that interests them – we include information aimed at them through the rest of the book – but we also include an insightful overview of the entire process, specifically with dads in mind, in the Appendix. Enjoy!

Icons Used in This Book

Like other books, this one has little icons in the margins to guide you through the information and zero in on what you need to find out. The following paragraphs describe the icons and what they mean.

This icon signals that we're going to delve a little deeper than usual into a medical explanation. We don't mean to suggest the information is too difficult to understand – just a little more detailed.

We flag certain pieces of information with this icon to let you know something is particularly worth keeping in mind.

This icon marks bits of advice we can give you about handling some of the minor discomforts and other challenges you encounter during pregnancy.

Throughout this book, we try to avoid being too alarmist, but there are some situations and actions that a pregnant woman clearly should avoid. When this is the case, we show you the Caution icon.

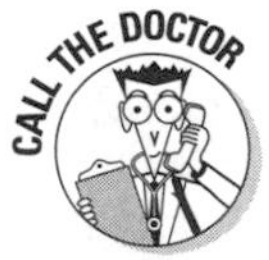

Many things you may feel or notice while you're pregnant will beg the question, 'Is this important enough for my practitioner to know about?' When the answer is yes, you see this icon.

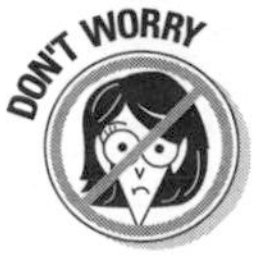

We know from experience that pregnancy can bring out the instinct to worry. Feeling a little anxious from time to time is normal, but some women go overboard working themselves up over things that really aren't a problem. We use this icon – more than any other one – to point out the countless things that you really need not fret about.

We're well aware that a dad's perspective and a mum's perspective are very different. That doesn't mean that dads are less important, or less well informed, and this icon helps dads-to-be (and their partners) to understand what's going on.

Where to Go from Here

If you're the particularly thorough type, start with Chapter 1 and end with the Appendix. If you just want to find specific information and then close the book, take a look at the table of contents or at the index.

Of course every mother, just like every pregnancy, is unique. Some women have particular risks because of their genetic make-up, their age, or their past medical history. Because of this, several sections of this book may be of no relevance to some pregnant women – the 'In this Chapter' list at the start of each chapter will help you to decide if you can skip certain sections.

Mark the pages that are especially interesting or relevant to you. Write little notes in the margins. Have fun and – most of all – enjoy your pregnancy!

Part I
The Game Plan

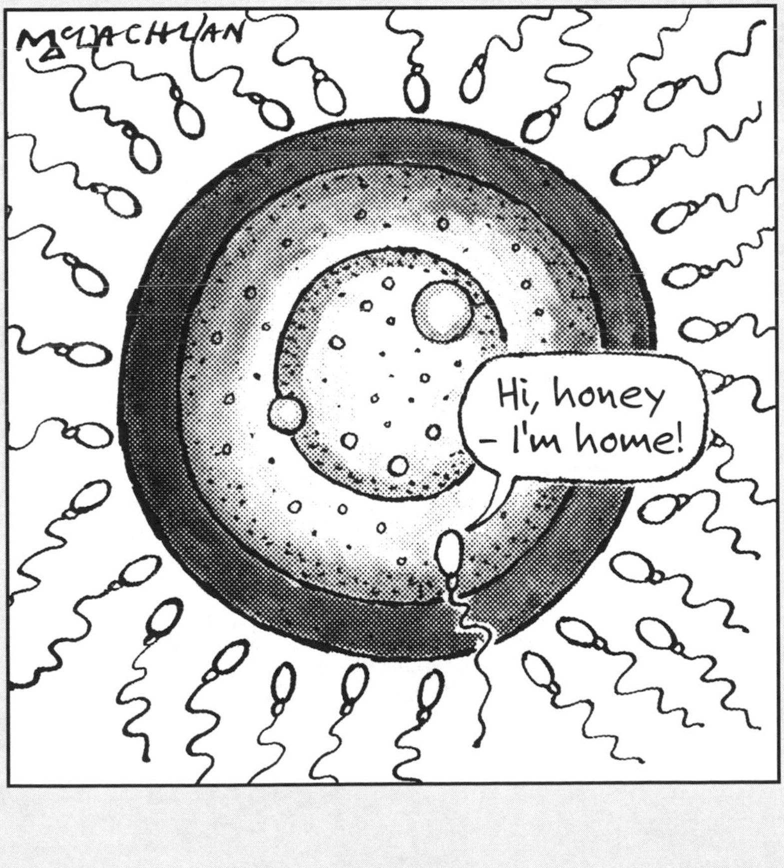

In this part . . .

I'm not sure I'm ready for this' is a normal reaction to finding out that you're pregnant, no matter how long you've been thinking about having a baby and no matter how long you've been trying to conceive. Suddenly, you're faced with the reality that your body is about to undergo some profound changes, and a baby is going to take shape inside you. Well, you may not *feel* ready, but preparing is easy enough. Ideally, your preparation begins with a visit to your GP a few months before you conceive. But even if you're not that far ahead of the game, this part tells you some of the many ways you can plan ahead for the very important, very interesting next nine months (plus).

Chapter 1

From Here to Maternity

In This Chapter

- Checking out your health and family history
- Preparing your body for pregnancy
- Making it happen: Conception made easy

Congratulations! If you're already pregnant, you're about to embark upon one of the most exciting adventures of your life. The next year or so is going to be filled with tremendous changes and (we hope) unbelievable happiness. If you're thinking about getting pregnant, you're probably excited at the prospect and also a little nervous at the same time.

And if your pregnancy is still in the planning stages, check out this chapter to find out what you can do to get ready for pregnancy – first by visiting your practitioner and going over your family and personal health history. Then you can discover whether you're in optimal shape to get pregnant, or if you need to take some time to gain or lose weight, improve your diet, quit smoking, or discontinue medications that could be harmful to your pregnancy. We also give you some basic advice about the easiest way to conceive, and we touch on the topic of infertility.

Getting Ready to Get Pregnant: The Preconception Visit

By the time you miss your period and discover you're pregnant, the embryo, now two weeks old or more, is already undergoing dramatic changes. Believe it or not, when the embryo is only two to three weeks old, it has already developed the beginnings of its heart and brain. Because your general health and nutrition can influence the growth of those organs, having your body ready for pregnancy before you get pregnant really pays off. Book what's called a *preconception visit* with your practitioner (usually your GP) to be sure your body is tuned up and ready to go.

Sometimes you can schedule this visit during a routine gynaecological appointment: When you go in for a well-woman check, mention that you're thinking about having a baby, and your practitioner will take you through the preliminaries. If you aren't due for one of these checks and you're ready to begin trying to get pregnant now, go ahead and book a preconception visit with your practitioner, and bring along the father-to-be, if at all possible, so both of you can provide health histories – and know what to expect from this adventure.

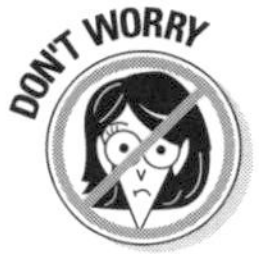

If you're already pregnant and didn't have a preconception visit, don't worry, because your practitioner will go over these topics at your first antenatal visit, which we discuss in Chapter 6.

Taking a look at your history

The preconception visit is a chance for your practitioner to identify areas of concern so that she can keep you and your baby healthy – even before you get pregnant. A multitude of factors come into play, and the practitioner is likely to ask you about the following:

- **Previous pregnancies and gynaecological history:** Information about previous pregnancies can help your practitioner decide how best to manage your future pregnancies. She will ask you to describe any prior pregnancies, any miscarriages or premature births, multiple births – any situations that can happen again. For example, knowing whether you had problems in the past, like pre-term labour or high blood pressure, is helpful for the practitioner. Your gynaecological history is equally important because information like prior surgery on your uterus or cervix or a history of irregular periods also may influence your pregnancy.
- **Your family history:** Reviewing your family's medical history alerts your practitioner to conditions that may complicate your pregnancy or be passed on to the developing baby. You want to discuss your family history because you can take steps before you conceive to decrease the chance that certain disorders, such as having a family history of neural tube defects (spina bifida, for example), will affect *your* pregnancy (see the sidebar 'Why the sudden hype on folic acid?' later in this chapter). In Chapter 9, we discuss in more detail different genetic conditions and ways of testing for them.

- **Looking at your ethnic roots:** Your preconception visit involves questions about your parents' and grandparents' ancestry – not because your practitioner is nosey, but because some inheritable problems are concentrated in certain populations. Again, the advantage of finding out about these problems before you get pregnant is that if you and your partner are at risk for one of these problems, you have more time to become informed and to check out all your options (see Chapter 6 for more on this topic).

Evaluating your current health

Most women contemplating pregnancy are perfectly healthy and don't have problems that can have an impact on pregnancy. Still, a preconception visit is very useful because it's a time to make a game plan and to find out more about how to optimise your chances of having a healthy and uncomplicated pregnancy. You can discover how to reach your ideal body weight and how to start on a good exercise programme; you can decide what you want to do about your alcohol intake; you can get help to stop smoking if you need it; and you can begin to take folic acid (see the sidebar 'Why the sudden hype on folic acid?' for more about this).

Some women, however, do have medical disorders that can affect the pregnancy. Expect your practitioner to ask whether you have any one of a list of conditions. For example, if you have diabetes, stabilising your blood sugar levels before you get pregnant and watching those levels during your pregnancy are important. If you usually take tablets to control your diabetes, you'll probably be advised to switch to insulin during your pregnancy. *Diabetes For Dummies* by Sarah Jarvis and Alan L. Rubin (Wiley) provides more information on how to handle diabetes and pregnancy.

If you're prone to high blood pressure (*hypertension*), your doctor will want to control it before you get pregnant, because controlling hypertension can be time-consuming and can involve changing medications more than once. If you have other problems – epilepsy, for example – checking your medications and controlling your condition are important. For a condition like *systemic lupus erythematosus* (SLE), your practitioner may encourage you to try to become pregnant at a time when you're having very few symptoms.

You can expect questions about whether you smoke, indulge in more than a drink or two a day, or use any recreational/illicit drugs. Your practitioner isn't interrogating you and is unlikely to chastise you, so be comfortable answering honestly. These habits can be harmful to a pregnancy, and dropping them before you get pregnant is best. Your practitioner can advise you on ways to kick these habits or refer you to help or support groups.

REMEMBER

Why the sudden hype on folic acid?

Folic acid was something your mother never thought about when she was expecting you. But within the past decade, folic acid has become a nutritional requirement for all pregnant women. The change came in 1991, when a British medical study demonstrated that folic acid (also known as folate, a nutrient in the B vitamin family) reduced the recurrence of birth defects of the brain and spinal cord (also called neural tube defects). This reduction occurred in cases where a mother's previous child was affected – by as much as 80 per cent. Subsequent studies have shown that even among women who have never had children with brain or spinal cord defects, those who consume enough folic acid can lower their baby's risk of *spina bifida* (a spinal defect) and *anencephaly* (a brain and skull defect) by 50 to 70 per cent.

Today, all women who are considering pregnancy are advised to consume 0.4 milligrams (that's 400 micrograms) of folate every day, starting at least 30 days before conception. You start early so that plenty of the nutrient is in your system at the time the neural tube is forming. If spina bifida, anencephaly, or similar conditions run in your family – especially if you ever carried a child with these problems – you should get ten times the usual amount (4 or 5 milligrams) every day.

The Food Standards Agency has been promoting the benefits of folic acid in the diet. Foods that are fortified with folic acid, including some breakfast cereals, are now marked with a folic acid flash – a blue circle containing a letter 'F'. Some foods, including green leafy vegetables, potatoes, eggs, yeast extract, and certain fruits, are naturally rich in folic acid. However, to make sure that you get enough folic acid during the crucial first trimester (the first 13 weeks) of pregnancy, you should take a supplement of at least 0.4 milligrams a day.

You also need to discuss any prescription or over-the-counter drugs you take regularly and your diet and exercise routines. Do you take vitamins? Do you diet frequently? Are you a vegetarian or a vegan? Do you work out regularly? Discuss all these issues with your practitioner.

If you are due for a cervical smear, your practitioner will probably recommend that you have it done during this preconception visit.

Answering Commonly Asked Questions

Your preconception visit is also a time for you to ask your practitioner questions. In this section, we answer the most common questions – about body weight, medications, vaccinations, and stopping birth control.

Getting to your ideal body weight

The last thing most women need is another reason to be concerned about weight control. But this point is important: Pregnancy goes most smoothly for women who aren't too heavy or too thin. Overweight women stand a higher-than-normal risk of developing diabetes or high blood pressure during pregnancy, and they're more likely to end up delivering their babies via caesarean section. Underweight women risk having too-small (low birth-weight) babies.

TIP

Try to reach a healthy, normal weight *before* you get pregnant. Trying to lose weight after you conceive isn't advisable, even if you're overweight. And if you're underweight to begin with, catching up on pounds when the baby is growing may be difficult. (Read more about your ideal weight and weight gain in Chapter 5.)

Reviewing your medications

Since the 1960s, very little research has been done on medicines during pregnancy, because of ethical problems. The Committee on Safety of Medicines (CSM) has set up a 'yellow card' system of reporting on suspected adverse drug reactions during pregnancy. The introduction of this system has allowed the medical authorities to build up a large database of drugs that have been used in pregnant women, and the effects of these drugs on these women.

Drugs used during pregnancy are divided into three main groups:

- Drugs known to be safe in pregnancy
- Drugs known (or suspected) to cause problems
- Drugs for which no side effects are known, but for which relatively little formal research has been done

For these last two groups, the *British National Formulary* – the bible for all health care professionals advising about drugs in pregnancy – often has entries such as 'manufacturer advises toxicity in animal studies' or 'manufacturer advises avoid unless potential benefit outweighs risk'. Your practitioner should have a full discussion with you about the potential risks and benefits of such drugs, leaving you in a position to make an informed decision about whether you wish to take the medicine. Find out more about the British National Formulary by visiting the publisher's Web site at `www.pharmpress.com` or `www.bmjbookshop.com`. Your local bookshop should be able to obtain a copy for you.

TIP

Pharmacists are a great source of advice about drugs: They're highly trained, and have the latest information on safety of medicines in pregnancy at their fingertips. Don't forget that even medications you can get without prescription need to be treated with caution in pregnancy. So let your pharmacists know whether you're pregnant if you're getting a non-prescription drug from them. Pharmacists are happy to advise you on any medications you're already taking, and whether you need to consult your doctor.

The following are some of the common medications that women ask about before they get pregnant:

- **Oral contraceptive pills:** Women sometimes get pregnant while they're on the Pill (because they missed or were late taking a couple of pills during the month) and then worry that their babies will have birth defects. But oral contraceptives haven't been shown to have any ill effects on a baby, and babies born to women using oral contraceptives are at no higher risk of birth defects.
- **Ibuprofen:** Occasional use of these and other *non-steroidal anti-inflammatory agents* during pregnancy (for pain or inflammation) hasn't been associated with problems in infants. However, avoid chronic or persistent use of these medications during pregnancy (especially during the last trimester), because they have the potential to affect platelet function and blood vessels in the baby's circulatory system.
- **Vitamin A:** This vitamin and some of its derivatives can cause miscarriage or serious birth defects if too much is present in your bloodstream when you get pregnant. The situation is complicated by the fact that vitamin A can remain in your body for several months after you consume it. Discontinuing any drugs that contain vitamin A derivatives – the most common is the anti-acne drug Accutane – at least one month before trying to conceive is important. Scientists don't know whether topical creams containing vitamin A derivatives – anti-ageing creams like Retin A and Renova, for example – are as problematic as drugs that you swallow, so consult your doctor about them.
- **Blood thinners:** Women who are prone to developing blood clots or who have artificial heart valves need to take blood-thinning agents every day. One type of blood thinner, warfarin, and its derivatives, can trigger miscarriage, impair the baby's growth, or cause the baby to develop bleeding problems or structural abnormalities if taken during pregnancy. Women who take this medicine and are thinking of getting pregnant should switch to a different blood thinner. Ask your practitioner for more information.
- **Drugs for high blood pressure:** Many of these medications are considered safe to take during pregnancy. However, because a few can be problematic, you need to discuss any medications to treat high blood pressure with your doctor (see Chapter 17).

- **Antiseizure drugs:** Some of the medicines used to prevent epileptic seizures are safer than others for use during pregnancy. If you're taking any of these drugs, discuss them with your doctor. Don't simply stop taking any antiseizure medicine, because seizures may be worse for you – and the baby – than the medications themselves (see Chapter 17).
- **Tetracycline:** If you take this antibiotic during the last several months of pregnancy, it may, much later on, cause your baby's teeth (and bones) to yellow.
- **Antidepressants:** Many antidepressants (like Prozac) have been studied extensively and are considered perfectly safe during pregnancy. If you are taking an antidepressant and planning to conceive, ask your doctor whether you'll be able to keep taking the medication while you're pregnant.
- **Antibiotics:** Many antibiotics, including penicillin, the cephalosporin group of antibiotics and erythromycin, are considered to be safe in pregnancy. Other antibiotics, such as trimethoprim, are fine in some stages of pregnancy but not in others. Your doctor can tell you when and what is safe.
- **Paracetamol:** Up to the full recommended dose, there's no evidence that paracetamol is harmful at any stage of pregnancy.

Considering herbal remedies and vitamin supplements

Many women choose to treat common ailments with over-the-counter plant extracts or other natural medications. Some of these medications are considered completely safe during pregnancy, but keep in mind that these agents may not be regulated nearly as closely as medicines available on prescription, and very few studies have evaluated their safety during pregnancy.

Most pharmacies and health food shops sell multivitamins targeted at pregnant women, often with a dose of folic acid built in. Health care professionals are divided on the benefits of these supplements. The Food Standards Agency recommends that most pregnant women don't need any vitamin supplements in early pregnancy except 400 micrograms of folic acid and 10 micrograms of vitamin D each day. The Food Standards Agency advise particular caution because some vitamins and supplements, such as vitamin A (see Chapter 4) and cod liver oil supplements, can be dangerous in pregnancy. To contact the Food Standards Agency in England, telephone 020 7276 8000, in Scotland 01224 285100, in Wales 02920 678999, and in Northern Ireland 02890 417700; or log on to their Web site at `www.foodstandards.gov.uk`.

Some herbal medications should not be used during pregnancy because they can cause uterine contractions or even miscarriage. A short list of agents that are not recommended during pregnancy includes mugwort, blue cohosh, tansy, black cohosh, Scotch broom, goldenseal, juniper berry, pennyroyal oil, rue, mistletoe, and chaste berry.

Recognising the importance of vaccinations and immunity

People are immune to all kinds of infections, either because they have previously suffered the disease (most of us are immune to chickenpox, for example, because we had it when we were children, causing our immune systems to make antibodies to the chickenpox virus) or because they have been vaccinated (that is, given an injection of something that causes the body to develop antibodies).

Rubella is a common example of an infection to which you may already be immune. Your practitioner can check to see whether you're immune to *rubella* (also known as *German measles*) by drawing a sample of blood and checking to see that it contains antibodies to the rubella virus. (*Antibodies* are immune system agents that protect you against infections.) If you are not immune to rubella, your practitioner is likely to recommend that you be vaccinated against rubella at least three months *before* becoming pregnant. However, getting pregnant before the three months are over is highly unlikely to be a problem. No cases have been reported of babies born with problems due to the mother having received the rubella vaccine even in early pregnancy. Many vaccines, including the flu vaccine, are safe to have even while you're pregnant. See Table 1-1 for information on several vaccines.

Most people are immune to measles, mumps, poliomyelitis, and diphtheria, and your practitioner is unlikely to check your immunity to all these illnesses. Besides, these illnesses aren't usually associated with significant adverse effects for the baby. The virus that causes chickenpox and shingles, on the other hand, does carry a small risk that the baby can contract the infection from her mother. While vaccination against chickenpox or shingles isn't routinely available in the UK, your doctor can give you an injection to protect you once you've been exposed to it if you aren't immune. If you don't know if you've ever had chickenpox, talk to your practitioner as soon as possible if you're in contact with someone who has chickenpox or shingles during your pregnancy.

Finally, if you're at risk of HIV infection, get tested before contemplating pregnancy. If you have contracted HIV, taking certain medications throughout pregnancy will decrease the chances that your baby also will contract HIV.

Table 1-1 Safe and Unsafe Vaccines during Pregnancy

Disease	*Risk of Vaccine to Baby during Pregnancy?*	*Immunisation*	*Comments*
Hepatitis B	None confirmed	OK	Used with immunogloblins for acute exposure, newborns need vaccine
Influenza	None confirmed	OK	
Measles	None confirmed	NO	Vaccinate after childbirth
Mumps	None confirmed	NO	Vaccinate after childbirth
Plague	None confirmed		Selected vaccination if exposed
Pneumococcus	None confirmed	OK, same as in non-pregnant women	
Poliomyelitis	None confirmed	Only if exposed	Get if travelling to endemic area
Rubella	None confirmed	NO	Vaccinate after childbirth
Rabies	Unknown	Indication same as for non-pregnant women	Consider each case separately
Smallpox	Possible miscarriage	NO	Unless emergency situation arises or foetal infection
Tetanus	None confirmed	OK if no childhood triple vaccines given or no booster in past 10 years	
Typhoid	None confirmed	Only for close, continued exposure or travel to endemic area	

(continued)

Table 1-1 *(continued)*

Disease	*Risk of Vaccine to Baby during Pregnancy?*	*Immunisation*	*Comments*
Varicella (chickenpox)	None confirmed		Immunoglobulins recommended in exposed non-immune women and should be given to newborn if exposed to disease around time of delivery
Yellow fever	Unknown	NO	Unless exposure is unavoidable

Quitting contraception

How soon can you get pregnant after you stop using birth control? It depends on what kind of birth control you use. The barrier methods – such as condoms, diaphragms, and spermicides – work only as long as you use them; as soon as you stop, you're fertile. Hormone-based medicines – including the Pill, Depo-Provera, NuvaRing, and the birth control patch (for example, Ortho-Evra) – take longer to get out of your system. You may ovulate very shortly after stopping the Pill (weeks or days, even). On the other hand, it can take three months to one year to resume regular ovulatory cycles after stopping Depo-Provera.

We know of no hard-and-fast rules about how long you should wait after stopping birth control before you start trying to conceive. In fact, you can start to try to conceive straight away. If you're Fertile Myrtle, you may get pregnant on the first try. But keep in mind that if you haven't resumed regular cycles, you may not be ovulating each month, and it may be more difficult to time your intercourse to achieve conception. (At least you can have a good time trying!) If you get pregnant while your cycles are irregular, it also may be harder to tell exactly what day you conceived and, therefore, to know your due date.

Some women use a hormone-releasing device called the Mirena or *intrauterine system* (IUS) for contraception. Although the risk of getting pregnant when you have one of these in place is tiny, it's not unknown. If this happens, you need to have your IUS taken out as soon as you can arrange it with your practitioner.

If you use an intrauterine device (also called a coil or IUD), you can get pregnant as soon as you have it removed. Sometimes a woman conceives with her IUD in place. If this happens to you, your practitioner may choose to remove the device, if possible, because getting pregnant with your IUD in place puts you at risk of miscarriage, *ectopic pregnancy* (a pregnancy that gets stuck in the fallopian tube), or early delivery. See Chapter 6 for more details.

DON'T WORRY

Getting pregnant with an IUD in place doesn't put the baby at increased risk of birth defects.

Introducing Sperm to Egg: Timing Is Everything

This book's title notwithstanding, we're going to assume that you know the basics of how to get pregnant. What many people don't know, though, is how to make the process most efficient, so that you give yourself the best chance of getting pregnant as soon as you want to. To do that, you need to think a little about *ovulation* – the releasing of an egg from one of your ovaries – which happens once each cycle (usually once per month).

After leaving the ovary, the egg spends a couple of days gliding down the fallopian tube, until it reaches the uterus (also known as the *womb*) (see Figure 1-1). Most often, pregnancy occurs when the egg is fertilised within 24 hours from its release from the ovary, during its passage through the tube, and the budding embryo then implants itself in the uterus's lining. In order to get pregnant, your job (yours and the father-to-be's) is to get the sperm to meet up with the egg as soon as possible (ideally, within 12 to 24 hours) after ovulation.

The absolute prime time to have sex is 12 hours prior to ovulation. Then the sperm are in place as soon as the egg comes out. Sperm are thought to live inside a woman's body for 24 to 48 hours, although some have been known to fertilise eggs when they are as much as seven days old. No couple should count on getting pregnant on the first try: On average, you have a 15 to 25 per cent chance each month. Roughly half of all couples trying to get pregnant conceive within four months, by six months, three-quarters of them make it, by a year, 85 per cent do, and by two years, the success rate is up to 93 per cent. If you've been trying unsuccessfully to conceive for a year or more, a fertility evaluation is warranted.

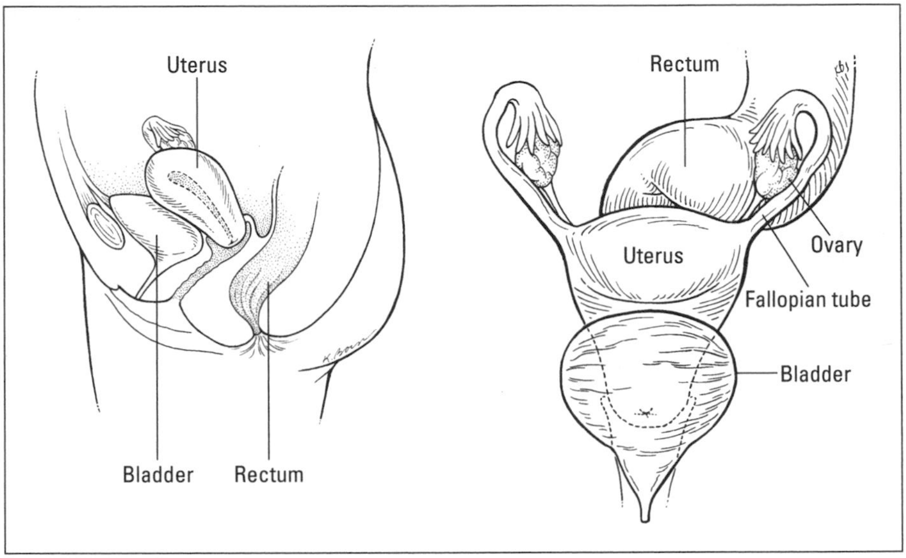

Figure 1-1: An overview of the female reproductive system.

Pinpointing ovulation

So when does ovulation happen? Typically, about 14 days before you get your period – that, if your menstrual cycles are 28 days long, is 14 days after the first day of your previous period. If you have a 32-day cycle, you probably ovulate on about the eighteenth day of your cycle. (Each cycle begins on the first day of a period.) To make sure that you get the sperm in the right place at the right time, have sex several times around the time of ovulation, starting five days before you expect to ovulate and continuing for two to three days afterward. How often? Once every two days is probably adequate, but why resist having sex every day if your partner has a normal sperm count?

DON'T WORRY

Doctors once thought that having sex daily resulted in a lower sperm count and reduced fertility. However, later medical studies found that this idea is true only in men who have a lower-than-normal sperm count to start with.

Monitoring your basal body temperature

Some women find that they can pinpoint their time of ovulation more easily if they keep track of their temperature, which rises close to the time of ovulation. To do this, you take your temperature (orally) each morning before you get out of bed. It typically reaches its lowest point right before your pituitary gland releases *luteinising hormone* (LH), which triggers ovulation. (Two days after the so-called *LH surge,* your temperature rises significantly – about a half to one degree above baseline – and stays elevated until you get your

Knowing when to see a doctor about infertility

Infertility is a problem that is affecting more couples than ever before, as people wait longer and longer to have children. One in ten couples older than 30 has trouble conceiving. After age 35, the ratio is one in five. Of course, age isn't a problem for everyone. Some women reportedly get pregnant even in their 50s. But face it: Spontaneous pregnancy in a woman's late 40s and 50s is rare.

When should you seek a doctor's help? Generally, after you've been trying unsuccessfully to get pregnant for the best part of a year. But if you have a history of miscarriages or difficulty conceiving, if you're older than 35, or if you already know that your partner has a low sperm count, you may want to get help before then. No matter what your situation, don't despair. Reproductive technologies become more sophisticated – and more successful – with each passing year. For a couple that has trouble conceiving right away, chances are better than ever that they will eventually become pregnant. Check out *Fertility For Dummies* by Jackie Meyers-Thompson and Sharon Perkins (Wiley) for more information.

Remember: If you're having trouble getting pregnant, and you're not sure whether it's time to see an infertility specialist, discuss it with your practitioner. On the NHS, most infertility clinics won't accept your case unless you've been trying to conceive, without success, for at least a year. However, if you go to see your GP before this, she may be able to get the ball rolling by carrying out preliminary tests.

period. If you get pregnant, it remains high.) You may want to invest in a special *basal body temperature* thermometer (sold in most pharmacies) because it has larger gradations and is easier to read.

Remember that a rise in your basal body temperature indicates that ovulation has already occurred. It doesn't predict when you will ovulate, but it does confirm that you're ovulating and gives you a rough idea when ovulation occurs in your cycle. Reading the signals can be hard because not all women follow the same pattern: Some never see a distinct drop in temperature, and some never see a clear rise.

Using an ovulation predictor kit

Another way to monitor the LH surge is to use a home ovulation predictor kit, which tests the amount of LH in urine. As opposed to basal body temperatures that we mentioned earlier in this chapter, the LH surge is useful in predicting when ovulation will occur during any given cycle. A positive test for any cycle tells you that you're ovulating and when. In general, these kits are very accurate and effective. The main drawback is the expense. At £15 to £20 per kit, they're more expensive than taking your temperature, especially if you have to check several times to find out when you were ovulating.

Taking an effective (and fun) approach

In most cases, parents-to-be are well advised to just relax and enjoy the process of trying to conceive. Don't get too anxious if it doesn't happen straight away. We often tell our patients: Think about stopping contraception a few months before you actually plan on getting pregnant – but only if getting pregnant straight away wouldn't be a disaster. This way, you have some carefree months of enjoying great sex without worrying each month if you're pregnant. And if you do conceive ahead of schedule, enjoy the nice surprise!

REMEMBER

If you've already been pregnant, don't assume it'll take the same time to get pregnant next time round. We've lost count of the number of patients who have become pregnant within a few months of their last delivery. Usually these patients tell us that because it took them six months (or a year, or however long) to conceive last time, they started trying a few months before they actually wanted to get pregnant on the assumption that it would take as long.

TIP

You can take a few steps to improve your chances of conceiving:

- If you smoke cigarettes or marijuana, quit.
- Avoid using K-Y Jelly or other commercial lubricants during sex, because they may contain spermicide. (Try olive oil or vegetable oil instead.)
- Limit your caffeine intake. Drinking more than three cups of coffee per day may decrease your chances of conceiving.

Chapter 2

I Think I'm Pregnant!

In This Chapter

- Noticing the signs that you may be pregnant
- Finding out: Taking a pregnancy test
- Choosing the right health care professional

So you think you may be pregnant. Or maybe you're hoping to become pregnant soon. Either way, you want to know what to look for in the early weeks of pregnancy so that you can know for sure as soon as possible. In this chapter, we take a look at some of the most common signals that your body sends you in the first weeks of pregnancy and offer advice for confirming your pregnancy and getting it off to a great start.

Recognising the Signs of Pregnancy

So assume it's happened: A budding embryo has nestled itself into your womb's soft lining. How and when do you find out that you're pregnant? Quite often, the first sign is a missed period. But your body gives off many other signals – sometimes even sooner than that first missed period – that typically grow more noticeable with each passing week.

- **Darling, I'm late!:** You suspect that you may be pregnant if you're late for your period. By the time you notice you're late, a pregnancy test will probably yield a positive result (see the upcoming section, 'Testing, Testing 1, 2, 3', for more on pregnancy tests). Sometimes, though, you may experience one or two days of light bleeding, which is known as *implantation bleeding* because the embryo is attaching itself to your uterus's lining.
- **You notice new food cravings and aversions:** The stories that you've heard about a pregnant woman's appetite are true. You may become ravenous for pickles, pasta, and other particular foods, yet turn up your nose at foods you normally love to eat. No one knows for sure why these changes in appetite occur, but experts suspect that these changes are, at least partly, nature's way of ensuring that you get the proper nutrients.

Crazy cravings

One day a couple of years after my first daughter was born, I (Joanne) found myself heading to the supermarket to buy pickles and ketchup, intent on mixing them together to make a lovely, tasty, green-and-red meal. I was craving it so much that it didn't even occur to me what an odd dish it is. In fact, it wasn't until I had cleaned up the dishes that I realised that pickles and ketchup had been my only craving during the early months of my first pregnancy. I had no other reason to think I was pregnant again; I hadn't even missed a period. But the next morning I tested myself, and sure enough, it was time for round two.

You may be very thirsty early in pregnancy and the extra water you drink is useful for increasing your body's supply of blood and other fluids. Lots of women also go off coffee and alcohol in the early stages of pregnancy.

- **Your breasts become tender and bigger:** Don't be surprised about how large your breasts grow early in pregnancy. In fact, large and tender breasts are often the first symptom of pregnancy that you feel, because very early in pregnancy, levels of oestrogen and progesterone rise, causing immediate changes in your breasts.

Testing, Testing, 1, 2, 3

Well, are you or aren't you? These days, you don't need to wait to get to your GP's surgery to find out whether you're pregnant. You can opt instead for self-testing. Home tests are urine tests that simply give a positive or negative result.

Getting an answer at home

Suppose you've noticed some bloating or food cravings, or you've missed your period by a day or two, and you want to know whether you're pregnant, but you aren't ready to go to a doctor yet. The easiest, fastest way is to go to the chemist and pick up a home pregnancy test. These tests are basically simplified chemistry sets, designed to check for the presence of *human chorionic gonadotropin* (hCG, the hormone produced by the developing placenta) in your urine. Although these kits aren't as precise as laboratory tests that look for hCG in blood, in many cases they can provide positive results very quickly – by the day you miss your period, or about two weeks after conception.

The unplanned pregnancy

If you're pregnant but weren't planning to be, the jumble of emotions you experience is likely to be confusing. Don't feel guilty about these mixed feelings – they're quite natural. If you make the decision to keep your baby, it's a good idea to write down your feelings (both for and against continuing with your pregnancy). That way, if you feel scared or full of doubt further down the line (and most women do, no matter how much they want a baby) you can remind yourself why the decision you've made is the best one for you.

If you weren't planning to get pregnant, you may not have taken folic acid before you conceived (refer to Chapter 1 for more on folic acid), or you may have smoked heavily, or drunk a lot of alcohol before you found out you were pregnant. Talk to your GP about these concerns, but don't worry too much. As long as you adopt a healthy lifestyle for the rest of your pregnancy (and tips are dotted throughout this book to help you), there's a good chance your baby will be just fine.

REMEMBER

The result of a home pregnancy test isn't a sure thing. You can get a *false negative* – a test that tells you you're not pregnant even when you are – although a positive test is highly unlikely to be wrong. If your test comes out negative but you still think you're pregnant, retest in another week or make an appointment with your doctor.

Going to your GP for answers

If you don't want to buy a pregnancy test kit yourself, you can get a test done either at your GP's surgery or at a local family planning clinic (look up their details in your local phone book). Your GP will send off a urine sample, or sometimes a blood test, to the lab, and you'll usually have to wait a few days for the result. Most family planning clinics can do a test and give you a result on the spot – but they'll then advise you to make an appointment with your GP to confirm the result.

Antenatal and Labour Care – What's Available?

Questions you hadn't thought of always exist, no matter how long you've waited to be pregnant. Some of them can wait until later in your pregnancy, and we cover most of them at the relevant stage in this book. But you do need to think at a very early stage about where you want to have your *antenatal care* (the check-ups of your health, and your baby's, that you get routinely during pregnancy). Even more surprising to many women is that you're likely to have to decide in the first few weeks of your pregnancy about where you want to have your baby (if you leave it too late, you may not be able to get booked into the hospital of your choice). Read on for tips on how to make a choice.

Where to have your baby

Your practitioner will be able to tell you which hospital or hospitals he can refer you to. You're smart to ask any parent friends you have about the options in your area, and to get some idea of the pros and cons.

Most babies are delivered in hospital, but over the last few years, maternity care has gone through a lot of changes. More and more options are becoming available for you to have your baby safely, but in a way you want. The available options vary across the country, so find out about the choices in your area from your GP. For more information, read the section 'Looking at your options: Private or NHS?' later in this chapter.

REMEMBER

In an ideal world, every woman would have the kind of delivery she wants – but don't set your heart on one kind of delivery until you know whether it's possible (and advisable) for you.

The most common places to give birth are

- **Hospital.** Not all hospitals have the same facilities, but all can deliver your baby by *caesarean section* (a surgical procedure used if vaginal delivery is not the best delivery option for you) if a problem arises, and have facilities for resuscitating your baby should something unfortunate happen. Some have *birthing centres* attached to them, providing home comforts in the hospital setting. You may find that your GP can refer you to more than one hospital in the area – which one you ask to be referred to will depend partly on your personal preference (or the recommendation of friends and your GP), but some of the questions you may want to ask before you decide include:
    - Does the hospital have facilities for providing epidural pain relief 24 hours a day (see Chapter 10)?
    - Does the hospital encourage natural childbirth, if that's your preference? Does it have a birthing centre, or facilities for a water birth?
    - Does the hospital have a special care baby unit (SCBU) for babies with medical problems, and do they have sophisticated facilities such as ventilators, in case your baby is born prematurely and needs help to breathe?

- **Midwife unit.** These centres are run entirely by midwives (see later in this chapter for more on midwives). If you have a midwife unit in your area, and you don't have medical problems, you should be able to go into the unit, instead of into the standard hospital labour ward, when you go into labour. Your baby should be delivered by one of the team of midwives who cared for you during your pregnancy. She, or a member of her team, can visit you at home after your delivery.
- **DOMINO scheme.** Domino stands for *domiciliary in-out.* This means that your midwife visits you at home; that you go into a midwife-led unit or hospital to have your baby; and that you go home soon afterwards. You can often be in and out within a few hours if all goes well.
- **GP unit.** In some areas, your GP can deliver your baby himself in a unit with midwives and hospital doctors attached. These are becoming uncommon, and you're unlikely to have one in your area unless you live in a very rural location.
- **Home birth.** Many doctors prefer women to deliver in hospital, in case there's an unexpected problem that requires urgent medical intervention. However, if you're healthy and have had a previous uncomplicated delivery, your risks are low. Many women prefer to be at home, feeling that it adds to the emotional experience of childbirth. You do have a right to have your baby at home, and to have a midwife attend your birth, even if your decision to have your baby at home is against medical advice (for example, if you're at high risk of complications, as we discuss in Chapters 13–15). Many areas now have teams of midwives working within the NHS, who can deliver your baby at home. Try to plan your home birth in advance – for a smooth delivery you'll need more than hot water and towels!

  TIP: If a home delivery interests you, start making enquiries as soon as possible, preferably at your booking appointment (see Chapter 6 for more on this appointment).

REMEMBER: In the UK, delivering a baby is illegal for anyone other than a midwife or doctor, except in an emergency.

Looking at your options: Private or NHS?

All UK citizens are eligible to have their baby delivered, without any costs, using National Health Service (NHS) facilities and staff. Most women in the UK do exactly this. However, some women prefer to register for fee-paying private antenatal care – either because it allows them more flexibility in timing their appointments, or because they want a particular consultant to look after them personally. Some women also choose private midwife-led care, and a few private hospitals offer a midwife-led service.

If you opt for a private delivery, your consultant will charge you for his services and the hospital will charge for your stay in hospital. If you need an anaesthetist (for an epidural or a caesarean section, for instance), he'll charge privately, too. Your consultant will deliver your baby personally. Even if you have private health cover, it's unlikely to cover you for a normal delivery – although some schemes will cover for caesarean sections, if your doctor confirms that the operation was needed on medical grounds.

Who's Who? The Varying Roles of Health Care Professionals

Throughout your pregnancy, you'll come into contact with a wonderfully skilled and varied bunch of professionals. But what do all these professionals do, and how do they fit into your pregnancy experience? The following sections explain the basics.

Your GP

Your first port of call when you think you're pregnant is to your General Practitioner (GP). Every resident in the UK is entitled to register with a GP, and over 98 per cent of people are. That means you probably already know your GP, and they may have looked after you for years (or occasionally even have delivered you!). If you don't have a GP, or you're looking for a new GP when you discover you're pregnant, you can find leaflets giving details about all the practices in your area in your local library, or you can contact your *Primary Care Trust* (who look after the nuts and bolts of general practice) for information – you can find their number in the phone book.

Your GP is responsible for general medical care outside of pregnancy, but he will often play a part in your antenatal care, too. *Shared care* is the most common form of antenatal care in the UK, meaning that at certain points in your pregnancy (don't worry, the hospital will tell you when these are) you'll have hospital appointments, but for other routine checks, you'll see your GP.

TIP

Until the late 1990s, most GPs were still responsible for their patients 24 hours a day, but they now have the right to opt out of complete 24-hour care. That doesn't mean you won't be able to talk to a GP out of hours – Primary Care Trusts have a duty to make sure there's an alternative in place. Since you're more likely to need advice or medical help out of hours during your pregnancy than you ever have been before, check with your GP as soon as you know you're pregnant what their arrangements for out of hours care are.

Your midwife

A *midwife* is a trained health care professional with a specialist qualification in midwifery, trained in looking after you and your baby before, during, and just after your delivery. If your pregnancy is normal, you may never meet a hospital doctor, but you will certainly meet at least one midwife during your pregnancy. Three-quarters of the babies in the UK are born with the help of midwives alone.

Most midwives tend to work in small teams. They may be based in hospital, in a midwifery unit, or attached to a GP's surgery. You may have a named midwife who leads and co-ordinates your care. In some areas, the same midwife may look after you during both pregnancy and labour, but in others, different midwives from the same team will attend to your needs.

Many women feel that getting to know their midwife well before she delivers their baby is very important. Our patients tell us, however, that it's almost impossible not to get to know someone when they're with you throughout your delivery, and that they build up a bond during labour, regardless of whether they knew the midwife beforehand.

Once you've had your baby, midwives will visit you at home until 10 (or occasionally 28) days after delivery. These midwives are usually not the same ones you meet before you have your baby; instead, they're from your local hospital (whether you had your baby there or not).

Independent midwives

A small number of midwives work privately, outside the NHS. These midwives charge for their services, but they do promise to provide continuity of care. Your private midwife will look after you throughout your pregnancy and labour – whether at home or in hospital. Most midwives are trained and experienced in water births and home births.

You can find out more about independent midwives by contacting the Independent Midwives Association through their Web site (`www.independentmidwives.org.uk`) or by phone on 01483 821104.

Your obstetrician

An obstetrician is a consultant doctor with special training in the complications of pregnancy and labour. If you're referred for hospital or shared (GP and midwife or hospital) antenatal care, you will usually have a named consultant. This consultant will be contacted if there are any problems before, during, or just after your labour. You may not need to meet your obstetrician if your pregnancy goes smoothly. If you go into hospital outside normal working hours, you may be under the care of the duty team at first – but your care will be transferred back to 'your' obstetrician as soon as possible.

You do have a right to see an obstetrician at your antenatal appointments or when you are in hospital – if you have concerns you think a specialist needs to answer, for instance. If you want to see an obstetrician – just ask.

Maternal-foetal medicine specialists

A maternal-foetal medicine specialist is an obstetrician with specialised training in high-risk pregnancies. If you have particular medical needs during your pregnancy, you may either be under the care of a maternal-foetal medicine specialist throughout, or referred to one later in your pregnancy. If you do need to see a maternal-foetal medicine specialist, you'll probably need to be referred to one of the big specialist or *tertiary referral* hospitals, which may be some distance from where you live, but that houses all of the necessary facilities.

Your paediatrician

A paediatrician is a doctor with special training in the care of sick babies and children; not, as hapless TV hotelier Basil Fawlty famously gaffed, a doctor who specialises in feet.

If your baby needs to be *resuscitated* – if it needs help to start breathing after it's born – or checked out straight after delivery, this is done by a paediatrician. A paediatrician examines your baby routinely before you leave hospital. If you have your baby at home, or go home soon after delivery, your GP may do this first baby check instead.

Your health visitor

Health visitors are nurses with further training in the care of children under five years old. They work in the community, and are usually attached to one or more GP's surgeries. Your health visitor is told about your baby's birth automatically by the hospital when you go home (or by your midwife, if you have a home birth), and visits you at home, usually when your baby is 2–4 weeks old. Health visitors carry out the routine child health surveillance checks your baby needs in its first few years of life. This surveillance includes regular checks of your baby's weight and development, most of which are carried out at the GP's surgery, until your 'baby' is five years old. Your health visitor is also an invaluable source of advice on everyday concerns about your baby.

Chapter 3

Preparing for Life during Pregnancy

In This Chapter

- Knowing when your baby is due
- Walking through a typical antenatal visit
- Anticipating big changes in your body
- Making decisions about lifestyle and medication issues
- Working while you're pregnant

Even though you're pregnant and your body is already undergoing miraculous changes, your day-to-day life goes on. How will you need to change your lifestyle in order to make your pregnancy go as smoothly as possible? What things in your life don't need to change, or need to be modified only slightly? You have a lot to consider: your job, the general level of stress in your life, what medications you take, whether you smoke or drink alcohol regularly, and what to do about routine things like going to the dentist or hairdresser. If you're like most normally healthy women, you'll probably find that for the most part, your life can go on largely as usual.

All the issues we mention are subjects for discussion with your practitioner. But in this chapter, and the next, we offer a general outline for how to plan your life during pregnancy. If you consider from the beginning how your daily habits and health practices interact with your pregnancy, you're likely to have an easier time getting used to your new state of being. The earlier you get started on the right diet, exercise, and overall health programme, the better (see Chapter 5 for more).

Working Out Your Due Date

For most parents-to-be, the *due date* (the date on which your baby should be born) is a very important date to be aware of. Having said that, only 1 in 20 women actually delivers on her due date – most women deliver anywhere from three weeks early to two weeks late. Nonetheless, pinpointing the due date as precisely as possible is important in order to ensure that the tests you need along the way are performed at the right time. Knowing how far along you are also makes it easier for your doctor to see that the baby is growing properly. What's more, it's just plain fun to know, of course!

The average pregnancy lasts 280 days – 40 weeks. Your due date – what doctors sometimes refer to as the *estimated date of delivery* (EDD) – can be calculated from the date on which your last menstrual period started. If your cycles are 28 days long, your EDD will be a full year later minus three months then adding seven days. So, if your last period started on 3 June, your EDD is the following 10 March (subtract three months and add seven days).

If your periods don't follow 28-day cycles, don't worry. You can establish your due date in other ways. If you've been tracking ovulation (refer to Chapter 1) and can pinpoint the date of conception, coming up with an accurate date is especially easy – just add 280 days to that date.

If you're unsure of the date your last period started and you haven't been tracking ovulation, never fear! An ultrasound scan gives you a good idea of your due date, and you'll be offered this scan when you go for your first hospital antenatal appointment.

A *first trimester* (taking place within the first three months of your pregnancy) ultrasound predicts your due date more accurately than one during your *second* or *third trimester* (taking place between 4–6 months and 7–9 months, respectively) – it's usually accurate to within one week. If you're not sure of

Weeks versus months

Most of us think of pregnancy as lasting nine months. But face it – 40 weeks is a little longer than 9 × 4 weeks; It's closer to ten lunar months (in Japan, they actually speak of pregnancy as lasting ten months) and a bit longer than nine 30–31-day calendar months. That's why your doctor is more likely to talk in terms of weeks.

Because you start counting from the date of the last menstrual period, you actually start the count a couple of weeks before you conceive. So when your doctor says you're 12 weeks pregnant, the foetus is really only ten weeks old!

your dates, or if your self-calculated due date is more than a week away from the due date predicted by your scan, your doctor will usually take the EDD from your ultrasound as the expected date to work on.

If maths isn't your strong point (or you have better things to worry about than adding and subtracting weeks!), your practitioner will work out your EDD for you.

Planning Antenatal Visits

After you finish celebrating the results of your positive pregnancy test, start thinking about what lies ahead. This stretch of time – from conception to birth – is known as the *antenatal* period (just for the record, after you've given birth is *postnatal*). The first thing to do is make an appointment with your GP. If you didn't have a preconceptional visit and you haven't been taking a folic acid supplement, go out and buy one straight away, even before you see your GP (see Chapter 1 for more about preconceptional visits and the benefits of folic acid).

Some things are consistent from trimester to trimester – like checking your blood pressure, urine, and the baby's heartbeat – so we cover these topics in this chapter. In Chapters 6, 7, and 8, we go over the specifics of what happens during antenatal visits for each trimester. See Table 3-1 for an overview of a typical schedule for antenatal visits.

Table 3-1 Typical Antenatal Visit Schedule

Stage of Pregnancy	*Frequency of Doctor Visits*
First visit to 28 weeks	Every four weeks
28 to 36 weeks	Every two weeks
36 weeks to delivery	Every week or two weeks

The National Institute of Clinical Excellence (NICE), a panel of experts looking at all sorts of medical treatments, has issued guidance on the ideal frequency of antenatal visits. For some women, especially those who've previously had a healthy baby and don't have any medical problems, NICE recommends only seven visits over the course of pregnancy. So if your practitioner says you don't need to be seen as often as Table 3-1 suggests, it means you're in good shape! If you develop problems during pregnancy or if your pregnancy is considered high risk (see the risk factors described in Chapter 2), your practitioner may suggest that you come in more frequently.

This schedule of antenatal visits isn't set in stone. If you're planning a holiday or need to miss an antenatal visit, tell your practitioner and reschedule your appointment. If your pregnancy is going smoothly, rescheduling usually isn't a big deal. However, because some antenatal tests have to be performed at specific times during pregnancy (see Chapter 9 for details), just make sure that missing an appointment won't affect any of these tests.

Antenatal visits vary a bit according to each woman's personal needs and each practitioner's style. Some women need particular laboratory tests or physical examinations. However, the following procedures are standard:

- **A doctor or midwife checks your blood pressure.** For more information on health issues, see Chapter 5.
- **You may – or may not – have your weight checked.** Pregnant women and their practitioners used to pay a lot of attention to weight gain. These days, weight gain is not recognised as a reliable indicator of how your pregnancy is proceeding, and other routine checks make weighing unnecessary for most women. What's more, deviations from the expected pattern of weight gain can cause unnecessary anxiety to women who don't have anything to worry about. So don't be surprised if your weight isn't checked at every appointment.
- **You give a urine sample (usually an easy job for most pregnant women!).** Your practitioner checks for the presence of protein or glucose to look for any signs of pre-eclampsia or diabetes (see Chapters 16 and 17). Some urine tests also enable your doctor to look for any signs that you have a urinary tract infection.
- **Starting sometime after 14–16 weeks, a midwife or doctor measures your fundal height.** This procedure is when a midwife or doctor uses a tape measure or her hands to measure your uterus to get a rough idea about how the baby is growing and whether you have an adequate amount of amniotic fluid (see Figure 3-1).

  The midwife or doctor is measuring the *fundal height,* the distance from the top of the pubic bone to the top of the uterus (the *fundus*). By 24 weeks, the fundus usually reaches the level of the navel. After 24 weeks, the height in centimetres roughly equals the number of weeks pregnant you are.

  The fundal height measurement may not be useful in women who are expecting twins or more, or in women who have large fibroids (in both cases, the uterus is much bigger than normal), or in women who are very obese (because it can be difficult to feel the top of the uterus).
- **A midwife or doctor listens for and counts the baby's heartbeat.** Typically, the heartbeat ranges between 120 and 160 beats per minute.

Most clinics use an electronic *Doppler device* (a small box with a microphone attached) to check the baby's heartbeat. With this method, the baby's heartbeat sounds a bit like horses galloping inside the womb. Sometimes, you can hear the heartbeat using this method as early as 8 or 9 weeks, but often it isn't clearly discernible until 12 to 14 weeks. A third way of checking the baby's heartbeat is by seeing it on ultrasound, where the heart can usually be seen at around six weeks.

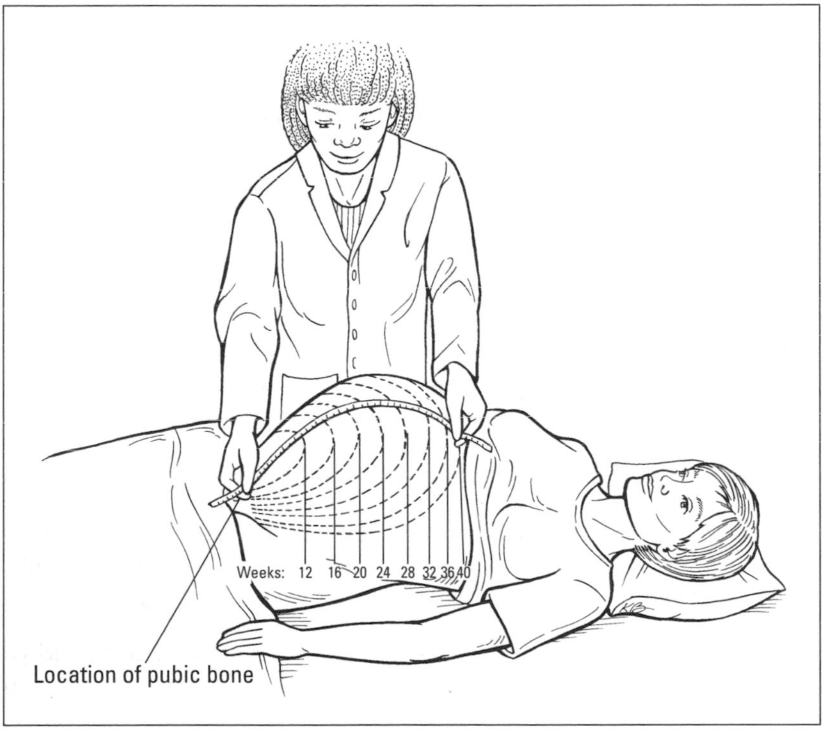

Figure 3-1: Your practitioner may measure your fundal height to check that your baby is growing properly.

Preparing for Physical Changes

When you're pregnant, your body is constantly changing. You can expect to experience changes such as mood swings, leg cramps, and stress. You've probably experienced these conditions before, just not with such intensity. The following sections cover these and other problems and let you know what you may be in for. Get your family and friends to read these sections, too – then tell them to consider themselves warned.

Spotting breast and bladder changes

You may have noticed at a very early stage (possibly before you knew you were pregnant) that your breasts were getting bigger. This is just one of the miraculous ways your body prepares for taking care of a baby, and it's all related to your hormones. You may also notice that you need to visit the loo more often. These frequent loo visits can be frustrating, but as long as you don't feel unwell, or have burning or stinging when you pass water, it's usually nothing to worry about.

Coping with mood swings

Hormonal shifts affect mood, as most women, especially those who suffer from PMS (premenstrual syndrome), already know. The hormonal fluctuations that support pregnancy are perhaps the most dramatic a woman experiences in her lifetime, so it's hardly surprising that emotional ups and downs are commonplace. And the fatigue that goes along with pregnancy can easily make these ups and downs more severe. Add to this biochemical mix the normal anxieties that the average expectant mother has about whether the baby will be healthy and whether she'll be a good mother, and you have plenty of fuel to produce good, old-fashioned mood swings.

Even those of us who consider we're well balanced are not immune from mood swings in pregnancy. They can hit at the most unlikely times – I (Sarah) could cope with almost anything that working as a GP threw at me, but would come home at night and burst into tears whenever I saw that cute little puppy on the toilet tissue advert on television!

REMEMBER

You're not alone. Moodiness is a normal part of pregnancy, and you're not the first or only woman to experience it. So don't blame yourself. Your family and friends will understand.

Living through leg cramps

Leg cramps are a common annoyance of pregnancy, and they're likely to become more frequent as the months go along.

The fact is that doctors aren't quite sure what really causes leg cramps. Because some doctors think leg cramps may be related to low levels of calcium or magnesium, supplementing with calcium or magnesium tablets has been suggested. However, the medical benefit of doing so has never been proven. Some doctors believe that leg cramps may be related to a decrease in circulation, which gets worse when you're sedentary and explains why leg cramps are more common at night. You may find that stretching and extending your legs and feet helps diminish the cramping.

TIP

Sometimes walking helps ease the pain of leg cramps. A foot or leg massage can also be useful – and leg cramps are a great excuse for getting frequent massages!

Noticing vaginal discharge

During pregnancy, your vaginal discharge normally increases substantially. Some women find that they need to wear thin panty liners every day. The discharge tends to be thin, white, and virtually odourless. Vaginal douches aren't a good idea because they may alter your natural ability to fight off vaginal infections.

CALL THE DOCTOR

If your vaginal discharge takes on a brown, yellow, or green colour, or if it develops a noxious odour, let your practitioner know. (Be sure to use your judgement about how much of an emergency this is – it isn't the sort of problem that requires a 3 a.m. phone call to the out-of-hours service.)

Pregnancy doesn't prevent you from getting a vaginal infection, and because of the high levels of oestrogen in your blood, you may be predisposed to developing a yeast infection (also known as *thrush*). A yeast infection usually produces a thick, white-yellow discharge, and it may in some cases cause itchiness or redness. Topical vaginal pessaries or creams should solve the problem, and they pose no risk to the foetus. Most over-the-counter preparations come in 1-, 3-, and 7-day preparations and are completely safe for the baby, as long as you don't push them in too enthusiastically. Avoid the oral treatment that you can buy from the pharmacist during your pregnancy.

TIP

During your pregnancy and for one year afterwards, you're entitled to free prescriptions, so you may prefer to get a prescription for thrush treatment from your GP. You don't necessarily need to make an appointment – if you've had thrush before and you're sure of the symptoms, your GP may well be happy to write you out a prescription on the basis of a telephone consultation. Alternatively, a few areas of the country now have pilot projects called *minor ailment schemes*, where your pharmacist can issue you with a prescription and get it signed up later by your GP. Ask in your GP's surgery or pharmacy to find out if you're in such an area.

Putting up with backaches

Backaches are a common complaint or symptom that many women experience during pregnancy. Back pain typically occurs in the latter part of pregnancy, although you may experience it earlier. The shift in your centre of gravity can be one cause; another can be the change in the curvature of your spine as the baby grows and the uterus enlarges. You may get some relief by getting off of your feet when you can, by applying mild local heat, and by taking paracetamol.

Some women experience pain extending from their lower back to their buttocks and down one leg or the other. This pain or, less commonly, numbness, is known as *sciatica,* which is due to pressure on the sciatic nerve, a major nerve that branches from your back, through your pelvis, to your hips, and down your legs. You can relieve mild cases of sciatica with bed rest, warm baths, or heating pads. If you develop a severe case, see your GP.

If your backache is troublesome, you may be able to get physiotherapy at your local hospital. You'll need to be referred to the physiotherapist by a doctor or midwife, so don't forget to ask at your antenatal appointment (see Chapter 6 for more about this appointment) or make a routine appointment with your GP.

Occasionally, preterm labour can present itself as low back pain. However, when it's preterm labour, the pain is more crampy, and it comes and goes, rather than being continuous.

Handling stress

Many women wonder whether stress has any effect on pregnancy. But that question is difficult to answer because stress is such an elusive concept. We all know what stress is, but each of us seems to handle it in her own way, and no one can really measure its intensity. We do know that chronic stress – day-after-day and unrelieved – can increase the levels of stress hormones circulating in the bloodstream. Many doctors think that such elevated levels of stress hormones can promote preterm labour or blood pressure problems during pregnancy, but few studies have been able to prove this idea.

While you're pregnant, pay attention to your own personal comfort and happiness. Everyone has her own way of relaxing – whether it's by getting a massage, going to the cinema, having dinner with friends, taking a hot shower or bubble bath, or just sitting back and putting her feet up. Take the time you need to be good to yourself.

Understanding the Effects of Medications, Alcohol, and Drugs on Your Baby

Alcohol, recreational drugs, and some medications that you take into your body can cross the placenta and get into your baby's circulatory system. Some of these substances are completely harmless, whereas others can cause problems. Knowing which substances you can safely use and which to avoid is crucial to your baby's health. The following sections outline which substances you can safely use and which you should avoid.

Taking medications

During your pregnancy, you'll probably experience at least a headache or two and an occasional case of heartburn. The question of whether you can safely take pain killers, antacids, and other over-the-counter medicines is bound to come up. Many women are afraid to take any medicine at all, for fear of somehow harming their babies. But most non-prescription drugs – and even many prescription drugs – are safe during pregnancy. During your first antenatal visit, go over with your practitioner what medications are okay to take during pregnancy – both over-the-counter medications and prescription medications. If another physician is treating you for a medical condition, let her know that you're pregnant, in case any adjustments need to be made.

Don't stop taking a prescription medication or change the dosage on your own without talking to your doctor first.

Many medications are labelled 'Don't take during pregnancy' because they haven't been adequately studied in pregnant women. However, this warning label doesn't necessarily mean that adverse effects have been reported, or that you can't use these medications. Whenever you have a question about a particular medication, ask your practitioner for advice. Don't be surprised if opinions vary between practitioners.

Certain medical problems, such as high blood pressure, pose more risk to the growing foetus than the medication you take to treat it does.

If you took any *teratogenic medications* (medicines known to be associated with foetal abnormalities) before you knew you were pregnant – or before you knew that the drugs could pose a problem – don't panic. In many cases, the drugs do no harm, depending on when during pregnancy you took them and in what quantities. Some medications can cause problems in the first trimester, but are totally safe in the third trimester, and vice versa. Relatively few substances are proven to be teratogenic to humans, and even those that are don't cause birth defects every time. Discuss with your practitioner what medications you've been taking, and what tests are available to check on your baby's growth and development.

Smoking

Unless you've been living on Mars for decades, you no doubt are aware that smoking is a health risk for you. When you smoke, you run the risk of developing lung cancer, emphysema, and heart disease, among other illnesses. During pregnancy, however, smoking poses risks to your baby as well.

The carbon monoxide in cigarette smoke decreases the amount of oxygen that your growing baby receives, and nicotine cuts back on blood flow to the foetus. Consequently, women who smoke stand an increased chance of delivering babies with low birth-weight, which may mean more medical problems for the baby. Babies born to smokers are expected to weigh a half-pound less, on average, than those born to non-smokers. The exact difference in birth-weight depends upon how much the mother smokes.

In addition to low birth-weight, smoking during pregnancy is associated with a greater risk of preterm delivery, miscarriage, placenta praevia (see Chapter 16), placental abruption (see Chapter 16), preterm rupture of the amniotic membranes, and even sudden infant death syndrome (SIDS) after the baby is born.

Giving up smoking can be extremely difficult. But keep in mind that even cutting back on the number of cigarettes you smoke is a benefit to your baby (and yourself).

If you give up smoking during the first three months you're pregnant, give yourself a pat on the back and be reassured that your baby is likely to be born at a normal weight.

Some women use nicotine patches, gum, or inhalers to help them kick the habit. The nicotine from these products is still absorbed into the bloodstream and can still reach the foetus, but at least the carbon monoxide and other toxins in cigarette smoke are eliminated. The total amount of nicotine absorbed from the intermittent use of the gum or inhalers may be less than the amount from the patch, which is used continuously. Talk to your GP about these different options. Newer approaches to smoking cessation, like the tablet Zyban, haven't been extensively studied in pregnant women. In women who smoke heavily, however, the benefits of this treatment may outweigh the possible risks.

Specialist smoking cessation clinics are now available on the NHS everywhere. You can get the details from your GP, your midwife, or by calling NHS Direct (0845 4647). These clinics give you the support – and, if necessary, prescribe the nicotine replacement therapy – that you need to help you stop smoking.

Drinking alcohol

Clearly, pregnant women who abuse alcohol put their babies at risk of foetal alcohol syndrome, which encompasses a wide variety of birth defects (including growth problems, heart defects, mental retardation, or abnormalities of the face or limbs). In addition, there's evidence that drinking more than about 10 *units* a week (a unit is a glass of wine or a half pint of normal strength lager) in the early stages of pregnancy can increase your risk of miscarriage. But controversy arises because medical science hasn't defined an absolute safe level of alcohol intake during pregnancy. Scientific data shows that daily drinking or heavy binge drinking can lead to serious complications, but no studies have consistently shown that an occasional glass of wine or an occasional drink will cause harm to your baby. If you do choose to have an occasional drink during pregnancy, avoid alcohol during the first trimester, when the baby's organ systems are forming, and after that limit your consumption to one to two drinks per week.

Using recreational/illicit drugs

Many studies have evaluated the effects of drug use during pregnancy. But the studies can be confusing because they tend to lump all kinds of users together, regardless of which drugs they use and how much they use. The mother's lifestyle also influences the degree of risk to the baby, which complicates the information even more. For example, women who abuse drugs are more likely to be malnourished than other women, they are typically of lower socioeconomic status, and they suffer a higher incidence of sexually transmitted diseases. All these factors, independent of drug use, can cause problems for your pregnancy and for your baby.

The following list tells the basics about the use of various recreational drugs and their effects on unborn babies:

- **Marijuana:** Marijuana is the illicit drug most frequently used during pregnancy. The data on marijuana use are controversial, but they do suggest that women who use marijuana when they're pregnant stand a higher-than-average risk of delivering their babies early or at low birthweight.

- **Cocaine and crack cocaine:** In a pregnant woman, the use of cocaine or crack can lead to severe high blood pressure, stroke, heart attack, and even sudden death. Cocaine use also raises the risk of problems with the baby's growth, preterm delivery, placental abruption (see Chapter 16), and foetal stroke. Women who use cocaine early in pregnancy put their babies at higher risk of developing a variety of birth defects. Also, infants born to women who use cocaine during pregnancy are at higher risk for behavioural and neurological problems, seizures, and sudden infant death syndrome (SIDS).
- **Narcotics and opiates (including heroin, methadone, codeine, Demerol, and morphine):** Narcotic addiction alone puts both the mother and the baby at a greater risk. Narcotic and opiate use is associated with foetal growth problems, preterm delivery, foetal death, and small head size. Perhaps even more important, narcotic addiction places the newborn at a high risk of complications (including death) due to withdrawal from the drug. If you're addicted to narcotics or opiates, beginning a treatment programme during your pregnancy can minimise the drugs' effects on your baby.

  We don't mean to imply that occasional short-term use of medications containing narcotics in therapeutic doses causes any problems. If you're undergoing a surgical or painful dental procedure during your pregnancy, for example, using such medications for short-term pain control may be perfectly acceptable – but to be on the safe side, do check with your GP first.
- **Amphetamines and other uppers (including crystal methamphetamine and blue ice):** Because these substances historically have not been used as widely as narcotics and cocaine, we have less information about their side effects during pregnancy. We do know that they decrease the user's appetite, which, in turn, could lead to poor foetal growth. Also, evidence shows that the drugs can increase the risk of foetal growth problems (including small head size), placental abruption (see Chapter 16), and foetal stroke or death.

Looking at Lifestyle Changes

Your lifestyle will inevitably change during your pregnancy. You may wonder whether it's still okay to do some of the things you may have done on a regular basis before you were pregnant. This section provides information on activities, such as whether you can safely colour your hair while you're pregnant, whether you can go into saunas and hot tubs, whether you can travel and when, and whether you can continue working. Your diet may also change – albeit only for the next nine months. Chapter 5 goes into more details on healthy diets for pregnant women.

Pampering yourself with beauty treatments

When your friends and relatives hear that you're pregnant, they'll probably tell you how beautiful you look or what a lovely maternal glow you have. And you may feel more beautiful, too, although some women feel the exact opposite. You may find that you're not happy with the physical changes that are happening to your body. Either way, if you're like most of our patients, you may wonder whether your customary beauty habits are safe to follow during pregnancy. In this section, we go over them one-by-one and let you know about any possible risks:

- **Botox:** The safety of botox therapy during pregnancy and breastfeeding is unknown. Our advice? Enjoy the beauty from your pregnancy glow while you're pregnant, and wait for the botox.
- **Chemical peels:** Alpha-hydroxy acids are the main ingredients in chemical peels. The chemicals work topically, but small amounts are absorbed into your system. We haven't found any data on whether chemical peels are safe during pregnancy and they're probably okay; but if you want to, discuss it first with your practitioner.
- **Facials:** You may notice that your complexion has changed over the past few months, because sometimes pregnancy hormones can wreak havoc on your skin. Facials may or may not help. But go ahead and have a facial anyway, if only to enjoy the time to sit back and relax! (See earlier comments about chemical peels.)
- **Hair dyes:** One of the first questions some of our patients bring up is, 'Can I have my hair dyed?' or 'Can I have my highlights done?' (Others wait until their roots have grown halfway down their heads and then plead for permission.) Using hair dyes during pregnancy is probably fine. No evidence suggests that modern hair dyes cause birth defects or miscarriage.
- **Hair waxing:** Waxing legs or the bikini line involves applying a heated wax preparation topically and then removing it along with the hair. Nothing in the wax preparations can lead to problems for your baby. So keep waxing away while you're pregnant to help you remain carefree and hair-free.
- **Laser hair removal:** The laser used for hair removal works by transmitting heat to the hair follicle, and stopping hair regrowth. Often anaesthetic creams are applied to the skin first to reduce pain. Although we can't find specific data on laser hair removal during pregnancy, we know of no reason that this therapy, which is applied locally, should cause any problem to your baby.

- **Manicures and pedicures:** Another frequently asked question is: 'Can I have a manicure/pedicure or have nail tips or acrylic nails placed while I'm pregnant?' Again, the answer is yes. Common sense suggests that if you go to a reputable salon where the equipment is properly cleaned and the area is well ventilated, the risk is nil.
- **Massages:** Massages are fine, and you'll find that many massage therapists offer special pregnancy massages aimed at accommodating your pregnant belly. Some use special tables with the centre cut out so that you can comfortably lie face down, especially in the latter part of your pregnancy.
- **Perms:** No scientific evidence suggests that the chemicals in hair perms are harmful to the developing baby. These preparations usually do contain significant amounts of ammonia, however, and for your own safety, use them in well-ventilated areas.
- **Wrinkle creams:** The two most common anti-wrinkle creams used today are Retin-A and Renova. Both of these preparations contain vitamin A derivatives. Substantial data exist to suggest that oral medications containing vitamin A derivatives can cause birth defects, but the information that's available on topical preparations such as Retin-A and Renova doesn't indicate a problem. Due to the significant effects of oral preparations, however, many practitioners are reluctant to recommend any medications containing these compounds – oral or topical – to their patients.

Relaxing in jacuzzis, saunas, or steam rooms

Using jacuzzis, saunas, or steam rooms when you're pregnant can be risky because of the high temperatures involved. In laboratory animals, exposure to high levels of heat during pregnancy has been known to cause birth defects or miscarriage. Studies involving humans suggest that pregnant women whose core body temperatures rise significantly during the early weeks of pregnancy may stand an increased risk of miscarriage or having babies with neural tube defects (spina bifida, for example).

However, problems typically occur only if the mother's core temperature rises above 39 degrees Celsius for more than ten minutes during the first seven weeks of her pregnancy.

In general, soaking in a warm, soothing bath is fine during pregnancy. Just make sure that the water temperature isn't too high, for the reasons just mentioned.

Common sense suggests that occasional use of jacuzzis, saunas, and steam rooms for less than ten minutes, and after the first trimester, is probably okay. However, remember to drink plenty of fluids to avoid dehydration.

Travelling

The main potential problem with travelling during pregnancy is that it puts distance between you and your practitioner. If you're close to your due date or if your pregnancy is considered high-risk, you probably shouldn't travel far from home. Your decision to travel, though, depends on what the risk factors actually are. If you have diabetes but it's well controlled, going on a trip is probably okay. But if you're pregnant with triplets, travelling to Timbuktu probably isn't a good idea. If your pregnancy is uncomplicated, travel during the first, second, and early third trimesters is usually okay.

Travelling by car poses no special risk, aside from requiring that you sit in one place for a long time. On long trips, stop every couple of hours to get out and walk around a bit. Wear your seat belt and shoulder strap; they keep you safe, and they won't hurt the baby, even if you're in an accident. The amniotic fluid surrounding the foetus serves as a cushion against any constriction from the lap belt. Not wearing restraints clearly poses a greater risk; studies show that the leading cause of foetal death in car accidents is death of the mother.

TIP

Wear your seat belt below your abdomen, not above it, and keep the shoulder strap in its usual position.

Most airlines allow women to fly short distances if they're less than 36 weeks pregnant, and long distances if they're less than 32 weeks pregnant. Many airlines require you to have a note from your practitioner indicating that she sees no medical reason why you shouldn't fly, especially after about 28 weeks of pregnancy. Check with the airline when you book, and give your GP a couple of days' notice to provide you with a certificate of fitness to fly. Your GP will charge you for providing this service.

Flying is perfectly safe, especially if you take a couple of precautions:

- **Get up from your seat occasionally during longer flights and walk around the plane.** Prolonged periods of sitting can cause blood to pool in your legs. Walking around keeps your circulation going.
- **Carry a bottle of water with you and drink from it frequently.** Aeroplane air is always very dry, so you can easily become dehydrated during long flights. Drinking extra water also ensures that you get up frequently to go to the loo, which keeps the blood from pooling in your legs.

You don't need to worry about airport metal detectors – or any other metal detectors – because they don't use ionising radiation. (The conveyor belt that carries your luggage after you check in does use ionising radiation, however, so we don't recommend that you climb onto the counter and send yourself through that machine.)

If you plan to visit tropical countries, where some diseases are particularly prevalent, you may want to be vaccinated before you go. But check with your doctor to see whether any vaccines you're considering are safe to have during pregnancy. (For more information on vaccines, see Chapter 1.)

Getting dental care

Most people see their dentist for routine cleanings every 6 to 12 months, which means you'll probably need to visit your dentist at least once during your pregnancy. Pregnancy itself shouldn't affect your dental health, but some recent studies have shown that pregnant women who suffer from *periodontal disease*, which is infection and inflammation of the gums, are at a higher risk for delivering small or premature babies.

Pregnancy causes an increase in blood flow to the gums. About half of all pregnant women develop a condition called pregnancy gingivitis, which is simply a reddening of the gums caused by this increased blood flow. In this condition, gums have a tendency to bleed easily, so try to be gentle when you brush and floss your teeth.

The good news is that while you're pregnant, and for one year after you deliver, you are eligible for free dental care on the NHS. Hooray. The bad news is that many areas of the country are very short of NHS dentists, and private dentists don't provide a discount. Boo.

If you need routine dental work – cavities filled, teeth pulled, crowns placed – don't worry. Local anaesthetics and most pain medications are safe.

Remember, if you plan on having extensive dental work that requires a general anaesthetic, make sure your anaesthetist knows that you're pregnant and has experience in giving anaesthetics to pregnant women.

Having sex

For most couples, having sex during pregnancy is perfectly safe. You may even find that sex during pregnancy is even better than before. However, you may have some issues to consider.

In the first half of pregnancy, because your body hasn't changed that noticeably, sex can usually continue as before. You may notice that your breasts are particularly sensitive to the touch, or even tender. Later, as the uterus grows, some sexual positions become more difficult. You and your partner may find that you have to be a little creative in making things work. If you find that intercourse is too uncomfortable, other forms of sexual gratification may work better for you and your partner.

Many women ask us whether having sex at the end of pregnancy is okay, even if the cervix is a little bit dilated. Having sex then is perfectly fine as long as your membranes haven't ruptured (your water hasn't broken).

CAUTION

Avoid intercourse if you're at a high risk for preterm labour. Most practitioners suggest refraining from intercourse because of the concern that it could introduce an infection into the uterus and because semen contains substances that are known to make the uterus contract. Additionally, if you have placenta praevia (see Chapter 16) in the third trimester, avoid intercourse. If you have a low-risk pregnancy, on the other hand, intercourse and orgasm isn't a risky business.

Another important aspect to consider is how each of you feels psychologically about having sex during pregnancy. You may find that your libido or sex drive has increased. Often, you may have vivid sexual dreams and that orgasm itself is heightened. Alternatively, you may find that your interest in sex is less than it was before you got pregnant. You may feel less attractive because of the physical changes that have taken place, which is perfectly normal.

JUST FOR DADS

As a father-to-be, you may also experience a changing desire for sex. You may be nervous that sex will hurt the baby (it won't), or you may simply be distracted by the prospect of being a dad. Don't worry – having a sneaking fear that the baby will know what you and mum are up to (she doesn't!), or not being able to keep your hands off your voluptuous wife are equally common and entirely natural!

Working during Pregnancy: A Different Type of Labour

More than 75 per cent of women work in the third trimester, and more than half work until a few weeks before delivery. For many women, working until the end of pregnancy keeps them happy and occupied, and helps them not to focus on the discomforts. In addition, many women don't have a choice to work or not, because they are the main income provider for their families, and their careers are top priority. Although most of the time, working throughout pregnancy doesn't cause any problems for the baby, there can be some exceptions. No matter what type of work you do, discuss your working conditions with your doctor.

Maybe your job requires minimal standing or walking, allows you to work regular hours, and never stresses you out. If that's the case, and if you have no previous medical problems, you may just as well skip this section (and let us know what your job is). But if you're like the rest of us, read on.

Stress-free, sedentary jobs are perfectly safe during pregnancy, but occupations that are physically demanding can be problematic. Most jobs fall somewhere in between, but even then the amount of stress varies according to the individual. If your pregnancy proceeds without complications, you probably can continue to work right up until delivery if you want to.

Stress in pregnancy, whether related to work or to home situations, isn't well studied. Some doctors believe that very high levels of stress may increase the risk of developing pre-eclampsia or preterm labour (both of which we discuss in Chapter 16). Too much stress obviously isn't good for anyone. Take whatever healthy measures you can to decrease the stress in your life.

If you work at a computer terminal, you may wonder if you're being exposed to anything harmful. But you have no need to worry – no evidence suggests that the electromagnetic field that computer terminals emit is a problem.

Some studies suggest that women who have jobs associated with physically demanding responsibilities, such as heavy lifting, manual labour, or significant physical exertion, may be at a slightly higher risk of preterm birth, high blood pressure, pre-eclampsia, or small-for-gestational-age babies. Long working hours however, have not been found to increase the chances for premature delivery. Other studies have also shown that jobs in which prolonged standing is required (more than eight hours a day) were associated with a greater chance for back and foot pain, preterm birth, and circulatory problems. The good news: The use of support tights, although not particularly attractive, is helpful in decreasing varicose veins.

Remember that your health and your baby's health are the highest priority. Don't feel that you're a wimp because you have to attend to your pregnancy. Some women believe that if they complain about certain symptoms or take time out from a busy schedule to eat or go to the loo, they will garner the disapproval of their superiors at work. Don't let yourself feel guilty about your special needs during this time, and don't let work cause you to ignore any unusual symptoms. If you need time off to deal with complications, take it, and don't feel bad about it. People who have never been pregnant don't completely understand the physical strains you're dealing with.

For more information about the benefits available and the rights you have when labouring through your labour, take a look at Chapter 4.

Chapter 4

Checking Out Your Rights and Welfare Benefits

In This Chapter

- Knowing your rights – you and the law
- Finding out about pregnancy's financial benefits
- Continuing to benefit as a new parent

Every pregnant woman in the UK needs the information in this chapter. Parents-to-be are entitled to hundreds of pounds worth of benefits, and understanding the basics is important if you want to make sure you get your full entitlement.

We've made this chapter as accurate and up to date as possible. However, benefits do change frequently, so check with your Jobcentre about the most up-to-date entitlements.

Two main groups of benefits exist for women:

- Entitlements during pregnancy
- Entitlements as a new parent

These entitlements are dealt with in separate sections in this chapter.

Reading through this chapter, you'll probably be either confused or a career statistician! Most people find the various entitlements confusing, but you don't have to find your way through the maze of jargon by yourself. You can ask for advice from your local Jobcentre Plus, Jobcentre or social security office (*Note:* When we talk about Jobcentres later in this chapter, we use the term 'Jobcentres' to include Jobcentre Plus, Jobcentre, or social security office.) Look for the number in your phone book, in the business numbers section. Alternatively, you can contact your local Citizens' Advice Bureau (CAB) – the number for your nearest location is also in the phone book.

Dads aren't forgotten when it comes to parental rights. You can find out about your rights as a father in the section 'Statutory Paternity Pay', later in this chapter.

Your Rights When You're Having a Baby

Financial benefits during pregnancy are important to understand, and are explained later in this chapter, but it's just as important to know about your rights as a pregnant woman. This section highlights your two most important rights: maternity leave, and the Sex Discrimination Act (1975).

Discrimination against pregnant women

Most cases of discrimination come about because someone believes they have been treated less favourably than someone else in a comparable situation. Until scientists work out how men can get pregnant (wouldn't *that* be fun to see), no direct male comparison for a pregnant woman exists. However, when you're pregnant you have something called *protected status*, meaning that if you're treated less favourably as a direct result of your pregnancy, you will automatically have a case of discrimination on the grounds of sex, under the Sex Discrimination Act.

Protected status lasts from the time your employer knows of your pregnancy until the end of your maternity leave (explained later in this chapter). If you feel that you've been discriminated against, talk to a solicitor or to your local Citizens' Advice Bureau.

Ordinary and additional maternity leave

Any woman having a baby is entitled to an ordinary maternity leave, or OML, of 26 weeks. You don't have to work for any particular length of time to qualify for OML. In fact, your OML can technically start from the first day of your employment, although you do need to give your employer notice of maternity leave before you start on an OML, unless doing so is not reasonably manageable. You can find out more about any exceptions, or about OML overall, from the Department of Trade and Industry booklet 'Maternity Rights', which you can get from your local Jobcentre or download from the Internet at `www.dti.gov.uk/er/maternity.htm`.

You can begin your OML at any time from the start of the eleventh week before your Expected Week of Confinement, unless your baby is born before then. Your *Expected Week of Confinement* (EWC) is the week your due date falls in. You must start your leave on whichever of the following scenarios happens earliest:

- You give birth.
- You start any pregnancy-related absence in the four weeks before your EWC.
- The date you've given your employer as your OML start date. (Remember, you need to notify your employer before the fifteenth week before your EWC, unless it's not reasonably manageable to do so.)

You're also entitled to additional maternity leave (AML) if you're already entitled to OML *and* have at least 26 weeks' service in your job by the end of the fifteenth week before your EWC. AML lasts for 26 weeks on top of OML, giving you up to a total of 52 weeks of maternity leave.

REMEMBER

Ordinary maternity leave and additional maternity leave are both unpaid periods away from work.

Financial Benefits during Pregnancy

The last thing you want to worry about during your pregnancy is money. Financial help is available, and this section helps you to get the best from it. You usually fall into one of the following benefits categories:

- You're employed, and earn enough to pay National Insurance (NI) Contributions – in this case, check out the section on Statutory Maternity Pay (SMP) in this chapter.
- You're employed, but earn less than the NI threshold – in this case, see the section on Maternity Allowance (MA) in this chapter.
- You aren't eligible for SMP, or have recently changed job or left work – head for the section on Maternity Allowance (MA) in this chapter.
- You're self-employed – the section on Maternity Allowance (MA) is for you, too.
- You can't get SMP or MA – you may be able to claim Incapacity Benefit. Talk to your Jobcentre for more details.

The payments you're eligible for sometimes depend on whether your earnings qualify you to receive National Insurance (NI). Working out your eligibility can be confusing, as you can be over this threshold even if you don't earn enough to be required to pay National Insurance contributions. Talk to your employer or your Jobcentre.

Statutory maternity pay

Statutory Maternity Pay (SMP) is claimed from, and paid by, your employer for up to 26 weeks. You can start claiming SMP at any time from the eleventh week before your expected date of delivery (EDD) until the day after your baby is born.

You should be entitled to SMP if:

- You're an employee in the week you start maternity leave.
- You have at least 26 weeks' continuous service by the end of the fifteenth week before your EWC and have been earning, over the eight weeks before you claim SMP, an average wage that is enough to be 'relevant' for National Insurance (NI) purposes. You can find out more about what's relevant from your Jobcentre.

The following provisos apply to SMP:

- You can't claim SMP and be paid for working.
- Tax and NI deductions apply to SMP.
- You need to let your employer know about your EWC at least four weeks before you intend to stop working, to qualify for SMP.
- You need a MAT B1 form to claim SMP (see the section 'You and your MAT B1', later in this chapter).
- You may need to apply for SMP from all your employers, if you have more than one.

Maternity allowances

You can start claiming Maternity Allowance (MA) at any time from the eleventh week before your EDD until the day after your baby is born, although you can't claim whilst you're still working. MA isn't taxable, and is paid for up to 26 weeks.

Ask about claiming for MA if you:

- can't get SMP (see above)
- are employed or self-employed and are paying NI contributions, or are earning more than an average of £30 a week

Sure Start Maternity Grants

If you, or your partner, are claiming Income Support, Income-based Jobseeker's Allowance, or some kinds of Working Tax Credit or Child Tax Credit, you may be eligible for a Sure Start Maternity Grant. This grant can be claimed from 11 weeks before your EWC until three months after you deliver. Designed to help with the cost of things for the new baby, you can find out more about Sure Start Maternity Grants at your Jobcentre or at the Department of Work and Pensions Web site: `www.dwp.gov.uk/lifeevent/benefits/sure_start_maternity_grant.asp`.

You and your Mat B1

You need a form Mat B1 to claim for several allowances, including SMP. The Mat B1 is a form confirming that you are pregnant, and also confirming your EDD. You can ask your practitioner for a form Mat B1 at any time from 20 weeks into your pregnancy.

Entitlements as a New Parent

After your baby is born the spending starts in earnest. Even the most conservative list of baby essentials is pretty long (see Chapter 13 for more details about what's needed). Fortunately, several sources of ongoing financial support are available. You should be sent details of these benefits automatically when you register your baby's birth (see Chapter 13). For more details on any of these benefits, contact your Jobcentre or nearest Inland Revenue enquiry centre (look for Inland Revenue in the business numbers section of the phone book). Alternatively, the Child Benefit Centre (0845 302 1444) can help with child benefit enquiries, and the Tax Credit Helpline (0845 300 3900) can tell you about tax credits.

Child benefit

As a parent, you're entitled to child benefit until your child is at least 16 years old. Child benefit is not affected by income or savings.

Working tax credit

If you and your partner (if you have one) are working, but your joint income is low, you may be eligible for working tax credit. This credit includes help with the costs of childcare. Working tax credit is paid to you if you are the main carer. The income level at which you stop being eligible depends on the number of children you have, but you won't be eligible under any circumstances if your family income is £60,000 a year or more.

Child tax credit

Child tax credit is a payment to support families with children until they are at leastage 16. You can claim child tax credit whether you're working or not, as long as your family income is under £58,000 a year. If you're receiving Income Support or income-based Jobseeker's allowance, you'll be given child tax credit automatically by the Department of Work and Pensions, without needing to apply. Otherwise, contact your Jobcentre, Inland Revenue Enquiry Centre, or Tax Credit Helpline.

Statutory Paternity Pay

As the father of a newborn baby, you may be entitled to up to two weeks Statutory Paternity Pay (SPP), paid by your employer. The employment and earning requirements are the same as those for SMP (see the section on 'Statutory maternity pay' earlier in this chapter). As with SMP, you can't claim for any week you're working, and you may have to make separate claims if you have more than one employer. You'll also need to tell your employer at least 15 weeks before you intend to claim SPP. You can start your SPP any day from your baby's birth, but it must be completed within eight weeks of your baby's EWC.

Chapter 5

Diet and Exercise for the Expectant Mother

In This Chapter

- Understanding healthy weight gain – yours and your baby's
- Thinking about what – and how much – you eat
- Knowing which foods to avoid
- Looking at special dietary considerations
- Staying fit, safely, during pregnancy

Through the ages, women have received all kinds of advice about what, and how much, to eat while they're expecting. Cultural traditions, religious beliefs, and scientific thinking have all had their influence. Your practitioner's advice is likely to depend on your particular health habits and your size when your pregnancy begins. Also, if you're carrying more than one baby, you're expected to gain more than the average number of pounds.

Health involves more than just eating well. Exercise is as important while you're pregnant as it was before, although what and how much you do to stay fit may change as your pregnancy progresses. This chapter provides you with the information you need in order to properly nourish yourself and your baby and to keep you exercising safely. If you want even more tips and advice, check out *Fit Pregnancy For Dummies* by Catherine Cram and Tere Stouffer Drenth (Wiley).

Looking at Healthy Weight Gain

Starting pregnancy at a healthy weight and gaining weight at a moderate pace throughout pregnancy can help ensure that your baby grows and develops normally, and that you stay healthy as well.

Determining how much is enough

The best way to figure out your ideal weight – and weight gain – is to look at a measurement that's known as *body mass index*, a number that takes into account both height and weight.

Find your body mass index by looking up your measurements on the chart in Figure 5-1. Locate your weight on the vertical line on the left-hand side of the chart and your height on the horizontal (bottom) line. (Alternatively, use the metric measurements on the top and right-hand side.) The place where those two points intersect on the chart is your body mass index (follow the diagonal lines until you find the BMI number).

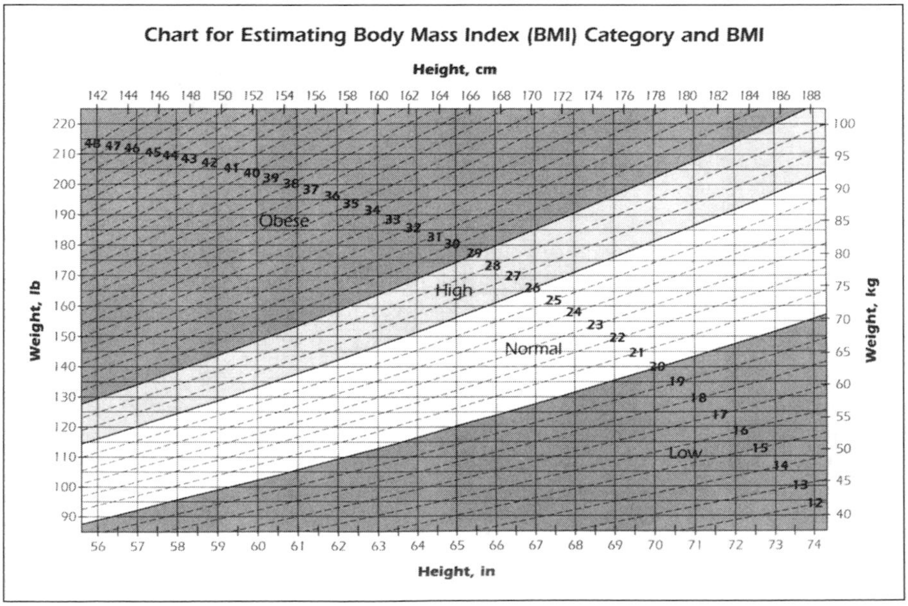

Figure 5-1: The body mass index chart.

Source: Nutrition During Pregnancy and Lactation, National Academy Press, 1992

After you know your body mass index, you can figure out your ideal weight gain during pregnancy by consulting Table 5-1. (But don't forget, this number refers to women carrying only one baby.)

Table 5-1 Figuring Out Your Ideal Weight Gain

Body Mass Index	*Recommended Weight Gain*
Less than 19.8 (underweight)	28 to 40 pounds (12.5 to 18 kilograms)
19.9 to 26 (normal weight)	25 to 35 pounds (11.5 to 16 kilograms)
26 to 29 (overweight)	15 to 25 pounds (7 to 11.5 kilograms)
29 or more (obese)	15 pounds (6 kilograms) or less

DON'T WORRY

Scientific research hasn't determined the optimal pattern of weight gain throughout pregnancy. Gaining very little weight early on (when you may be in the throes of morning sickness) may have less effect on foetal growth than does poor weight gain in the late second or third trimesters. Some women gain weight inconsistently, putting on a large number of pounds early and then much less later on. Nothing is necessarily unhealthy about this pattern. That's why (as mentioned in Chapter 3) you may find that you don't get weighed regularly at your antenatal appointments.

Avoiding weight obsession

Use the charts of optimal weight gain as a guide, but don't become fanatical about how much you weigh. Even if the amount you gain is not going to plan, as long as your doctor says that the baby is growing normally, you have nothing to worry about. Women who gain more than average can still have healthy babies, and so can women who gain very little. The size of your 'bump' is, on the whole, a much more accurate predictor of your baby's wellbeing – and your practitioner keeps a regular eye on this.

REMEMBER

The bottom line is that you want to do all you can to improve your baby's chances of optimal growth and development, but not at the expense of driving yourself crazy.

Where does the weight go?

The good news is the weight you gain during pregnancy doesn't all go to your thighs. Then again, the weight doesn't all go to the baby. A pregnant woman typically adds a little to her own body fat. That you can tell by a woman's pattern of weight gain – more in the hips or more in the belly – whether she's going to have a boy or a girl is a myth, however. (See Chapter 20 for some other myths regarding determining your baby's sex.)

Look at this realistic view of your weight gain – assuming it's 27 pounds, which is fairly average:

Baby	7 pounds (3,180 grams)
Placenta	1 pound (455 grams)
Amniotic fluid	2 pounds (910 grams)
Uterus	2 pounds (910 grams)
Breasts	1 pound (455 grams)
Fat stores	7 pounds (3,180 grams)
Body water	4 pounds (1,820 grams)
Extra blood	3 pounds (1,360 grams)

Understanding your baby's weight gain

Although your weight gain may follow a path all its own, your baby's own bulking-up pattern is likely to progress slowly at first, and then pick up at about 32 weeks, only to slow again in the last weeks before birth. At 14–15 weeks, for example, the baby puts on weight at about 0.18 ounces (5 grams) per day, and at 32–34 weeks, 1.06 to 1.23 ounces (30–35 grams) per day (that's about half a pound or 0.23 kilograms each week). After 36 weeks, the foetal growth rate slows, and by 41–42 weeks (you're overdue at this point), minimal or no further foetal growth may occur. Check out Chapter 7 for more about how your baby grows.

In addition to your diet and weight gain, the following factors affect foetal growth:

- **Cigarette smoking.** Smoking can reduce the birth-weight by about half a pound (about 200 grams).
- **Diabetes.** If the mother has diabetes, the baby can be too big or too small.
- **Genetic or family history.** In other words, rugby players usually don't have children who grow up to be professional jockeys!
- **Foetal infection.** Some infections affect growth.

- **Illicit drug use.** Drug abuse can slow foetal growth.
- **Mother's medical history.** Some medical problems, like hypertension or lupus, can affect foetal growth.
- **Multiple pregnancy.** Twins and triplets are often smaller than single babies.
- **Placental function.** Placental blood flow that's below par can slow down the baby's growth.

Your practitioner keeps an eye on your baby's growth rate, most often by measuring fundal height (see Chapter 3 for more on this). If your fundal height measurements are abnormal, or if something in your history puts you at risk for growth problems, your practitioner is likely to send you for an ultrasound scan to assess the situation more accurately.

Taking Stock of What You're Taking In

Sticking to a well-balanced, low-fat, high-fibre diet is important not only for your baby but also for your own health. Consuming adequate protein is important, because protein carries out many of the body's functions. The fibre in your diet helps to prevent or reduce constipation and haemorrhoids (piles). By not consuming too much fat, you help keep your heart healthy, and also avoid putting on extra pounds that may be difficult to shed. By avoiding excessive weight gain, you also decrease the chances of developing stretch marks. To read more about stretch marks, see Chapter 8.

If your diet is balanced and not too heavy in sugar or fat, you don't need to modify the way you eat dramatically. During pregnancy, take in roughly 300 *extra* calories a day, on average.

Your growing baby – and your changing body – need more than just extra calories. They also need more vitamins and minerals, so make sure your 300 extra calories come from the healthy options in the section that follows, no matter how tempted you are by that extra piece of chocolate cake.

Using a healthy eating pyramid

No single food can satisfy all your important nutritional needs. A *healthy eating pyramid* (see Figure 5-2) is a general guideline that illustrates the relative proportions of servings you should eat in each group.

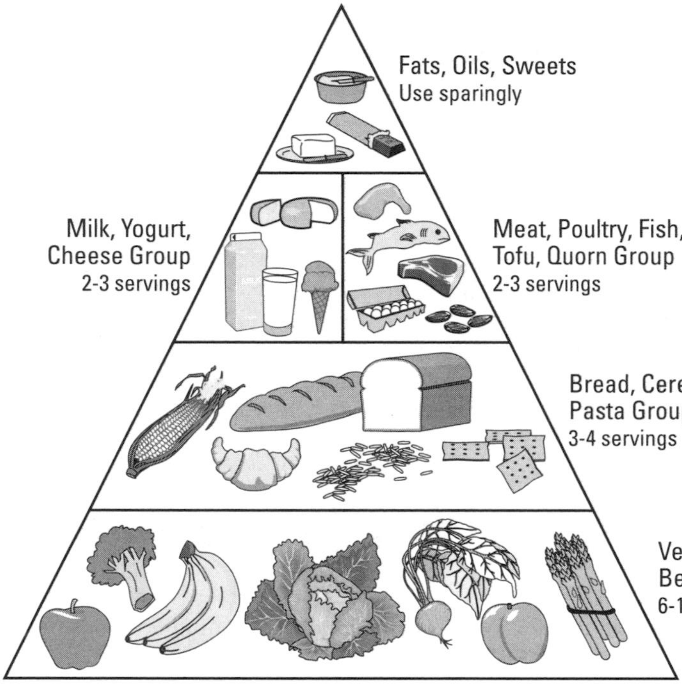

Figure 5-2: Use a healthy eating pyramid to help you eat healthily during pregnancy.

Even though the pyramid may seem to contain a lot of food, satisfying this requirement is easier than you think. For example, one slice of bread, a few biscuits, or half a cup of pasta each makes up just a single serving – so a full meal for most of us will include several such servings.

REMEMBER

Fruit and vegetables are not only a good source of vitamins and minerals but they also provide fibre, which is very important during pregnancy to help reduce constipation.

DON'T WORRY

Experiencing morning sickness during the first trimester is very common (see Chapter 6). If you're experiencing this nausea and can't eat a well-balanced diet, you may wonder whether or not you're getting enough nutrition for you and the baby. Actually, you can go for several weeks not eating an optimal diet without any ill effects on the baby. You may find that the only foods you can tolerate are foods heavy in starch or carbohydrates. If all you feel like eating are potatoes, bread, and pasta, go right ahead. Keeping something down is better than starving.

Your body can build stores of some vitamins, such as A and D. Other vitamins, like folic acid and vitamin C, can't be stored and need to be eaten regularly. So when you do feel like eating, try to opt for foods with a high level of folic acid and vitamin C.

Is caffeine safe during pregnancy?

Although some people think that the only food that contains caffeine is a strong cup of coffee, you can find caffeine in many of the other things you eat and drink on a daily basis: tea, many fizzy drinks, cocoa, and chocolate. Most studies suggest that it takes more than 300 milligrams (mg) of caffeine a day to affect the foetus (a mug of coffee contains between 40–150 mg, and a bar of chocolate between 30–60 mg). While no evidence suggests that caffeine causes birth defects, consuming caffeine above this level can raise the risk of low birth-weight and miscarriage. To be on the safe side, though, it's worth sticking to a total caffeine consumption of under 300 mg a day. Since the average caffeine consumption in the UK is about 400 mg a day, you're likely to have to think about cutting your caffeine intake a bit. If you have a history of miscarriage, or if your practitioner is concerned that your baby is growing too slowly, consider cutting out caffeine altogether.

TIP

If you earn a low income, you may be among the 800,000 people in the UK who are eligible for free healthy eating vouchers. These vouchers can be exchanged for healthy foods in local shops. Ask your practitioner for details.

REMEMBER

As your pregnancy progresses, your body needs a lot of extra fluid. Early on, some women who don't drink enough liquid feel weak or faint. Later in pregnancy, dehydration can lead to premature contractions. Make a point of drinking plenty of water (or milk or juice) – about 6 to 8 glasses a day, and a bit more if you are carrying more than one baby.

Supplementing your diet

If your diet is healthy and balanced, you naturally get most of the vitamins and minerals you need – with the exception of folic acid, iron, calcium, and possibly vitamin D (refer to Chapter 1). Some countries routinely recommend vitamin supplements for all pregnant women, but in the UK, most practitioners suggest that you pay more attention to your diet and not rely on such supplements.

TIP

If you are hungrier than usual, try to fill up on healthy foods like fruit, wholemeal bread, and low-fat cheese rather than the empty calories found in sweets, cakes, and biscuits. Eating healthily doesn't need to cost a fortune – baked beans on toast, or a baked potato filled with tinned tuna and sweetcorn are about as healthy as you can get.The following sections give you advice on some of the harder to source vitamins during your pregnancy.

Folic acid

You might have heard about the importance of folic acid in the development of your baby's nervous system before you ever get pregnant. If not, don't worry – just start taking a folic acid supplement of 400 micrograms a day as soon as you can in the first trimester. You can find out more about folic acid in Chapter 1.

Calcium

Calcium is essential for healthy teeth and bones – for both you and your baby. You need about 1,200 mg of calcium every day while you're pregnant. Most women actually get much less. If you're already starting out somewhat calcium deficient, the calcium requirements of the developing baby will only make matters worse for you. A foetus can extract enough calcium from its mother, even if it means getting it at the expense of the mother's bones. So the extra calcium needed during pregnancy is really aimed at protecting you and your health.

Getting enough calcium from your diet alone is possible if you really pay attention. You can get what you need from three to four servings of calcium-rich foods, such as milk, yoghurt, cheese, green leafy vegetables, and canned fish with bones (if your stomach can take it).

Iron

Iron is an essential component of red blood cells. You need more iron when you're expecting, because both you and the baby are making new red blood cells every day. On average, you need 30 mg of extra iron every day of your pregnancy, which is what most antenatal vitamins contain. Blood counts can easily drop during pregnancy, because your body is gradually making more and more blood *plasma* (fluid) and *relatively* fewer red blood cells (which is called *dilutional anaemia*). If you do develop anaemia, you may need to take an extra iron supplement.

Foods rich in iron include chicken, fish, red meat, green leafy vegetables, beans, nuts, and enriched or whole-grain breads and cereals. You can raise the iron content of foods by cooking them in cast-iron pots and skillets.

Vitamin C

Vitamin C is essential in everybody's diet, to help combat the risk of a condition called scurvy. Your body doesn't store vitamin C very well, so try to eat or drink some daily. Fruit and vegetables are particularly good sources of vitamin C, as well as fibre and minerals. Fruit juice is high in vitamin C.

Vitamin D

Your body needs vitamin D to use the calcium it gets through your diet more effectively. Most dairy products provide a good source of vitamin D.

Diet isn't the only source of vitamin D available; you can also get vitamin D from sunlight, which isn't an excuse to become a sun worshipper and give yourself skin cancer in later life. Unless you have dark skin and cover up completely, you should get enough vitamin D from day-to-day exposure without sunbathing.

Determining Which Foods Are Safe

When our patients ask us about nutrition and which foods to avoid, certain items come up again and again. Some of the foods we're most often asked about should be avoided, and others are unlikely to cause harm.

Debunking popular food myths

Many of the foods that have at one time or another been thought dangerous for pregnant women aren't likely to harm you or your baby.

Although you don't have to avoid the following foods, eat them in moderation.

- **Cheeses:** Most people believe that processed and pasteurised cheeses aren't only safe, but they're also a great source of both protein and calcium. See the section 'Identifying potentially harmful foods' for information about unpasteurised cheeses and soft cheeses with skins.
- **Fish:** Most fish is perfectly safe to eat during pregnancy. Fish is a great source of protein and vitamins, and is also low in fat. The high levels of protein, omega-3 fatty acids, vitamin D, and other nutrients make fish an excellent food for pregnant mothers and their developing babies. However, certain fish – tuna, shark, marlin, and swordfish – contain high levels of mercury, which may lead to certain childhood developmental delays or problems with fine motor skills. To be on the safe side, limit or avoid fish with high levels of mercury when you're pregnant. The Food Standards Agency recommends no more than one tuna steak or two cans of tuna a week, but you can still enjoy salmon, haddock, cod, and sole worry-free.
- **Sushi:** Raw fish carries a small risk of a parasitic infection (which can make you feel sick), whether you're pregnant or not. Pregnancy doesn't increase the danger, and your foetus is unlikely to suffer any harm from such an infection. Make sure that the fish comes from a reliable source.
- **Smoked meats or fish:** Many pregnant women worry about eating smoked meats and fish because they've heard that these foods are high in nitrites or nitrates. Although these foods do contain these substances, they won't hurt your baby if eaten in moderation.

Identifying potentially harmful foods

Most of the infections you can get through food during pregnancy are very rare, despite occasional media scaremongering. However, a few infections that can be passed on through food are worth knowing about and taking measures to avoid; we've listed them in this section. The good news is that you can still have an excellent and varied diet if you exclude all the potential sources of infection below – so it shouldn't be a great sacrifice to cut them out.

Listeriosis

Listeriosis is caused by bacteria (germs or bugs) called *Listeris monocytogenes* (listeria). In its mild form listeriosis causes a flu-like illness, but during pregnancy it can cause miscarriage, stillbirth, or severe illness in your newborn baby.

Luckily, listeriosis is a very rare disease, occurring in about 1 in 30,000 births in the UK. What's more, listeriosis is easy to avoid, simply by not eating certain foods that have been linked to high levels of the bacteria. To avoid the risk of listeriosis, avoid:

- soft cheeses with skins
- blue-veined cheeses
- unpasteurised cheeses
- any kind of pâté
- microwave meals or ready-cooked poultry, unless thoroughly heated and piping hot

You don't need to avoid these foods before you know that you're pregnant for sure, or after the baby is born; you just need to avoid them during your pregnancy.

Toxoplasmosis

Toxoplasmosis is caused by an infection called *Toxoplasma gondii* (which is found in raw meat and cat faeces). Of course, nobody deliberately eats cat faeces, but your hands and food can easily be contaminated if you don't take a few simple precautions. Like listeriosis, toxoplasmosis is rare – approximately 1 in 50,000 total births.

If you get toxoplasmosis when you aren't pregnant, the symptoms resemble a mild flu-like illness. If you get toxoplasmosis during pregnancy, however, you may experience serious problems with your vision and central nervous system.

To avoid toxoplasmosis:

- Avoid eating any raw or undercooked meat.
- Always wash your hands after handling raw meat.
- Wash salad and vegetables thoroughly.
- Avoid drinking goat's milk while you are pregnant, unless pasteurised, sterilised, or UHT (ultra-heat-treated).
- Wash your hands after handling cats or kittens, no matter how clean they may seem.
- Get someone else to clean out cat litter trays regularly if possible, and always wash your hands afterwards if you do have to touch them.
- Always wear gloves when gardening, and wash your hands after gardening even if you have worn gloves.
- Avoid going near sheep or lambs at lambing time (see the sidebar 'Sheep and lambing – why the fuss?').

Chlamydiosis

Chlamydiosis is a very rare disease, but can cause you to miscarry if you're pregnant. Only pregnant women who come into close contact with sheep and newborn lambs at lambing time are at risk from this infection (see the sidebar 'Sheep and lambing – why the fuss?' for more on this).

Sheep and lambing – why the fuss?

It's hard to imagine lambs being anything other than cute and cuddly, isn't it? Well, they are most of the time. However, if you're pregnant, close contact with sheep or lambs can pose the threat of several infections, including listeriosis, toxoplasmosis, and chlamydiosis. For all these reasons, we recommend that if you're pregnant, you should not help with lambing, or milk ewes that have recently given birth, or touch the afterbirth, or come into contact with newborn lambs.

This sound advice might just seem for rural mums-to-be, but when I (Sarah) first started work as an inner city GP, one of my patients picked up on the sheep-safety section in a leaflet I gave her, and explained that her parents lived on a sheep farm in Wales, where she was planning to spend all her free time. Since then, I've lost count of the number of pregnant women who don't consider themselves at risk, but who hadn't realised that visiting a children's petting farm with their older children might pose a threat to their present pregnancy. The moral of this story is don't ever assume it won't happen to you!

Milk-borne infections

Milk that hasn't been heat-treated (pasteurised, sterilised, or UHT) can carry harmful germs that can affect your pregnancy. In the UK, all such milk has to carry the warning 'This milk has not been heat-treated and may therefore contain organisms harmful to health.'

Considering Special Dietary Needs

Try as you may to follow all the rules of healthy nutrition, you may encounter certain problems with digestion such as constipation or heartburn. Or you may find that you need to tailor the rules to fit your particular eating habits – for example, if you're a vegetarian. In this section, we address some of the issues that arise for women with special nutritional considerations and for all women who may experience any digestive problems.

Eating right, vegetarian-style

If you're a vegetarian, rest assured that you can produce a healthy baby without eating steak. But you do have to plan your diet more carefully. Vegetables, whole grains, and legumes (peas and beans, to you or me) are rich in protein, but most don't have complete proteins. (They don't contain all the essential amino acids that your body can't produce by itself.) To get all your protein, you can combine whole grains with legumes or nuts, rice with kidney beans, or even peanut butter with whole-grain bread. The combination doesn't have to occur at the same meal, only on the same day.

If you don't eat any animal products, including milk and cheese, your diet may not provide enough of six other important nutrients: vitamin B12, calcium, riboflavin, iron, zinc, and vitamin D. Bring up the topic with your doctor, and you may want to discuss your diet with a dietician.

Combating constipation

Progesterone, a hormone that circulates freely through your body during pregnancy, can slow down your digestive system and thus cause constipation. Women who are on bed rest because of pregnancy complications are at particular risk of constipation because they're so inactive. If you need to take iron because you're anaemic, this only makes matters worse.

You can counteract constipation by drinking plenty of fluids, by eating adequate fibre (in the form of fruits, vegetables, beans, bran, and other whole grains), and, if possible, by getting exercise every day (you can find out more later in this chapter). You may experience abdominal discomfort, bloating, or wind from eating too much of foods high in fibre, so use a little trial and error to see which fibre-rich foods you tolerate best.

Dealing with diabetes

If you have diabetes or if you develop diabetes during pregnancy, adjust your diet so that it includes specific quantities of proteins, fats, and carbohydrates to ensure that you maintain a normal level of blood glucose (sugar). We discuss diabetes in more detail in Chapter 17.

If you need more detailed information, check out *Diabetes For Dummies* by Sarah Jarvis and Alan L. Rubin (Wiley).

Working Out for Two

During pregnancy, exercise helps your body in many ways: It keeps your heart strong and your muscles in shape, and it relieves the basic discomforts of pregnancy – from morning sickness to constipation to achy legs and backs. The earlier in pregnancy you get regular exercise, the more comfortable you are likely to feel throughout the 40 weeks. Regular exercise may even make for shorter labour, too.

So if you're in good health and not at risk for obstetric or medical complications, by all means go ahead and continue with your exercise programme – unless your programme calls for climbing Ben Nevis, bungee jumping, or some other superstrenuous activity. If you have any queries, go over your exercise programme with your practitioner.

As good as exercise is for most pregnant women, we don't advise it for everyone. If you have any of the following conditions (see Chapters 15 and 16 for more detail), you may be better off not working out – at least not until you discuss the situation with your doctor:

- Bleeding
- Incompetent cervix
- Intrauterine growth restriction

- Low volume of amniotic fluid
- Placenta praevia (late in pregnancy)
- Pregnancy-induced hypertension
- Premature labour or preterm rupture of the membranes
- Triplets or more

You can find out many more tips for safe and healthy exercise in *Fit Pregnancy For Dummies* by Catherine Cram and Tere Stouffer Drenth (Wiley).

Adapting to your body's changes

Even if you work out in moderation, remember that pregnancy causes your body to undergo real physical changes, which can affect your strength, stamina, and performance. The following list details some of those changes:

- **Cardiovascular changes:** When you're pregnant, the amount of blood that your heart pumps through your body increases. That increase in blood volume usually has no effect on your workout. But if you lie flat on your back, especially after about 16 weeks of pregnancy, you may find yourself feeling dizzy or faint (or even nauseous), through pressure from your uterus on your major blood vessels. It happens even more readily if you're carrying a multiple pregnancy and your uterus is that much heavier.

  If you're doing any exercises that require you to lie on your back (and also if you're accustomed to sleeping on your back), put a small pillow or foam wedge under the right side of your back or your right hip. The pillow tilts you slightly sideways and effectively lifts your uterus off the blood vessels.

- **Respiratory (breathing) changes:** Your body is using more oxygen than usual to support the growing baby. At the same time, breathing is more work than it used to be because the enlarging uterus presses upward against the diaphragm. For some women, this difficulty makes performing aerobic exercise a little harder.
- **Structural changes:** As your body shape changes – bigger abdomen, larger breasts – your centre of gravity shifts, which can affect your balance. You notice this shift in gravity especially if you dance, cycle, ski, surf, ride horses, or do anything else (walk tightropes, maybe?) where balance is important. Pregnancy hormones also cause some laxness in your joints, which also can make balance more difficult and may increase your risk of injury.

- **Metabolic changes:** Pregnant women use carbohydrates faster than non-pregnant women do, which means that they're at a higher risk of developing *hypoglycaemia* (or low blood sugar). Exercise can be very useful in helping lower and control blood sugar levels, but it also increases the body's need for carbohydrates. So if you exercise, make extra sure that you're eating an adequate amount of starch.
- **Effects on the uterus:** One study of women at *term* (far enough along to deliver) showed that their contractions increased after moderate aerobic exercise. Another study indicated that exercise is associated with a lower risk of early labour. But most studies have shown that exercise has no effect either way, and does not pose a risk of preterm labour in healthy pregnant women.
- **Effect on birth-weight:** Some studies have shown that women who work out strenuously (at high intensity) during pregnancy have lighter-weight babies. The same effect appears to occur in women who perform heavy physical work in a standing position while they're pregnant. But this decrease in birth-weight seems to be due mainly to a decrease in the newborn's subcutaneous fat – more exercise has no effect on the foetus's normal growth.

Exercising without overdoing it

Your changing body is going to demand a changing exercise routine. Don't beat yourself up if you find that pregnancy makes it harder to continue the workouts you're accustomed to. Modify your programme according to what you can reasonably tolerate.

Listen to your body. If weightlifting suddenly hurts your back, lighten up. You may find it easier to perform non-weight-bearing exercises like swimming or cycling. No matter what your particular exercise regimen may be, keep in mind the basic rules for working out during pregnancy:

- If you have a moderate exercise routine, keep it up. If you've been pretty sedentary, don't suddenly plunge into a strenuous programme; ease in slowly to avoid putting too much strain on your body.

  Remember that keeping up a regular schedule of moderate activity is better than engaging in infrequent spurts of intense exercise, which are more likely to cause injury.
- Avoid overheating, especially during the first six weeks of pregnancy.
- Avoid exercising flat on your back for long periods of time; it may reduce blood flow to your heart.

- Try not to overheat or become dehydrated, and if you feel fatigued, dizzy, faint, or nauseous, stop. On very hot or humid days, don't exercise outdoors.
- Avoid anything that puts you at risk of being hurt in the abdomen, like cycling.
- Steer clear of high-impact, bouncy exercises that can tax your loosening joints.
- Throughout the nine months, low- or moderate-impact workouts make more sense than high-impact ones.
- Carry a bottle of water to every exercise session and stay well hydrated.
- Eat a well-balanced diet that includes an adequate supply of carbohydrates (see 'Taking Stock of What You're Taking In' earlier in this chapter).
- Talk to your practitioner about what your peak exercise heart rate should be. (Many practitioners suggest 140 beats per minute as the upper limit.) Then measure your heart rate regularly at the peak of your workout to make sure that it's at a safe level.

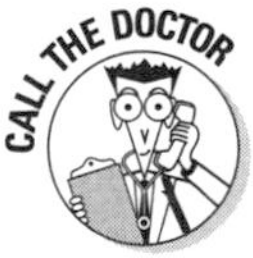

- Stop exercising and talk to your doctor if you experience any of these symptoms:
  - Shortness of breath out of proportion to the exercise you're doing
  - Vaginal bleeding
  - Rapid heartbeat (that is, more than 140 beats per minute)
  - Dizziness or feeling faint
  - Any significant pain

Comparing forms of exercise

Now isn't the time to go for that Ms Fitness title, but that certainly doesn't mean you can't exercise. Because your pregnant body demands you take new precautions, choose your style of exercise carefully.

Working your heart: Aerobic exercise

Weight-bearing exercises like running, walking, aerobics, and using a step machine are great, as long as you don't do too much. These exercises require you to support all your weight – which is ever-increasing. Because your joints are loosening at the same time, you run a slightly higher risk of injuring yourself. Remember to do only what you know you can do rather than setting off on a new exercise routine that is too demanding for your current state of fitness, not to mention your pregnancy.

The hormone changes you experience during pregnancy increase your risk of overstretching your muscles and ligaments. Any exercise that involves impact on your joints – especially high impact exercises like running, aerobics, and step classes – can jolt the small joints and ligaments of your spine. Wearing well-designed, cushioned sports shoes can help absorb the impact and prevent problems.

If you choose to take aerobics classes, look for those designed specifically for pregnant women. If no classes are available, talk to the instructor to find modifications for exercises that are inappropriate.

You may find it easier, particularly later in pregnancy, to perform non-weight-bearing exercises, such as cycling (especially on an exercise bike) or swimming. Because your weight is supported, you have less chance of injuring yourself, and your joints aren't stressed. If you're new to exercise, a low-intensity workout in the pool or on an exercise bike is ideal.

Downhill skiing, water skiing, and horseback riding put you at risk of falling with significant impact, which could injure you or your baby. Although these activities may be fine early in pregnancy, talk to your doctor before doing them in your second or third trimester. Cross-country skiing is less risky, especially if you're experienced.

Strengthening your muscles

You won't get a great cardiac benefit from weightlifting, yoga, or body sculpting, but you can improve your muscle tone and flexibility, which comes in handy during labour and delivery.

Weightlifting machines may be preferable to using free weights because you know you won't drop the weights onto your abdomen. Use free weights only with caution, preferably with the help of a trainer or a skilled friend. A trainer can also show you the proper way to exhale and inhale during lifting. Breathing well is important because it lessens the chance that you might *bear down* (otherwise known as *valsava,* or increase your abdominal pressure), which can reduce blood flow, raise your blood pressure, and stress your heart.

Avoid using very heavy weights, which can cause injury to your joints and ligaments.

Yoga, which is a great choice for pregnant women, isn't only an excellent form of exercise, but may also be helpful in mastering breathing and relaxation techniques. Yoga is particularly useful in strengthening lower back and abdominal muscles and increasing stamina and physical endurance – all of which make you better equipped to handle the rigours of pregnancy.

Specific yoga classes exist for pregnant women. See the sidebar 'Practising safe yoga' for more about this form of exercise.

Practising safe yoga

Yoga can be a wonderful and relaxing way to work out while you're pregnant, but only if you exercise caution. Follow these tips when doing yoga during pregnancy:

- If you're new to yoga, take a beginners' class to ease yourself into a new exercise regime.
- Be careful about positions that stretch your muscles too much. Due to elevated levels of progesterone and relaxin (hormones produced during pregnancy), you can easily overstretch your muscles and ligaments.
- When bending forward, try to bend from the hips, not from the back. Also, try to lift your chest high to avoid putting extra pressure on your abdomen.
- After the mid second trimester, try to avoid performing poses that require you to lie flat on your back for extensive periods of time, because pressure from a pregnant uterus may decrease blood return both to your heart and to the baby.
- As a general rule for any exercise, if you feel any pain or discomfort, stop and rest.

Part II

Pregnancy: A Drama in Three Acts

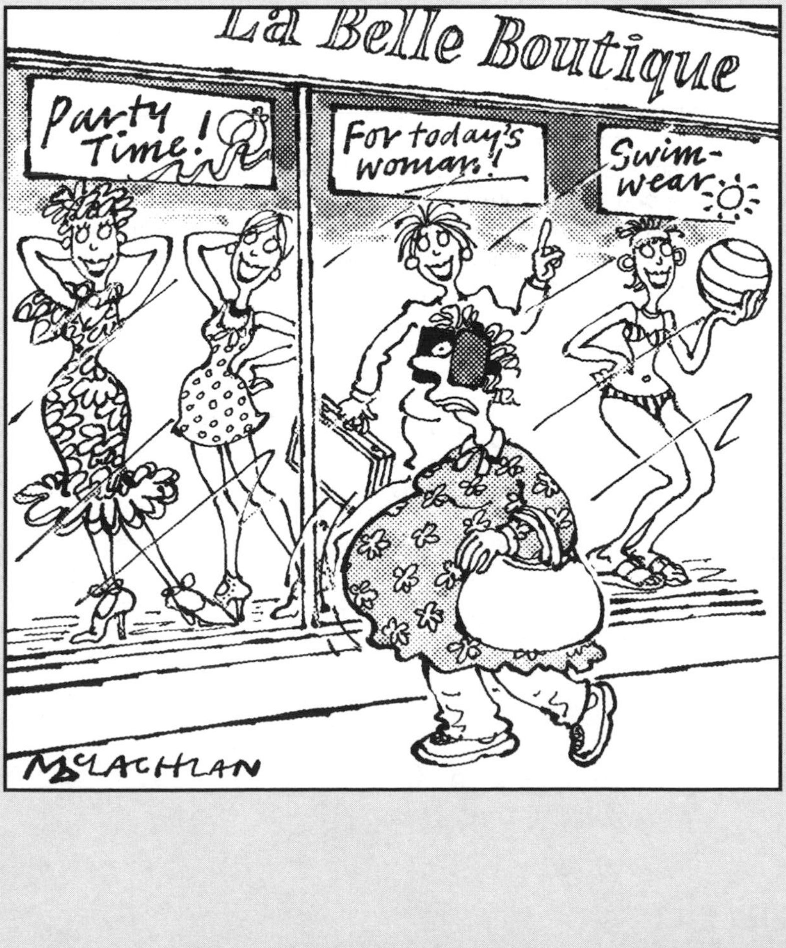

In this part . . .

If you're like most women, you're likely to become a bit calendar-conscious during pregnancy. It's 40 weeks. It's nine months (plus). But perhaps the most useful way to think of pregnancy is to divide it, as your practitioner does, into three trimesters, each about three months long. They do this because your baby's growth, as well as the changes going on in your body, happen in these three fairly distinct stages. In this part, we let you know what's likely to happen – how your baby develops, how you're likely to feel, and how your practitioner takes care of you – in each trimester. We also share some good ideas on preparing for labour.

Chapter 6

The First Trimester

In This Chapter

- Understanding the way your baby develops from conception through the first trimester
- Preparing yourself for physical changes
- Anticipating tests and questions at your antenatal visits
- Recognising some of the signs that things may not be going smoothly

The first trimester of your pregnancy (refer to Chapter 3 for more on trimesters) is an exciting time, full of many changes for you and especially for your baby, which in just 12 short weeks grows from a single cell to a tiny being with a beating heart and functioning kidneys. With all that change going on in your baby, you can certainly expect many changes in your own body – from fatigue and nausea to newly voluptuous (va-va-voom!) but tender breasts. As you experience these changes you need to know what's normal and what's worth a call to your practitioner, whom you begin visiting regularly at this point.

A New Life Takes Shape

Pregnancy begins when the egg and sperm meet, which happens in the fallopian tube. At this stage, the egg and sperm together form what we refer to as the *zygote* – a single cell. The zygote divides many times into multiple cells called a *blastocyst,* which travels down the fallopian tube and into the *uterus* (also called the *womb*), shown in Figure 6-1. When it reaches the uterus, both you and your baby begin to experience major changes.

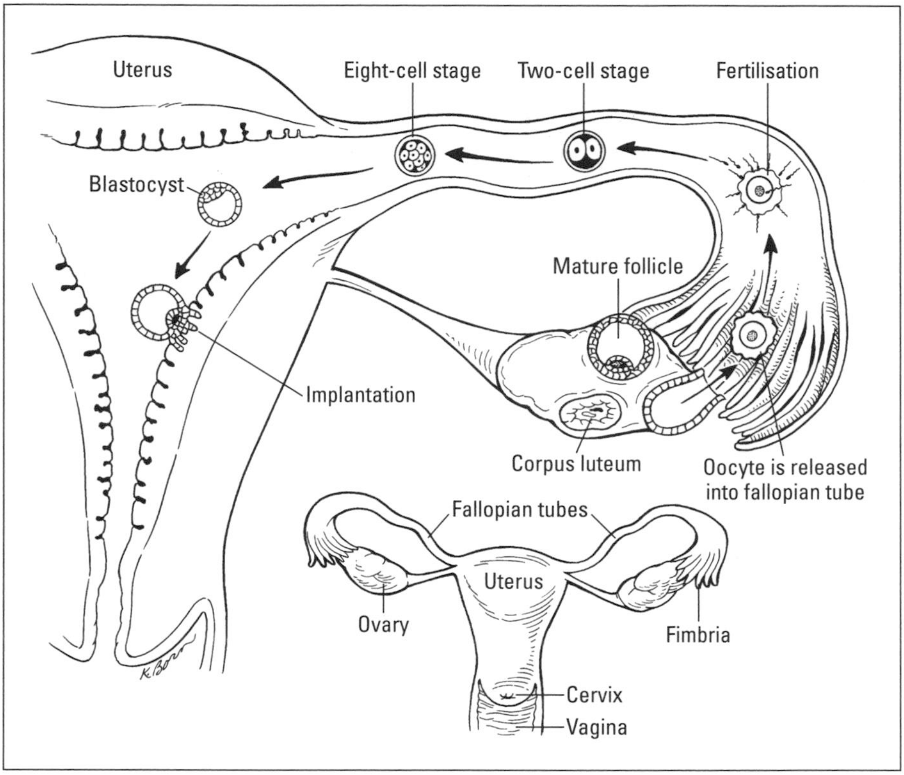

Figure 6-1: The female reproductive system in action.

On or about the fifth day of development, the blastocyst attaches to the blood-rich lining of the uterus during a process called *implantation*. Part of the blastocyst grows to become the *embryo* (the baby in the first eight weeks of development), and the other part becomes the *placenta* (the organ that implants into the uterus to provide oxygen and nourishment to the foetus and eliminate its waste products).

Your baby grows within the *amniotic sac* in the uterus. The amniotic sac is full of clear fluid – the *amniotic fluid*. The balloon actually comprises two thin layers of membrane called the *chorion* and *amnion* (which are together known as the *membranes*). When people talk about water breaking, they're referring to the rupturing of those membranes that line the uterus's inner walls. The baby swims in this fluid and is attached to the placenta by the umbilical cord. Figure 6-2 shows a diagram of an early pregnancy, including a developing foetus and the *cervix*, which is the uterus's opening. The cervix opens up, or *dilates*, when you're in labour.

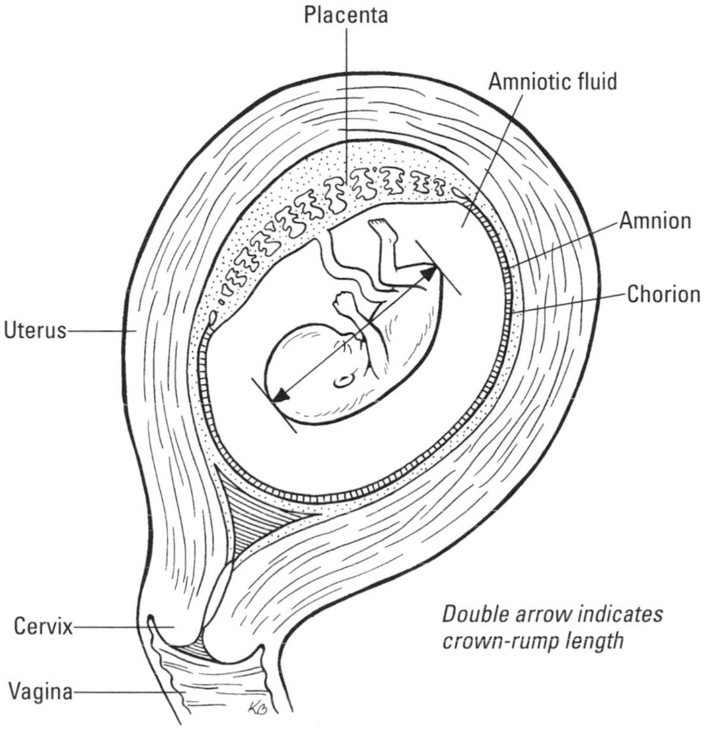

Figure 6-2: An early pregnancy.

The placenta begins to form soon after the embryo implants in the uterus. Maternal and foetal blood vessels lie very close to one another inside the placenta, which allows various substances (such as nutrients, oxygen, and waste) to transfer back and forth. The mother's blood and the baby's blood are in close contact, but they don't usually mix. (You can read about a few exceptions in Chapter 15.)

The placenta grows like a tree, forming branches that in turn divide into smaller and smaller branches. The tiniest buds of the placenta are called the *chorionic villi,* and it's within these *villi* that small foetal blood vessels form. About three weeks after fertilisation, these blood vessels join to form the baby's circulatory system, and the heart begins to beat.

After eight weeks into your pregnancy, the developing embryo is referred to as a *foetus.* Amazingly, by this time almost all the baby's major organs and structures are already formed. The remaining 32 weeks allow the foetus's structures to grow and mature. The brain, although also formed very early, continues to develop as well as grow throughout the pregnancy (and even into early childhood).

REMEMBER

When we refer to weeks, we mean menstrual weeks, which means weeks from the last menstrual period, not weeks from conception. So at eight weeks, the baby is really six weeks from conception.

By the end of the eighth week, arms, legs, fingers, and toes begin to form and the embryo begins to perform small, spontaneous movements. If you have an ultrasound examination performed in the first trimester, you can see these spontaneous movements on the screen. The brain enlarges rapidly, and ears and eyes appear. The external genitalia also emerge and can be differentiated as male or female by the end of the twelfth week, although sex differences are not yet detectable by ultrasound.

By the end of the twelfth week, the foetus is about 10 centimetres (4 inches) long and weighs about 28 grams (1 ounce). The head looks large and round, and the eyelids are fused shut. The intestines, which protruded slightly into the umbilical cord at about week 10, are now well inside the abdomen. Fingernails appear, and hair begins to grow on the baby's head. The kidneys start working during the third month. Between 9 and 12 weeks, the foetus begins to produce urine, which you can see within the small foetal bladder on ultrasound.

Adapting to Pregnancy: Body Changes in the First Trimester

Your baby isn't the only one growing and changing during your pregnancy (not that we have to remind you of that). Your own body also has to adjust, and the adjustments it makes aren't always the most pleasant and comfortable for you. Being prepared for what lies ahead can help ease your mind. So in the following sections, we let you know what is in store for you during the first trimester.

DON'T WORRY

If you don't get any of the changes mentioned in this section, don't panic. No changes for you doesn't mean there's a problem with your baby. For example, fewer than half of pregnant women vomit in the first trimester, and over a third get no nausea at all. Some women simply aren't troubled by tiredness or other symptoms – and go on to deliver perfectly healthy babies. We've listed the changes so that you won't worry if they do occur; if you don't experience them, stop worrying and celebrate feeling well!

Breast changes

One of the earliest and most amazing changes in your body happens to your breasts. Even during the first month of pregnancy, most women notice that their breasts grow considerably larger and feel very tender. The nipples and *areolae* (the circular areas around the nipples) also grow bigger and may begin to darken. Breast changes are caused by the large amounts of oestrogen and progesterone your body produces during pregnancy. These hormones cause the glands inside your breasts to grow and branch out, in preparation for milk production and breastfeeding after the baby is born. Blood supply to the breasts also increases markedly. You may notice large, bluish blood vessels coursing along your breasts, but this is nothing to worry about.

TIP

Plan to go through several bra sizes while you're pregnant – and don't skimp on buying new bras. Good support helps reduce stretching and sagging later on. Get yourself fitted for bras, rather than trusting to guesswork – most maternity shops and shops with a baby section will have an assistant trained to advise you on the best bra for you. Although some women like the way they look with larger breasts, others feel more self-conscious. Whichever way you feel, we guarantee that other pregnant women feel the same way, so don't feel embarrassed about it.

Fatigue

During the first trimester, you're likely to feel overwhelming fatigue. This fatigue may be a side effect of all the physical changes your body is experiencing, including the dramatic rise in hormone levels. Rest assured that your exhaustion will probably go away somewhere around the twelfth to fourteenth week of your pregnancy. As your fatigue lessens, you'll probably feel more energetic and almost normal, until about 30–34 weeks into your pregnancy, when you may tire out again. Remember that fatigue is nature's way of telling you to get more rest. If you can, try to take a short nap during the day and go to bed earlier than usual at night.

JUST FOR DADS

Many a mother-to-be feels more exhausted in the first trimester than at any other stage of pregnancy – yet she may not have told anyone except you about the happy news, and will be expected to behave normally at work to prevent her colleagues becoming suspicious. She won't have reached that obvious stage of pregnancy where people give up their seat on the tube for her, either. So now is a particularly important time for you to be aware of her needs, and to give her all the help and encouragement you can.

Tips for keeping nausea at bay

Unfortunately, we can't tell you how to make your nausea totally disappear. But you can try a few things to make it better. Here are a few suggestions:

- Eat small, frequent meals, so that your stomach is never empty.
- Don't eat just before bedtime.
- Don't worry too much about adhering to a balanced diet; just eat whatever appeals to you during this relatively short period of time.
- Avoid perfume counters, active kitchens, smelly taxis, or other places where odours may be strong.
- Wear loose, baggy clothes that don't constrict you at the waist – there's plenty of time to get back into those size 10 jeans once the baby's born.
- Keep crackers by your bedside – some women find that eating them before getting out of bed in the morning helps to decrease the nausea.
- Ginger (in the form of tea or tablets, for example) may help some women.
- You may notice that your nausea worsens when you brush your teeth. Switching toothpaste brands may help.
- Try eating dry toast, digestive biscuits, whole-wheat crackers, potatoes, and other bland, easy-to-digest carbohydrates.
- If you're bothered by the accumulation of saliva in your mouth, sucking on lemon drops or acid drops may be helpful.
- Acupressure wristbands, sold in pharmacies and health food stores, give some women relief.
- Relaxation exercises and even hypnosis work for some women.

Any-time-of-day sickness

For some women, the nausea that can strike during the first trimester is worse in the mornings, maybe because the stomach is empty at that time of day. But ask anyone who's had morning sickness, and she'll tell you: It can hit any time it wants. It often starts during the fifth or sixth week (that is, three to four weeks after you miss your period – we describe how doctors calculate the timing of pregnancy in Chapter 3) and goes away, or at least becomes much less severe, by the end of the eleventh or twelfth week. It can last longer, though, particularly in women who are expecting twins or more, because multiple placentas release more human chorionic gonadotropin (hCG), a hormone released by the placenta.

The cause of morning sickness isn't absolutely clear, but it appears to be related to the rise in hCG.

You may hear some women say that morning sickness is a sign that you're experiencing a normal pregnancy, but that claim is a myth – and so is the reverse. If you're not having morning sickness, or if it suddenly disappears, don't worry that your pregnancy isn't normal; just enjoy your good fortune. You may hear that the severity of your queasiness indicates whether you're having a girl or a boy – but that's also a myth, so don't buy those pink or blue outfits just yet (and turn to Chapter 20 for even more myths about determining the sex of your bundle of joy).

If you're experiencing nausea, we sympathise. Even when nausea doesn't actually cause you to vomit, it can be extremely uncomfortable and truly debilitating. Certain odours – from foods, perfumes, or musty places – can make it worse. Look in the nearby sidebar called 'Tips for keeping nausea at bay' for recommendations on how to minimise morning sickness.

If you experience extreme nausea with or without vomiting, talk to your doctor about medicines that may be helpful. Some women find relief from medicines called metoclopramide, cinnarizine, or promethazine – but most doctors advise that you use non-drug measures, like the ones described above, to control your symptoms if you can.

Occasionally, the nausea and vomiting are so severe that you develop a condition called *hyperemesis gravidarum.* The symptoms include dehydration and weight loss. If you develop hyperemesis gravidarum, you may need to be given fluids and medications intravenously.

If your queasiness gets out of control – if you experience weight loss, if you find that you can't keep down food or liquids, or if you feel dizzy or faint – call your doctor.

Don't compound the problem by worrying about it. The nausea is harmless – to you and the baby. Your optimal weight gain for the first three months is only 2 pounds. Even losing weight probably isn't a big problem.

Bloating

Well before the baby is big enough to stretch out your stomach, your belt may begin to feel uncomfortable and your tummy may look bloated and distended. This side effect of the hormone shift starts happening as soon as you conceive. *Progesterone,* one of the two key pregnancy hormones, causes you to retain water. Progesterone also slows down the bowels, causing them to enlarge and thus increase the size of the abdomen. *Oestrogen,* the other key pregnancy hormone, causes your uterus to enlarge, which also makes your abdomen feel bigger. This effect is often more pronounced in second or third pregnancies because the first pregnancy causes your abdominal muscles to relax to a greater degree.

Frequent urination

From early on in your pregnancy, you may feel as if you're spending your whole life in the loo. During pregnancy, you need to urinate more frequently for a variety of reasons. At the beginning of your pregnancy, your uterus is inside your pelvis. But toward the end of your first trimester (at around 12 weeks), your uterus expands enough to rise up into your abdominal cavity. Your enlarging uterus may compress your bladder, which both decreases its capacity and increases the feeling that you need to urinate. Also, your blood volume rises markedly during pregnancy, and that means the rate at which your kidneys produce urine also increases.

You can't do much about your need to urinate frequently, except use common sense. Before going out for long (or even short) trips, empty your bladder so that you don't find yourself needing facilities when none are available. Drink plenty of fluids during pregnancy to avoid dehydration, but try to drink more during the day and less in the evening, so that you aren't up all night going to the loo.

If you find yourself urinating even more than your pregnancy norm, or if you feel any discomfort or burning, or notice blood during urination, talk to your practitioner. When you're pregnant, bacteria in your urine are more likely than usual to cause a urinary tract infection (see Chapter 17).

Headaches

Many pregnant women notice that they get headaches more often than they used to. These headaches may be the result of nausea, fatigue, hunger, the normal physiologic decrease in blood pressure that starts to occur at this time, tension, or even depression. Paracetamol, in recommended doses, is perfectly fine to take for occasional headache relief. Some women find that a little caffeine can also alleviate symptoms of a headache (but also see Chapter 5 for more on caffeine in pregnancy).

Food and rest can usually cure headaches that are caused by nausea, fatigue, or hunger. So try eating and getting some extra sleep. If neither of those tactics works, something else is probably causing your headache.

Simple pain relievers like paracetamol are often the best treatment for headaches, including migraines. If over-the-counter medications don't relieve your headache, talk with your practitioner about alternatives.

Base your decision on whether to use migraine medications on the severity of your problem. If your headaches are chronic or recurrent, you may need to take medications, despite their effects on your foetus. Consult with your practitioner before taking these medications.

Avoid taking regular doses of aspirin unless recommended by your practitioner, because adult doses of aspirin can affect platelet function (important in blood clotting).

Constipation

About half of all pregnant women complain of constipation. When you're pregnant, you may become constipated because the large amount of progesterone circulating in your bloodstream slows the activity of your digestive tract. The iron in supplements for anaemia in pregnancy can make matters worse. Try these few suggestions to deal with the problem:

- **Eat plenty of high-fibre foods.** Bran cereals, fruit, and vegetables are all good sources of fibre. Some women find it helpful to eat some popcorn, but choose the low-fat kind, without all the butter and added oil. Check the fibre content on package labels and choose foods with a higher fibre content.
- **Drink plenty of water.** Staying well-hydrated helps keep food and waste moving through the digestive tract. Some juices (especially prune juice) may help, while others (such as apple juice) may only exacerbate the problem.
- **Exercise as regularly as you can.** Exercise helps constipation, so enjoy some safe exercise (even if it's only walking).

Cramps

You may feel a vague, menstrual-like cramping sensation during the first trimester – this is a very common symptom, so don't worry. The cramping is probably related to your uterus growing and enlarging.

If you experience cramping along with vaginal bleeding, give your practitioner a call. Although the majority of women who experience bleeding and cramping go on to have perfectly normal pregnancies, sometimes these two symptoms together are associated with miscarriage. Cramping alone, without bleeding, is unlikely to be a problem.

Booking Baby In: Your First Antenatal Appointments

Most women make an appointment with their GP within the first six or eight weeks after their last menstrual period – this means within four to six weeks of the baby being conceived (refer to Chapter 3 for more details).

The questions and tests GPs carry out when you first go to see them vary enormously across the country, and even between doctors in the same practice. However, your GP should give you tips on diet (see Chapter 5), and refer you for your *hospital booking appointment* (your first hospital antenatal appointment).

Who you see at the hospital will depend on the type of care you've opted for (midwife-led, shared care or hospital-only care – refer to Chapter 2) and whether or not you have any risk factors. The booking appointment is also usually your longest hospital appointment – so take a good book and set aside half a day for it. You may have your first ultrasound scan at this appointment.

TIP

If possible, bring the father-to-be for this initial visit. His family medical history and ethnic roots are important, too. Also, he should have a chance to ask questions, address his concerns, and find out what to look forward to in the coming months.

Understanding the consultation

At your booking appointment, you'll be asked a number of questions. At some hospitals, you'll be sent a questionnaire asking these questions in advance – take the completed form to your booking appointment. The questions you may be asked are outlined in the following sections

The starting date of your last menstrual period, and the length of your menstrual cycle

Answering both of these questions helps to determine your due date. (For more information on calculating your due date, refer to Chapter 3.) If you don't know exactly the date that your last period began, try to remember the exact date of conception. If you're unsure about either of these dates, don't worry – your ultrasound scan can tell, to the nearest week, when your baby is due.

Details of any previous pregnancies or gynaecological problems

Your history can help determine how best to manage this pregnancy. For example, if you have a history of preterm labour (see Chapter 16) or gestational diabetes (Chapter 17), knowing that history prepares your practitioner for the possibility that it may happen again.

Whether you've conceived after infertility treatment

Most of the impact of infertility treatment on pregnancy outcomes is related to the higher incidence of multiple pregnancies – twins and more. Couples who have gone through *in-vitro fertilisation* (see Chapter 15) generally have babies that are as healthy as those who were conceived spontaneously.

Your past medical history

Your practitioner may also ask you about any medical problems you've had and any surgeries you've undergone, including problems that aren't gynaecological in nature. Certain medical conditions may affect pregnancy, and others won't, so tell him everything and let him work out what's significant.

Your family medical history

The family medical histories of both you and the baby's father are important for two reasons. First, your practitioner can identify pregnancy-related conditions that can recur from generation to generation, like having twins or exceptionally large babies. The other reason is to identify serious problems within your family that your baby can inherit. Some of these problems, such as cystic fibrosis, can be screened for by blood tests. Other inherited medical conditions are covered later on in this section, under 'Your ethnic background'.

If you have a family history of a particular condition, you'll ideally have discussed the issue with your GP before you conceive. If you haven't consulted your doctor in advance, it's essential to find out as much as you can about conditions that run in your family as soon as you know you're pregnant, and to let your doctor know immediately.

In the UK, if you have a condition that could be inherited, you'll usually be referred to a specialist genetic counselling clinic. Here, you'll find a doctor with special training in clinical genetics, supported by a team of nurse counsellors. These specialist doctors aren't based in every hospital (they're usually only found in the big *tertiary referral centres*, which are large, often specialised hospitals that deal with patients at high risk). Clinics may, however, be run in your local hospital, where you can discuss the sort of tests that are available to find out if your baby is affected by an inherited condition.

Screening for cystic fibrosis

Cystic fibrosis (CF) is one of the most common genetic diseases in the UK, with an incidence of about 1 in 2,000. CF is a recessive condition, which means that both parents need to be carriers to place the baby at risk for having the disease. More than 1,000 different genetic mutations have been associated with CF. Screening for the 25 most common mutations will pick up 57 to 97 per cent of carriers of CF, depending on ethnic background. For example, screening detects 97 per cent of carriers among the Ashkenazi Jewish population and 80 per cent of carriers in the Northern European Caucasian population. If anyone in your family is affected, speak to your doctor about CF screening during your first antenatal visit.

If you are referred to a tertiary referral centre, try to attend with the baby's father – the team will need information from both sides of the family.

Your ethnic background

Even if your and your partner's family history is free of any known genetic disorders, your ethnic backgrounds are important because some genetic disorders occur more frequently in one ethnicity than others. People of Afro-Caribbean extraction, for example, are more likely to carry the gene for the blood disorder sickle cell anaemia, and people of Southern European extraction may be more likely to carry the gene for thalassaemia. A simple blood test can usually determine whether you're a carrier of these diseases.

Some people don't know very much about their ethnic background or family medical history, perhaps because they were adopted or haven't had much contact with their biological families. If this situation is true in your case, don't worry. Keep in mind that the chances that both you and your partner carry a gene for a particular disorder are extremely low, unless you both come from one of the high-risk groups detailed in the following list:

- **Inherited genes.** We inherit characteristics and conditions from our parents through our genes – a genetic code that tells our body how to function. Some conditions, called *hereditary conditions*, can be passed on through our genes. Two of the most common forms of inheritance are *autosomal dominant* and *autosomal recessive*. An autosomal dominant gene is one that gives you the disease, even if you only inherited the gene for that disease from one parent. An autosomal recessive gene is one that can be passed on through the generations with few or no symptoms, and which only gives rise to the disease if a baby inherits the same gene from both parents. Someone who has one gene, but not both, is called a *carrier*.

- **Sickle cell anaemia.** Sickle cell anaemia is inherited in an autosomal recessive manner, which means that both parents need to be carriers to place the baby at risk for having the disease. If you have one gene for sickle cell and one normal gene, you are a sickle cell carrier (sometimes known as having sickle cell trait). Sickle cell trait is extremely common in parts of Africa, probably because having the sickle cell trait reduces your chance of getting malaria. This means that in the past, people with the sickle cell trait would have been more likely to survive than their compatriots without it. You're also more likely to have sickle cell trait if you have an Indian, Mediterranean, or Middle Eastern background.

  The symptoms of sickle cell anaemia can range from quite mild to severe and life-threatening. The disease causes *anaemia* (see Chapter 5) and can make your baby more prone to infection.

- **Alpha- and beta-thalassaemia.** People whose ancestors come from Italy, Greece, and other Mediterranean countries are at elevated risk of having – and passing to their children – genes for the blood disorder *beta-thalassaemia*, also known as *Mediterranean anaemia* or *Cooley's anaemia.* Asians may suffer from a similar blood problem named *alpha-thalassaemia.* Both of these disorders produce abnormalities in *haemoglobin* (the protein in red blood cells that holds onto oxygen) and result in varying degrees of anaemia. Like sickle cell anaemia, thalassaemia is inherited in an autosomal recessive manner. This means that both parents have to carry the gene for there to be a risk that their baby has the disease.

- **Tay-Sachs disease.** Tay-Sachs affects the nervous system that is usually fatal in early childhood. This disease is inherited in a *recessive* manner, which means that both parents need to be carriers to place the baby at risk for having the disease. Being a carrier doesn't mean that you have Tay-Sachs yourself, only that you carry a gene for it.

REMEMBER

If you do belong to one of these groups, talk to your practitioner about getting tests done.

Other health and lifestyle questions

Your practitioner may ask about several other aspects of your lifestyle. This information helps your practitioner to work out if any particular problems need to be monitored. We give more ideas about why these issues are so important in Chapter 3, but here's a brief list of the sort of things you may be asked about:

- Any medicines you've taken since you became pregnant
- Any allergies (especially to medicines)
- Whether you smoke
- Whether you drink alcohol

Considering the physical examination

As well as asking you lots of questions at your booking appointment, your practitioner needs to examine you. Routine checks include:

- Your weight (this may only be done at your booking appointment – refer to Chapter 5 for reasons why)
- Your heart and lungs (to check your general health)
- Your tummy (to check your baby's growth – see Chapter 8)
- Your blood pressure (which can make you feel light-headed if it's low, and can cause serious problems if it's too high – see the section on pre-eclampsia in Chapter 16, and high blood pressure in Chapter 17)
- Your blood and urine, and an ultrasound scan (see the next section, 'Looking at standard tests', for more on these)

Looking at standard tests

Brace yourself: You're probably going to be pricked with a needle and made to pee in a cup during your first antenatal visit. Here's a look at the standard procedures, including blood and urine tests.

Urine test

Your urine will usually be checked for sugar and protein at every appointment. Sugar in your urine can be a sign of diabetes (see Chapter 17), and protein can indicate a urine infection or a condition called pre-eclampsia (see Chapter 16). Take a small sample with you in a clean, rinsed container.

Standard blood tests

Blood tests are used to check a number of things:

- **Haemoglobin.** Your blood is tested to check if you are anaemic (see Chapter 5). If you are, you may be offered iron and folic acid tablets, and you may need more frequent blood tests.
- **Blood group and antibodies.** This test tells whether your blood group is O, A, B, or AB. The test also looks for a substance in your blood called the *Rhesus factor*. If you don't have this substance – and one in four or five women don't – you are known as R*hesus negative*. If you're Rhesus negative and your baby is Rhesus positive, your body can occasionally become *sensitised* to your baby. This means that your body will see a

future baby as an intruder and try to fight it off, the way it fights off infections. This can cause a problem in your baby's blood when born (for more about this, see the section on blood incompatibilities in Chapter 15).

- **Rubella antibodies.** Your blood is checked to see if you're immune to German measles. This is usually a mild illness if you're not pregnant, but can damage your baby if you catch it in the early stages of pregnancy. Most women are immune to German measles, but if you aren't, your practitioner will advise you to be very careful to avoid contact with anyone who has the illness. You'll also be advised to get vaccinated against rubella soon after you deliver, so you won't be susceptible in later pregnancies.
- In the UK, every baby is offered immunisation via the MMR injection. Until a few years ago, most babies were vaccinated, and cases of German measles had become very rare. However, a high profile media debate highlighted possible dangers from the MMR jab, and some parents have chosen not to vaccinate their children, even though very strong evidence suggests that the benefits of the MMR jab outweigh any risks. This means that more cases of German measles have been seen, and the risk of coming into contact with someone with the illness has increased.
- **VDRL.** VDRL (standing for *Venereal Disease Research Laboratory*, not that you'd necessarily wish to know that) is a very accurate test to check for syphilis (a sexually transmitted disease that can cause abnormalities in your baby or even stillbirth). This test can sometimes produce a *false positive result* – one that says you're affected when you aren't. To confirm the diagnosis of syphilis another, more specific, blood test should be performed. Because syphilis must be adequately treated, all antenatal clinics offer this test.
- **Hepatitis B.** You can carry this infectious disease of the liver without knowing you've got it. If you have the disease, you can pass it on to your baby, so it's important to be tested.
- **Glucose screening.** Glucose screening identifies women who may have gestational diabetes. The test involves two blood samples, taken before and after drinking a glucose mixture (which tastes like a flat fizzy drink). If this test shows that you have gestational diabetes, you need to control your diet carefully, and more antenatal checks will be necessary. To find out more, see Chapter 17, or pick up a copy of *Diabetes For Dummies* by Sarah Jarvis and Alan L. Rubin (Wiley). Some hospitals don't do this test unless your weight is outside the ideal range, but your urine will be checked for sugar anyway.
- **Double or triple test.** This test is an investigation for foetal abnormalities. The test gives an idea of your risk of having a baby affected by *Down's syndrome* or *spina bifida*, and can tell whether you're at low or

high risk; but the test doesn't give you an absolute answer. For more details on the tests and these conditions, see the section on testing for foetal abnormalities in Chapter 9.

- **HIV antibodies.** This test is completely voluntary. However, if you are affected, knowing this early can help staff to reduce your chances of passing the infection on to your baby. You can find out more in Chapter 17.
- **Other tests.** If you are at risk of inherited conditions like thalassaemia or sickle cell anaemia (discussed earlier in this chapter), more tests can be made on your blood. Speak to your practitioner about these tests.

Ultrasound

You are normally offered an *ultrasound* examination at your booking appointment. This test uses sound waves to check your baby, and is completely safe and painless for both of you. The scan can check how many babies you have, their size, and their growth. Later in pregnancy – at about 20 weeks – you may be offered another ultrasound scan. At this stage you're likely to see your baby in much more detail. This scan can check for problems with your baby's spine, limbs, heart, and other organs. More details about ultrasound scans can be found in Chapter 9, and some very pretty pictures of scans are shown in Chapter 22.

In some hospitals, every pregnant woman is offered two ultrasound scans – one at about 12–14 weeks of pregnancy, and one at about 20 weeks. In other hospitals, only one scan is offered routinely, usually at 13–16 weeks. If you're at high risk for any reason (if you have a past family history of Down's syndrome, if you're over 35 or 37, or if a potential abnormality is picked up at your first scan or antenatal appointment), you'll be invited for more ultrasound scans. We cover all the features these scans routinely look for later, even though they may not be done before 20 weeks.

The following information is evaluated during a first trimester ultrasound examination:

- **The accuracy of your due date:** An ultrasound can show whether the foetus is any larger or smaller than the date of your last menstrual period would suggest. An ultrasound in the first trimester is actually more accurate than a later ultrasound in confirming or establishing your due date.
- **Foetal abnormalities:** Although a complete ultrasound examination to detect structural abnormalities in the foetus usually isn't performed until 15–20 weeks, some problems may already be visible by 11–12 weeks. Much of the brain, spine, limbs, abdomen, and urinary tract structures may be seen with transvaginal ultrasound.

- **Foetal number:** An ultrasound shows if you're carrying more than one foetus. We go into greater detail about this topic in Chapter 15.
- **The condition of your ovaries:** An ultrasound can also reveal abnormalities or cysts in your ovaries. Sometimes an ultrasound shows a small cyst, called a *corpus luteal cyst*. This is a cyst that forms at the site where the egg was released. Over the course of three or four months, the cyst gradually goes away. Two other types of cyst, called *dermoid cysts* and *simple cysts,* are unrelated to the pregnancy and may be found incidentally during an ultrasound examination. The size of the cyst and any symptoms you may be having determine if and when it needs removing.
- **The presence of fibroid tumours:** Also simply called *fibroids,* these are benign overgrowths of the muscle of the uterus. We go into more details about these in Chapter 17.
- **Location of the pregnancy:** Occasionally, the pregnancy may be located outside the uterus, which is called an *ectopic pregnancy* (see the 'Ectopic pregnancy' section later in this chapter for more information).

Your booking appointment – now it's your turn!

Your booking appointment is a good chance to ask the questions you want answers to. Areas you may have queries about may include:

- What are your choices for antenatal care?
- Is a home birth possible – or safe – for you and your baby?
- Will the pregnancy have any effects on any medical problems you have?
- What sort of exercise can you do during pregnancy?
- What antenatal classes are offered by the hospital?
- What other antenatal classes are available in your area?

Of course, many other questions may occur to you. If you have a pre-existing medical condition (more on those in Chapter 17), you'll want to know what sort of extra monitoring you should have. For example, some hospitals have doctors who specialise in the care of pregnant women with medical conditions, because the treatment needed for the condition may be different during pregnancy.

Make a list in advance of any questions you may want to ask. Seeing your baby for the first time on the ultrasound scan is emotional stuff, and it may knock every other thought out of your head. You may also find that questions occur to you along the way. For example, you may want to know more about the hospital's policy on carrying out prenatal testing for foetal abnormalities (see Chapter 9). Don't hesitate to ask – your practitioner will be happy to provide any answers he can, and should be able to give you written information, or point you in the direction of someone who can answer your queries if he doesn't know the answer himself.

Recognising Causes for Concern

In each trimester, a few things may go less than smoothly. The following sections describe some of the things that can happen during the first trimester of your pregnancy and what they may mean to you.

Bleeding

Early in pregnancy, around the time of your missed period, experiencing a little bleeding from the vagina isn't uncommon. The amount of bleeding is usually less than what you would expect with a period and lasts for only one or two days – it's called *implantation bleeding*, and it happens when the fertilised egg attaches to the uterus's lining. Bleeding due to implantation isn't a cause for concern, but many women may be confused by it and mistake it for their period.

In some cases, bleeding can be the first sign of an impending miscarriage (see the next section for more information). In this case, the bleeding often accompanies abdominal cramping. Keep in mind, however, that the vast majority of women who experience bleeding go on to have a completely normal pregnancy.

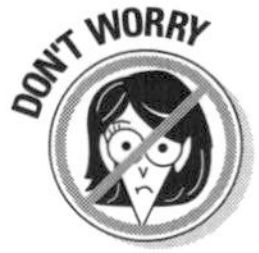

Bleeding also may occur later in the first trimester, but it doesn't necessarily indicate a miscarriage. About one-third of women experience bleeding during the first trimester, and the majority of them go on to have perfectly healthy babies. Bleeding is especially common in women carrying more than one foetus – and again, most go on to have normal pregnancies. Bright red bleeding usually indicates active bleeding, while dark staining usually indicates old blood that is making its way out from the cervix and vagina. An ultrasound examination generally doesn't show any evidence of the source of the bleeding. However, sometimes a collection of blood, known as a *subchorionic* or *retroplacental collection*, is visible and indicates an area of bleeding from behind the placenta. This blood is reabsorbed over several weeks and during this time, some dark blood continues to pass out through the cervix and vagina.

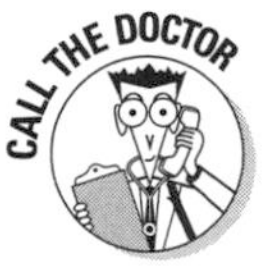

If you notice some bleeding, let your practitioner know. If the bleeding is a small amount and not associated with a lot of abdominal cramping, it isn't an emergency. If you're bleeding very heavily (much more than a period), call your practitioner immediately. Your practitioner may want to perform a pelvic examination, and refer you for an ultrasound scan to investigate the cause of the bleeding and see whether the pregnancy is still viable and located inside the uterus. Your practitioner can generally do very little about the bleeding. Some doctors may suggest that you rest at home for a few days and avoid exercise and sex. No scientific data supports these instructions, but given that no really good alternatives exist, they certainly don't hurt.

Miscarriage

The great majority of pregnancies proceed normally. But about one in five end in early miscarriage, often before a woman even knows she's pregnant. A *miscarriage* is the loss of a pregnancy up to 28 weeks from conception. The vast majority of miscarriages happen in the first trimester. If a miscarriage occurs early in a pregnancy, you may mistake it for a normal menstrual period. About half the time, chromosomal abnormalities in the embryo cause the miscarriage. In another 20 per cent of cases, the embryo may have structural defects that are too small to be detectable by ultrasound or pathological examination.

You're going to be tempted to shout the amazing news of your pregnancy from the rooftops – or at least whisper it around the office. Try to be patient, at least until you're into the second trimester and have had an ultrasound scan. By all means let your partner and parents know, but remember that if something does go wrong, well-meant comments by people who don't know can be extremely distressing.

By five to six weeks into your pregnancy, an ultrasound (which you may be referred for if you suffer vaginal bleeding in the first trimester) can detect a foetal heartbeat. After a foetal heartbeat is identified, the risk of miscarriage drops significantly (to about 3 per cent). Prior to five weeks, the foetus itself may not be visible; instead, the ultrasound may show only the gestational sac. If you've had a threatened miscarriage in the first few weeks of pregnancy and an ultrasound doesn't show a heartbeat, don't worry too much. The foetus simply may not be well enough developed yet and you'll be asked to return for another scan a week or so later.

Miscarriage may lead to cramping and bleeding. You may feel abdominal pains that are stronger than period pains, and you may pass foetal and placental tissue. In cases where all the tissue is passed, your practitioner doesn't need to do anything else. Often, though, some tissue remains in your uterus, and you may need to have a D&C (*dilation and curettage*) procedure, designed to empty the uterus. If your doctor thinks you're at risk of a miscarriage, you'll be referred to the hospital. At the hospital, an ultrasound will give a better idea of whether you need a D&C. If you do, you'll have to have a general anaesthetic while the doctor *dilates* (gently opens) the cervix with surgical instruments and empties the remaining contents of the uterus with a suction device. You'll likely go home later the same day, or at least the next morning. Sometimes, you may have no overt signs of miscarriage. Your practitioner may discover during a routine antenatal visit that the foetus is no longer alive, which is known as a *missed miscarriage.* If you have a missed miscarriage very early in your pregnancy, a D&C may not be necessary; but if it happens later in the first trimester, you may need to have a D&C to reduce the risk of heavy bleeding or incomplete passage of tissue.

Unfortunately, most miscarriages can't be prevented. Many, if not most, miscarriages may simply be nature's way of handling an abnormal pregnancy. Having a miscarriage doesn't mean that you can't have a perfectly normal pregnancy in the future. Even in women who have had two consecutive miscarriages, the chances are very good (about 70 per cent) that the next pregnancy will be successful, even without any special treatment.

Any woman who experiences three or more consecutive miscarriages may have some underlying condition that can be identified and possibly treated. She should have a complete physical examination and undergo special tests to look for causes. Some women who have even two miscarriages may want to be examined. If you miscarry, discuss with your practitioner the possibility of undergoing certain tests – or sending foetal or placental tissue to a laboratory for chromosomal analysis.

Ectopic pregnancy

An *ectopic pregnancy* occurs when the fertilised egg implants outside the uterus – in one of the fallopian tubes, the ovary, the abdomen, or the cervix. An ectopic pregnancy is a serious problem and a threat to the mother's health.

Fortunately, ultrasound has advanced to the point that it can detect ectopic pregnancies very early. However, as ultrasound scans in pregnancy aren't routinely carried out before about 12 weeks of pregnancy, you're likely to have developed symptoms before this stage. If you have an earlier scan for any reason, you may not have any symptoms but your doctor will still identify the condition during an ultrasound.

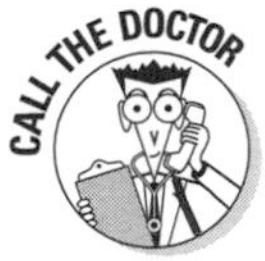

Signs of an ectopic pregnancy include vaginal bleeding, abdominal pain, dizziness, and feeling faint. The abdominal pain may be severe and is usually on one side. The bleeding may start just after you have missed your period – sometimes before you even know you are pregnant. You'll need to have an operation to remove the embryo or foetus, but unfortunately, a doctor can't move it to the uterus so that the pregnancy can continue as normal.

Chapter 7

The Second Trimester

In This Chapter

- Taking a look at your baby's development
- Looking – and feeling – like you're going to have a baby
- Knowing when to be concerned

The second trimester, which encompasses the three months between week 13 and week 26, is often the most enjoyable part of pregnancy. The feelings of nausea and fatigue so common during the first trimester are usually gone, and you feel more energetic and comfortable. The second trimester is a very exciting time because you can feel the baby moving within you and you're finally starting to show. During the second trimester, blood tests, antenatal tests, and ultrasound can confirm that the baby is healthy and growing normally. And many women find that they can finally grasp the concept that they'll soon be having a baby. The second trimester is often the time you start sharing the exciting news with family, friends, and colleagues.

Discovering How Your Baby Is Developing

Your baby grows rapidly during the second trimester, as you can see in Figure 7-1. The foetus measures about 8 centimetres long (3 inches) at 13 weeks and by 26 weeks, it's about 35 centimetres (14 inches) and weighs about 1,022 grams (2¼ pounds). Somewhere between weeks 14 and 16, the limbs begin to elongate and start to look like arms and legs. Co-ordinated arm and leg movements are observable on ultrasound, too. Between 18 and 22 weeks, you may begin to feel foetal movements, although they don't necessarily occur regularly throughout the day.

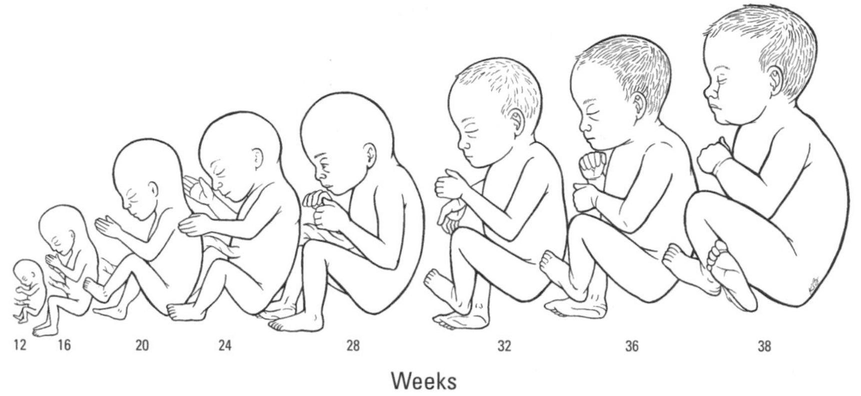

Figure 7-1: Notice that during the second trimester (13–26 weeks), your baby grows and develops at an astounding rate.

The baby's head, which was large in relation to the body during the first trimester, becomes more in proportion as the body catches up. The bones solidify and are recognisable on ultrasound. Early in the second trimester, the foetus looks something like an alien (think E.T., but without the glowing finger), but by 26 weeks, it looks much more like a human baby.

The foetus also performs many recognisable activities – it not only moves, but also undergoes regular periods of sleeping and wakefulness and can hear and swallow. Lung development increases markedly between 20 and 25 weeks. By 24 weeks, lung cells begin to secrete *surfactant,* a chemical substance that enables the lungs to stay expanded. Between 26 and 28 weeks, the eyes – which had been fused shut – open, and hair (called *lanugo*) appears on the head and body. Fat deposits form under the skin, and the central nervous system matures dramatically.

At 23 to 24 weeks, the foetus is considered *viable,* which means that if it were born at this time, it would have a reasonable chance of surviving in a neonatal unit experienced in caring for very premature babies. A premature baby born at 28 weeks (nearly three months early) and cared for in an intensive care unit has an excellent chance of survival.

Most mothers begin to feel their babies move at about this time. Knowing for sure when you first feel your baby moving inside you is difficult. Many women sense fluttering movements (called *quickening*) at about 16 to 20 weeks. Not every woman can tell that sensation is actually the baby moving; some think they just have wind (and maybe you *did* eat too much curry). Around 20 to 22 weeks, the foetal movements are much easier to identify but

Clothing yourself in maternity garb

Thank goodness the fashion industry has recognised that women continue to care about looking chic and professional when they're pregnant – which doesn't necessarily mean wearing those choir-boy blouses with big bows at the neck. Many women look forward to shopping for maternity clothes, while others aim to stay in their usual clothes for as long as possible. Keep in mind that you only need maternity clothes for a few months, and they're not cheap. Here are a few suggestions:

- Don't plan too far ahead; buy clothes only as you need them. When you do shop, buy clothes that fit comfortably but have enough room to accommodate further growth.
- Don't be shy about accepting hand-me-downs. Women rarely wear out their maternity clothes. Your friends are probably happy to see their clothes get more use.
- Look for charity shops, and National Childbirth Trust (NCT) car boot sales (advertised in the local press) – they're good places to find inexpensive maternity clothes.
- If you have trouble finding maternity clothes in your style, remember that you can often go a long way through your pregnancy in regular leggings and big shirts or sweaters.
- Perhaps the most important items to buy are comfortable shoes and roomier bras. Both shoe size and bra size can increase during pregnancy.
- You don't have to wear special maternity underwear – unless you find it especially comfortable. Many kinds of regular underwear fit well under a bulging belly.

they still aren't consistent. Over the course of the next four weeks, the movements fall into a more regular pattern.

Different babies have different movement patterns. You may notice that your baby tends to move more at night – perhaps to prepare you for all the sleepless nights you'll have after she is born! Or you may simply be more aware of the baby's movements at night because you're more sedentary at that time. If this is your second (or third or fourth . . .) child, you may start to feel movements a couple of weeks earlier.

If you haven't felt your baby move at all by 22 weeks, let your practitioner know. She may recommend an ultrasound, especially if you haven't had one already, to check the baby. A common explanation for not feeling the baby's movements is that the placenta is implanted on the anterior (front) wall of the uterus between the baby and your skin. The placenta acts as a cushion and delays the time when you first feel movements.

Understanding Your Changing Body

By 12 weeks, your uterus begins to rise out of your pelvis. Your practitioner can feel the top of the uterus through your abdominal wall. By 20 weeks, the top of your uterus reaches the level of your navel. Then each week, your uterus grows by about one centimetre (½inch). Your practitioner may run a tape measure from your pubic bone to the top of your uterus to measure the *fundal height* (refer to Chapter 3) to see that your uterus and the baby are growing appropriately. Many women begin to show at 16 weeks, although looking pregnant varies a great deal. Some women look pregnant at 12 weeks; others aren't obvious until 28 weeks.

Many of the changes you experience have little to do with your belly's size. Rather, the changes involve your baby's development and your body's continuing adaptation to pregnancy. You may experience some, none, or all of the symptoms in this section.

Women in their second pregnancies often think something's wrong, because they are so much bigger than in their first pregnancy. Not so – different sizes in different pregnancies is perfectly normal. Six weeks into her second pregnancy Sarah was wearing maternity gear that she hadn't even bought until eighteen weeks into her first!

Forgetfulness and clumsiness

Until she was pregnant, Joanne never would have believed that misplacing keys, bumping into furniture, and dropping things could be real side effects of pregnancy. We don't know of any medical explanation for these effects, but some women do feel that they're more scatterbrained and clumsy. If it happens to you, don't worry. You're not losing your mind. Look at it this way: Now you have an excuse for having forgotten your best friend's birthday! And rest assured that you'll go back to being your brilliant, co-ordinated self after your baby is born.

Wind

You may find that you develop an annoying and embarrassing tendency to burp and pass wind at inopportune times during this trimester. (Now you can duel it out with your husband.) You're not the first pregnant woman to run into this problem; unfortunately, though, you can do very little about it – besides getting a dog to blame it on. Try to avoid becoming constipated (refer to Chapter 6) because that can make things worse.

Hair and nail growth

Your fingernails and toenails may become stronger and grow at an unprecedented rate while you're pregnant. Manicures are safe when done in a reputable, clean salon – and often relieve stress – so sit back and enjoy your beautiful nails.

Pregnancy also speeds up hair growth. Unfortunately, some women find that hair also begins growing in unusual places – on their face or stomach, for example. Waxing, plucking, or shaving the unwanted hair is safe, but hair removal creams (depilatories) contain chemicals that haven't been extensively studied. Because safer alternatives are readily available, we suggest avoiding these creams. Take comfort in the likelihood that the unwanted hair disappears after your baby is born.

Heartburn

Heartburn – the burning sensation you feel when stomach acids rise into your oesophagus – is common during pregnancy. Heartburn has two basic causes (neither of which validates the old myth that heartburn means your baby will have a lot of hair). First, the high level of progesterone that your body is producing can slow digestion and relax the sphincter muscle between the oesophagus and the stomach, which normally prevents the upward movement of stomach acids. Second, as the uterus grows, it presses upward on the stomach, which can push stomach acids into the oesophagus. (See Figure 7-2.)

TIP

You may get relief from heartburn by following these suggestions:

- Eat small, frequent meals rather than large ones.
- Carry an antacid liquid or tablet when you're away from home (ask your GP to prescribe them – prescriptions are free when you're pregnant).
- Carry a packet of dry biscuits to munch on when you feel heartburn. They may neutralise the gas.
- Avoid spicy, fatty, and greasy foods.
- Avoid eating just before bedtime, because heartburn occurs most readily when you lie down. Also, try sleeping with your head elevated on several pillows.

Lower abdominal/groin pain

Between 18 and 24 weeks, you may feel a sharp pain or a dull ache near your groin on either or both sides. When you move quickly or stand, you may notice it worsen, and it may fade if you lie down. This pain is called *round ligament pain*. The round ligaments are bands of fibrous tissue on each side of the uterus that attach the top of the uterus to the labia. The pain occurs because as the uterus grows, the ligaments stretch. The pain can be quite uncomfortable, but it's normal and usually goes away or at least lessens considerably after 24 weeks.

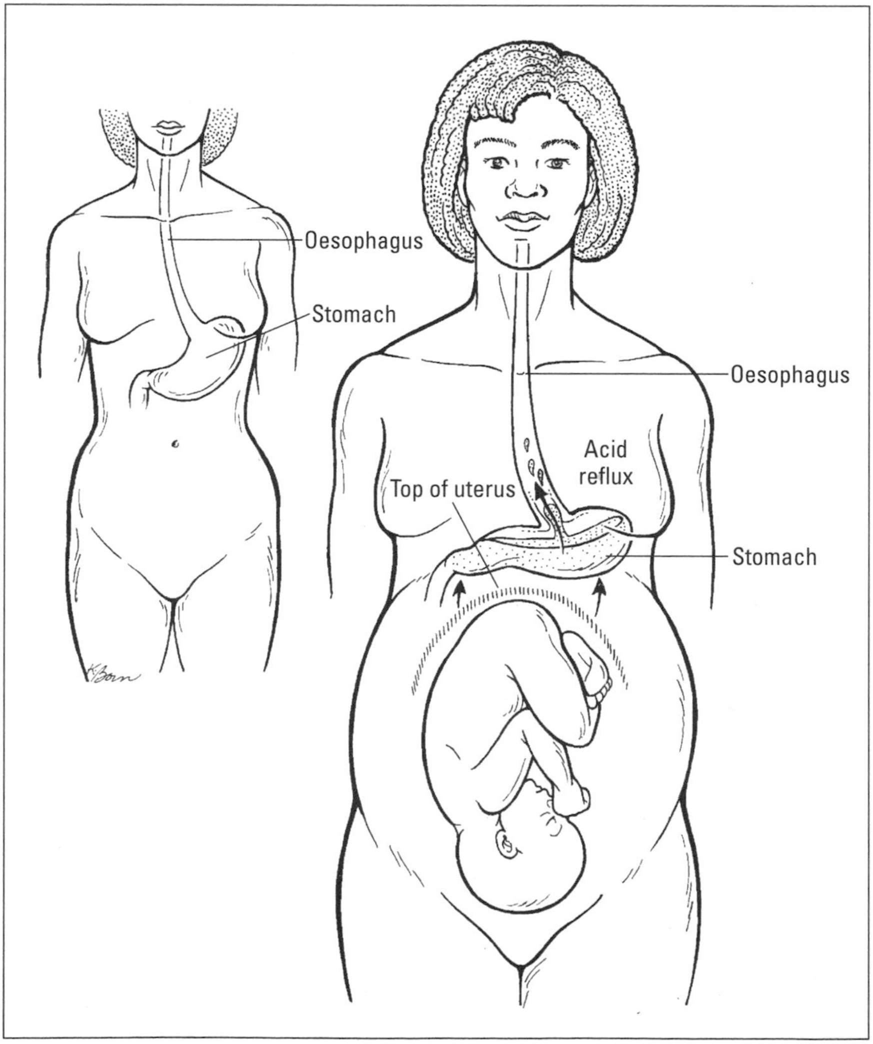

Figure 7-2: As your baby grows, your uterus expands, pushing upward on your stomach and oesophagus, sometimes leading to heartburn.

Sometime in the middle of the second trimester (the exact time varies) you may start to feel mild, short-lived contractions or cramps. These are referred to as *Braxton-Hicks contractions* and are nothing to worry about. Braxton-Hicks contractions often are more noticeable when you're walking or physically active and then go away when you get off your feet. If these contractions become uncomfortable and regular (more than six in an hour), call your practitioner.

Nasal congestion

The increased blood flow that occurs during pregnancy can cause stuffiness and some swelling of the mucous membranes inside your nose, which in turn can lead to postnasal drip and, ultimately, a chronic cough. Nasal saline drops may provide some relief and are perfectly safe to use during pregnancy. Keeping the air in your home or office well humidified also helps. Your pharmacist or GP may be able to advise you on a nasal spray that works (steroid sprays can be effective and most are safe in pregnancy). You (or your partner, more specifically) may notice that suddenly you're snoring like never before. This common symptom again relates to the increase in nasal congestion. Our advice? Buy your partner a good set of earplugs!

Nosebleeds and bleeding gums

Because of the higher volume of blood coursing through your body to support your pregnancy, you may experience some bleeding from small blood vessels in your nose and gums. This bleeding usually stops by itself, but you can help by applying slight pressure to the point of bleeding. If bleeding becomes particularly heavy or frequent, call your doctor.

TIP

Using a softer toothbrush may help to minimise bleeding when you brush your teeth.

Skin changes

The hormones coursing through your body at soaring levels may make strange things happen to your skin. These changes, illustrated in Figure 7-3, don't occur in all women, and if they do happen to you, rest assured that they usually fade away after the baby is born.

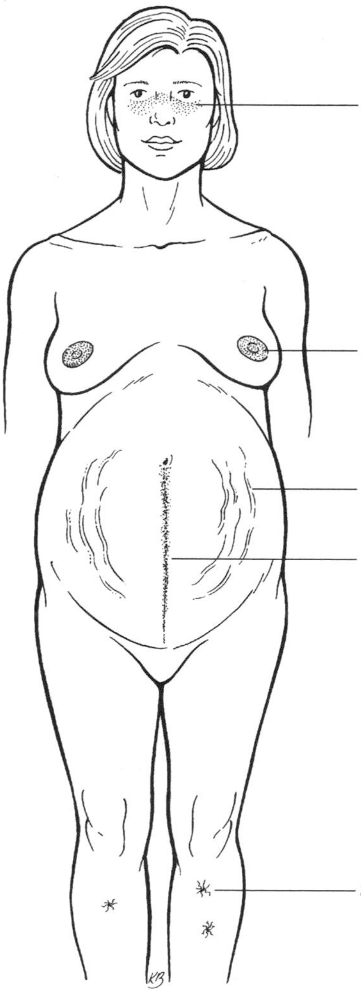

Figure 7-3: Some common skin changes associated with pregnancy.

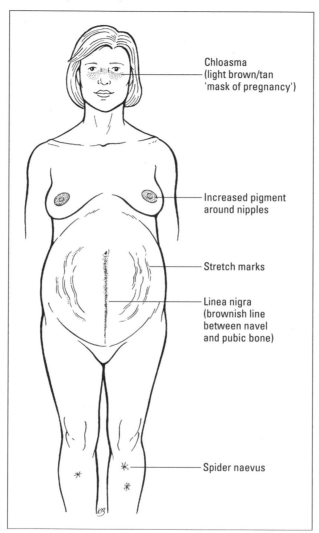

- You may notice a dark line, called the linea nigra, on your lower abdomen, running from your pubic bone up to your navel. This line may be more noticeable in women with relatively dark skin. Fair-skinned women often don't develop this line at all.
- The skin on your face may also darken in a mask-like distribution around your cheeks, nose, and eyes. This darkening is called *chloasma*, or the *mask of pregnancy.* Sun exposure makes it even darker.
- Red spots, called *spider naevi,* may suddenly appear anywhere on your body. Press on them, and they probably turn white. These spots are

concentrations of blood vessels caused by the high level of oestrogen in your body and they'll probably disappear after delivery.

- Some women notice a reddish colouring on the palms of their hands. Known as *palmar erythema*, this colouring is another oestrogen effect, and it, too, will go away.
- *Skin tags* are also a common occurrence, although it isn't totally clear why they develop. Fortunately, these tags, too, fade away or disappear after pregnancy.

Many of the skin changes noticed during pregnancy are also seen in alcohol abusers. But don't worry, your practitioner won't think you're secretly hitting the bottle – these changes are very common in pregnancy.

Checking In: Antenatal Visits

In the second trimester, you're likely to see your practitioner every four to six weeks. You'll be given a shared care antenatal booklet in your second trimester, containing details of all your consultations – take it with you to all your appointments, whether at hospital or at your GP's surgery. This booklet includes dates when you should make a GP or hospital appointment. If your care is shared between the hospital and your GP (and you can find out more about the types of care offered in Chapter 2), all your appointments may be with your GP in the second trimester, except for a blood test and ultrasound (which take place at hospital). At each visit, your GP checks your blood pressure, your urine, the size of your 'bump', the foetal heart rate, and sometimes your weight. You may want to ask questions about foetal movement, childbirth classes, your weight gain, and any unusual symptoms or discomforts you may experience.

Your practitioner routinely performs a number of tests during your second trimester to find out whether you're at risk for such complications as diabetes, anaemia, or birth defects. You may also have an ultrasound examination. Check out Chapter 9 for more information on second-trimester antenatal tests.

Recognising Causes for Concern

In this section, we talk about certain problems that can develop during the second trimester and symptoms that you should discuss with your practitioner.

Bleeding

Some women experience bleeding in the second trimester. Possible causes of bleeding include a low-lying placenta (*placenta previa*), premature labour, cervical incompetence, or placental abruption (all covered in Chapter 16). Sometimes the doctor can't find a cause for the bleeding. If you do experience bleeding, it doesn't necessarily mean that you will have a miscarriage (see Chapter 6 to find out more about miscarriages), but you should call your doctor – she'll probably recommend that you have an ultrasound and be monitored to make sure that you're not contracting. Bleeding may increase the risk for premature delivery, so your doctor may recommend that your pregnancy come under extra-close surveillance.

Foetal abnormality

Although the vast majority of pregnancies proceed normally, about 2 to 3 percent of infants are born with some abnormality. Most of these abnormalities are minor, although some do lead to significant problems for the newborn. Some abnormalities are due to chromosomal problems, and others stem from abnormal development of organs and structures. For example, some newborns may have heart defects or abnormalities of the kidneys, bladder, or gastrointestinal tract. Many of these problems, though not all of them, can be diagnosed on an antenatal ultrasound (see Chapter 9). If you are confronted with any such problem, gather all the available information about it, so that you know what to expect and what the treatment options are.

Incompetent cervix

During the second trimester, usually between 16 and 24 weeks, some women develop a problem known as an *incompetent cervix.* The cervix opens up and dilates, even though the woman feels no contractions. This condition may lead to miscarriage (read more about miscarriage in Chapter 6) – indeed, an incompetent cervix is most often diagnosed after the miscarriage occurs. A woman who develops this condition ordinarily doesn't notice any symptoms, although sometimes she may report feeling pelvic heaviness or pressure that's out of the ordinary, or she may notice some spotting. Most women who experience an incompetent cervix do so for no identifiable reason. Other women may have one of the following risk factors:

- **Cervical trauma:** Some evidence suggests that multiple *D&Cs* (dilation and curettage) or procedures called *cervical cone biopsy* or *LEEP* (in which a cone-shaped portion of the cervix is removed in the diagnosis or treatment of cervical abnormalities) can lead to cervical incompetence. A significant tear of the cervix during a prior delivery may also increase the risk for cervical incompetence.

- **Multiple gestations:** Some obstetricians believe that carrying multiple babies, especially triplets or more, may increase the risk for an incompetent cervix – but this is a very controversial issue. Some obstetricians recommend placing a *cerclage* (a stitch in the uterus – see the explanation that follows) in all patients with triplets or more, but others perform the procedure only in patients that they think are at high risk for incompetent cervix.
- **Prior history of incompetent cervix:** After you have had an incompetent cervix, your risk of having it again in a subsequent pregnancy is increased.

In cases in which an incompetent cervix is diagnosed before the pregnancy is lost, the woman's cervix can be held shut with a cerclage around the cervix. The cerclage is usually placed at 12 to 14 weeks, although it's occasionally performed as an emergency procedure later in the pregnancy. Doctors most commonly perform the procedure in the hospital under spinal or epidural anaesthetic, but the woman is usually discharged later the same day.

Some women with a cerclage notice that they have a heavy discharge throughout pregnancy. If you need to have a cerclage, talk to your doctor about how active you can be – if you can have sex and how much exercise is advisable. Complications associated with *elective* cerclage (not emergency cerclage) are unusual but can include infection, contractions, rupture of membranes, bleeding, and miscarriage.

Identifying other potential problems

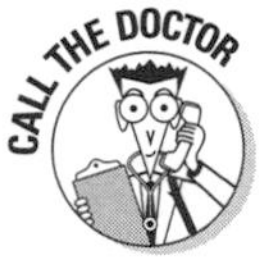

Below is a list of second-trimester symptoms that require some attention. If you experience any of them, call your practitioner:

- Bleeding
- An unusual sense of pressure or heaviness
- Regular contractions or strong cramping
- A lack of normal foetal movement
- High fever
- Severe abdominal pain

Chapter 8

The Third Trimester

In This Chapter

- Preparing to enter the real world – your baby wants out!
- Dealing with your changing body
- Planning for the main event
- Knowing when to be concerned
- Getting ready to go to the hospital

You're finally ready for the third act – your pregnancy's final trimester. By now, you're probably accustomed to having a bulging tummy, your morning sickness is long gone, and you've come to expect and enjoy the feeling of your baby moving around and kicking inside you. In this trimester, your baby continues to grow, and your practitioner continues to monitor your and your baby's health. You also begin making preparations for the new arrival, which may mean anything from getting ready to take a leave of absence from your job to taking childbirth classes (and other ways of finding out what to expect during labour and delivery).

Your Baby Gets Ready for Birth

At 28 weeks, your baby measures about 14 inches (about 35 centimetres) and weighs about 2½ pounds (about 1.14 kilograms). But by the end of the third trimester – at 40 weeks, your due date – it measures about 20 inches (50 centimetres) and weighs 6 to 8 pounds (about 2.7 to 3.6 kilograms) – sometimes a bit more, sometimes a bit less. The foetus spends most of the third trimester growing, adding fat, and continuing to develop various organs, especially the central nervous system. The arms and legs get chubbier, and the skin becomes thicker and smoother.

During the third trimester, your baby is less susceptible to infections and to the adverse effects of medications, but some of these agents may still affect its growth. The last two months are usually spent getting ready for the transition to life in the world outside the uterus. The changes are less dramatic than they were early on, but the maturation and growth that happen now are very important.

By 28 to 34 weeks, the foetus generally assumes a head-down position (called a *vertex presentation*), as shown in Figure 8-1. In this position the buttocks and legs (the bulkiest parts of the foetus's body) occupy the roomiest part of the uterus – the top part. In about 4 per cent of singleton pregnancies, the baby may be positioned buttocks-down (breech) or lie across the uterus (transverse). (See the section 'Recognising Causes for Concern', later in this chapter, for more on breech presentation.)

By 36 weeks, growth slows, and the amniotic fluid volume is at its maximum level. After this point, the amount of amniotic fluid may start to decline because blood flow to the baby's kidneys decreases as the placenta ages, and the baby produces less urine (and therefore less amniotic fluid).

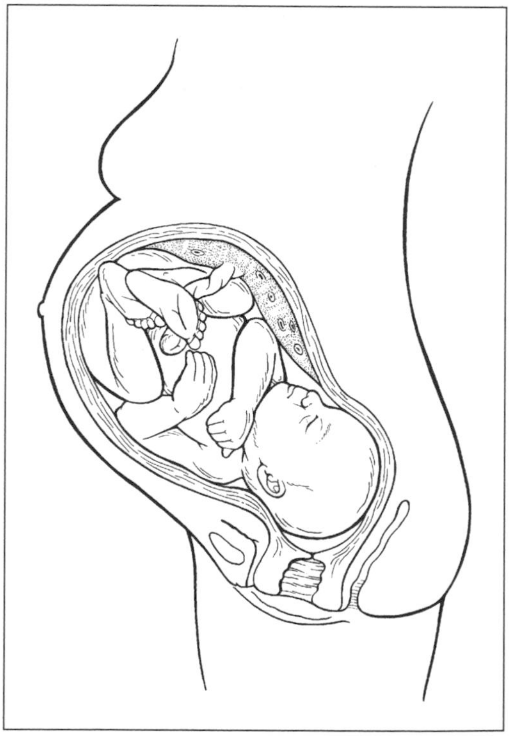

Figure 8-1: How your baby may look inside your uterus during the third trimester.

Movin' and shakin': Foetal movements

Look down at your belly during times of foetal activity during the third trimester, and it may appear that an alien from outer space is doing an aerobic dance inside you. Although foetal movements don't actually reduce as your due date approaches, the timing and quality of the movements change. Toward the end of pregnancy, foetal movements may feel less like jabs and more like tumbles or rolls, and you notice longer periods of quiet between movements. The foetus is adapting to a more newborn-like pattern, taking longer naps and having longer active cycles.

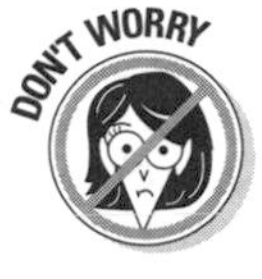

Friends and family may inundate you with well-meaning advice about how much your baby should be moving. You may also hear scare stories about mothers who fail to pick up signs that their babies are in trouble, because the mother ignored a lack of foetal movements. And if this isn't your first pregnancy, this baby's pattern of movements may be different from your last. But most babies are just fine, and every baby has a different pattern of waking, sleeping, and being active. Getting to know your baby's personal pattern of activity is important, so you can recognise any changes.

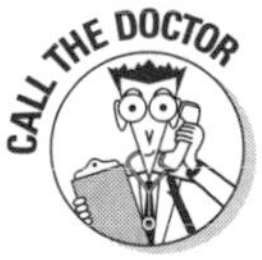

To help you learn to recognise your baby's particular pattern of movements, you are given an information leaflet about the 'Cardiff Count to Ten' kick chart at your antenatal appointment (head to Chapter 6 for more on this appointment). If you don't have this chart, ask your practitioner for one. You don't have to use the chart, but some women find it reassuring, especially in the last few weeks of pregnancy, when there's not so much room for your baby to move and he might seem less active. The 'Cardiff Count to Ten' kick chart helps you in recognising and recording ten individual foetal movements over 12 hours every day. If you don't feel ten movements in the 12-hour period, call your labour ward to arrange for a cardiotocograph test (CTG) to monitor the baby's heartbeat (see Chapter 9).

Flexing the breathing muscles

The foetus undergoes what are called *rhythmic breathing movements* from 10 weeks onward, although these movements are much more frequent in the third trimester. The foetus doesn't actually breathe, but its chest, abdominal wall, and diaphragm move in a pattern that is characteristic of breathing. You don't notice these movements, but a doctor can observe them with ultrasound. Many doctors believe these movements are signs that the baby is faring well. During the third trimester, the amount of time a foetus spends performing the breathing movements increases, especially after meals.

Hiccupping in utero

At times you may feel a quick, rhythmic pattern of foetal movements, occurring every few seconds. These movements are probably hiccups and are completely normal. Some women feel foetal hiccups several times throughout the day; others sense them only rarely. These hiccups feel strange, but standing on your head and drinking water, which we hear is a great cure, probably isn't your best option now.

Keeping Up with Your Changing Body

As the baby grows, so does your belly. Although big is beautiful, it can become uncomfortable. You may notice that your uterus pushes up on your ribs, and sometimes you notice kicking in one spot in particular – that is probably where the baby's extremities are, either feet or arms. If you're pregnant with twins or more, the discomforts are, of course, even more pronounced. Women with twins may feel one baby move more than the other, which is usually related to the babies' positions – one position is more noticeable than the other. Whether you have one, two, or more babies inside, moving around like you used to becomes more and more difficult as you get bigger.

TIP

If you find rising after lying on your back is difficult and no one is around to help, try turning on your side first and then pushing yourself up to a sitting position (see Figure 8-2).

A pregnant woman knows no strangers

You may find that your belly has suddenly become public property. Perfect strangers feel compelled to put their hands on your abdomen and tell you how pleased they are that you're about to have a baby. Although some women find this kind of behaviour caring and supportive, others find it annoying, embarrassing, and that it makes them uncomfortable.

What's more, many people – who would never dream of commenting on your size if you weren't pregnant – appear to have no qualms about discussing your weight gain, hip size, or the shape of your bump. Suddenly, you're surrounded by people who think they have a fail-safe method of telling you whether you're carrying a boy or a girl, or telling you how difficult getting rid of your excess weight after delivery is.

The best advice we can offer is not to pay any attention to these people's advice – politely if possible (although pregnancy is a great excuse for just wandering off in mid conversation because you can always put your inattentiveness down to hormones!). If some comments raise question marks in your mind, look up the topics in this book or talk to your practitioner for reassurance.

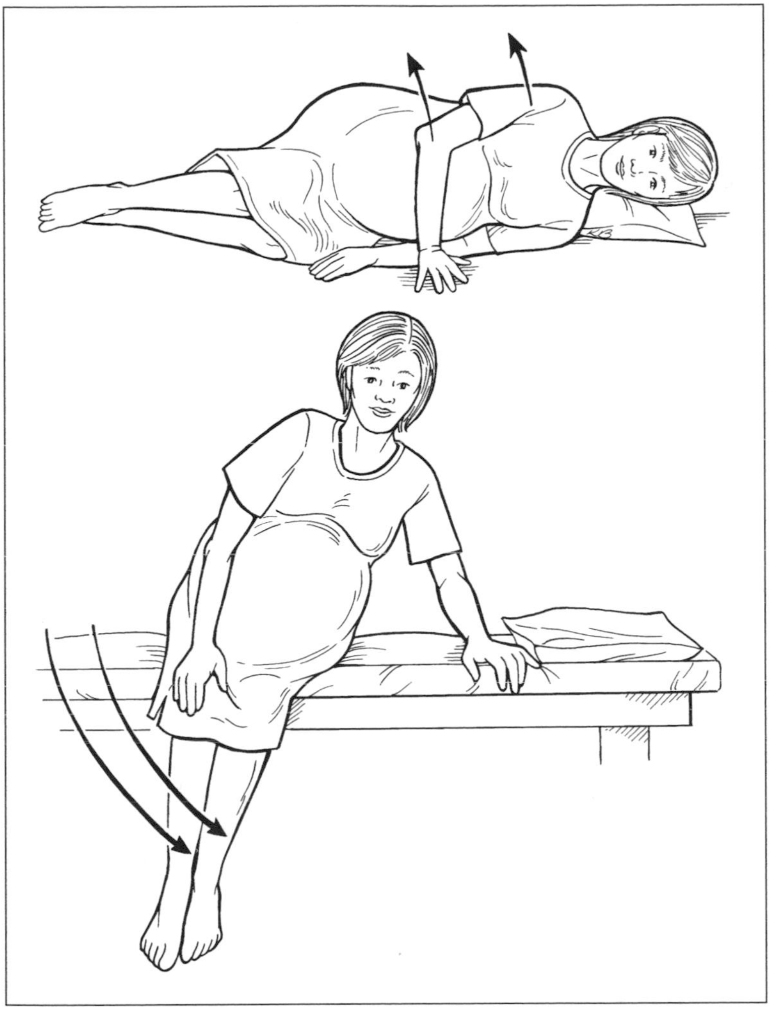

Figure 8-2: Make it easy on your back: Before trying to get up from lying down, first roll over to your side and then push yourself up while swinging your legs down.

Accidents and falls

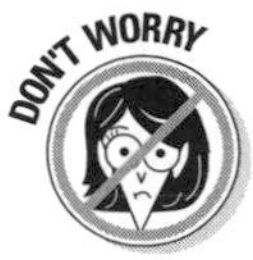

Being pregnant may make you more cautious about taking obvious risks, but it doesn't prevent you from stumbling or otherwise having an occasional mishap. If you do fall, don't worry. Chances are good that the baby remains well protected within your uterus and within its sac of amniotic fluid, which is an excellent natural cushion. If you do have an accident, let your practitioner know; he may want you to come in to check that the baby is fine.

Braxton-Hicks contractions

In the late second trimester or beginning of the third trimester, your uterus may, from time to time, become momentarily hard or feel as though it's turning into a hard ball. You are probably experiencing Braxton-Hicks contractions – not the kind you have in labour – which are like practice contractions.

Braxton-Hicks contractions are usually painless, but at times they may be uncomfortable, and they may occur with more frequency when you are active and subside when you rest.

If you're less than 36 weeks along and you experience contractions that are persistent, regular, and increasingly painful, call your doctor to make sure that you're not in premature labour.

Carpal tunnel syndrome

If you feel numbness, tingling, or pain in your fingers and wrist, you're probably experiencing *carpal tunnel syndrome.* Swelling in the wrist puts pressure on the *median nerve*, which runs through the *carpal tunnel* from the wrist to the hand, creating these sensations. One or both hands can be affected, and the pain may be worse at night or upon awakening.

If carpal tunnel syndrome becomes persistent or bothersome, discuss it with your practitioner, who may be able to refer you to a physiotherapist. Wrist splints, available by referral from your practitioner, can relieve the problem. Try not to be discouraged if the pain doesn't seem to get better, though, because it usually improves (often quite suddenly) after delivery.

Fatigue

The fatigue that you felt early in your pregnancy may return in the third trimester. You may feel as if you're just slowing down. You're tired all the time, you're carrying around more weight, you're not very comfortable much of the time, and you may feel that you can't accomplish everything you need to. Women may find their second or third pregnancies more tiring than the first because they also have to care for one or more older children.

Try to be realistic about what you can do, and don't feel guilty about what you can't manage. No one wants you to be Superwoman. Take time out for yourself and get as much rest as you can. Delegate tasks: Let other people help with household chores and other responsibilities. Take advantage of the quiet times: Rest as much as you can now, because after delivery, the work really picks up!

At this late stage of pregnancy, your partner is carrying a large amount of extra weight (see Chapter 13 if you don't believe us) and is going through all sorts of physical changes. As if this weren't enough, she's probably nervous about what labour has in store. Now's the perfect time for you to pamper your partner – after all, she deserves the fuss, and once your baby is born you'll both have other things on your minds.

Piles

No one wants to talk about them, but *piles* – dilated, swollen veins around the rectum – are a common problem for pregnant women. Piles are varicose veins of the rectum (we talk about varicose veins later in this section). The uterus causes piles by pressing on major blood vessels, which leads to pooling of blood, and ultimately makes the veins enlarge and swell. Progesterone relaxes the veins, allowing the swelling to increase. Constipation makes piles worse. Straining and pushing hard during bowel movements puts added pressure on the blood vessels, causing them to enlarge and possibly protrude from the rectum.

Piles can cause bleeding of bright red (not dark) blood when you open your bowels. As long as this blood is on the paper or spattered in the toilet pan, and you're happy it's coming from you bottom and not your vagina, don't be concerned. This bleeding doesn't harm the pregnancy, but if it becomes frequent, or your piles are painful, talk to your GP. Meanwhile, you can try the following:

- **Avoid constipation.** Straining to push out a hard stool can make piles worse. Refer to Chapter 6 for advice on how to avoid constipation.
- **Exercise.** Activity increases the natural action of the bowel, so the stool doesn't get too hard.
- **Get off your feet when you can.** This relieves extra pressure on your veins.
- **Try over-the-counter topical medications.** Your pharmacist can tell you what's safe.
- **Take warm baths two to three times a day.** Soaking in warm water can help relieve the muscle spasms that most often cause the pain.

Pushing during the second stage of labour can make piles worse or make them appear where they weren't before. But, most of the time, piles go away after delivery.

Insomnia

During the last few months of pregnancy, many women find sleeping difficult. Finding a comfortable position when you're eight months along isn't easy. You feel a little like a beached whale. Getting up five times a night to go to the loo doesn't make things any easier. However, you may find relief in the following:

- **Drink warm milk with honey.** Warming the milk releases *tryptophan*, a naturally occurring amino acid that makes you sleepy; the honey causes you to produce insulin, which also makes you drowsy.
- **Exercise during the day.** Activity helps to tire you out, which means you'll fall asleep sooner.
- **Limit your liquid intake after 6 p.m.** Don't limit it to the point that you become dehydrated, however.
- **Stock up the bed with pillows.** Turning over may be a hassle when you have to rearrange the pillows, but pillows between your legs and under your bump can make you much more comfortable.
- **Take a warm, relaxing bath before going to bed.** Many women say a bath helps make them feel sleepy.

Feeling the baby engage

Many women look forward to the engagement of the baby's head. But you don't need to start choosing a ring. *Engagement* means that the foetal head has reached the *ischial spines*, which are bony landmarks in your pelvis that your practitioner can feel during an internal examination (see Figure 8-3). Engagement marks the point at which the widest part of the baby's head has passed through the narrowest part of your pelvis. After engagement occurs, your pelvis should then be big enough for the baby's head to pass through in labour. The chance that your labour will go smoothly also increases.

DON'T WORRY

In your first pregnancy, the baby's head engaging increases your chance of having a normal labour, but even if your baby's head doesn't engage at all, you can still have a perfectly normal delivery. In first pregnancies, the baby's head usually engages two to three weeks before delivery. In subsequent pregnancies, it's perfectly normal for the head not to engage until you're actually in labour. So don't be concerned if your baby's head hasn't engaged – it doesn't mean that a caesarean section is inevitable.

After your baby's head is engaged, you have more space under your ribs, which generally makes breathing a lot easier. Unfortunately, however, the baby has to go somewhere when its head engages, and that somewhere is right on top of your bladder, so you may find that your trips to the loo are even more frequent than before (hard to believe, we know). You may also feel a pressure or heaviness, or even sharp twinges, in your vagina. Don't worry – this is all part of the baby's passage through your pelvis.

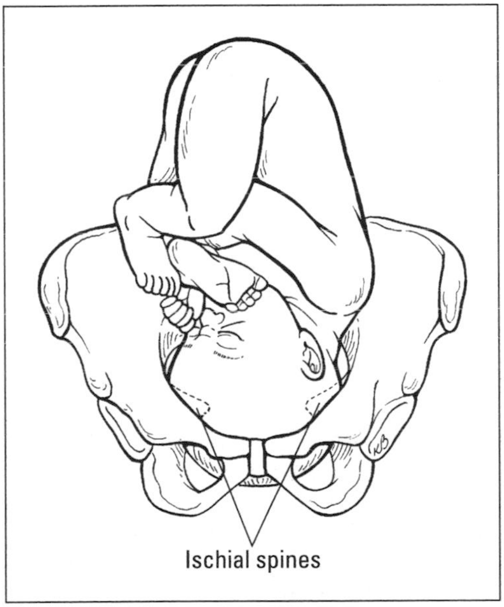

Figure 8-3: The baby's head reaches the bony ischial spines in your pelvis and is engaged.

Pregnancy rashes and itches

Pregnant women are subject to the same rashes that non-pregnant women get. One rash is unique to pregnancy, however – *Pruritic Urticarial Papules of Pregnancy*, or PUPP. Although PUPP sounds scary, it's really more of a nuisance than anything else because the rash can cause some intense itching. PUPP is pretty common, occurring in about 1 in 160 pregnancies (more often during a first pregnancy and in women having twins or more).

PUPP tends to occur about 36 weeks into pregnancy, although it can start at any time from 17 weeks of pregnancy to 1 week after delivery. PUPP is characterised by red patches that first appear in the stretch marks on your tummy. These patches can spread to other areas on the abdomen and to the legs, arms, chest, and back. They almost never spread to the face. (Thank heaven for small mercies.)

PUPP may look dramatic, but poses no risk to your baby. However, if you develop PUPP, your doctor is likely to recommend some blood tests to check that you don't have any other conditions associated with itching.

The only sure-fire way to make PUPP go away is to deliver. Some women tell us that the itching goes away within hours of giving birth. Before delivery, however, unscented moisturisers or calamine cream can be very soothing. If these treatments don't do the trick, your GP may prescribe mild topical steroid cream or antihistamine tablets. Even if you don't have a rash, you may notice that you itch a lot, especially where stretch marks develop. This itching is very common and usually is caused by the stretching of your skin as the baby gets bigger.

One in 50 pregnant women develop *cholestasis of pregnancy*, or *obstetric cholestasis*, a condition affecting your liver. This condition usually starts after 20 weeks into pregnancy, when an increase of bile acids (from your liver) in your blood causes itching. The itching tends to start on your torso and your lower legs and arms, becoming more intense as it progresses, but disappearing after delivery. You won't usually see any changes in your skin to account for the itching. If the itching is mild, you can treat it with skin moisturisers, topical anti-itching medications, or oral antihistamines (ask your GP or pharmacist). If the itching is severe, your doctor may recommend oral medications that help to clear the bile acids from the bloodstream. Your practitioner also monitors your baby more closely, possibly with regular Cardiotocograph tests (CTGs) and ultrasound examinations (see Chapter 9), because of the increased risk of foetal distress or premature delivery.

Preparing for breast-feeding

Contrary to popular belief, every mother does not take to breast-feeding like a duck to water. Breast-feeding (see Chapter 14) can be incredibly rewarding for you, as well as for your baby, but the technique can take a lot of practice to get right. So before you deliver, you want to toughen up your nipples to reduce the chance of cracked, sore nipples when you're breast-feeding. You can do this by rubbing your nipples gently with your fingers or with a flannel, or by wearing a nursing bra with the flaps down, to let your nipples rub against your clothes.

Don't be too vigorous with your nipple stimulation – pummelling your nipples too vigorously can make your uterus contract, and can even bring on premature labour.

Some women worry that they don't have the right type of breasts for breast-feeding, but no breast type is right or wrong. Breasts both large and small can produce adequate milk. Some women with retracted or inverted nipples can make breast-feeding easier by massaging their nipples so that they protrude more. (See Chapter 14.) Some maternity shops and chemists sell special breast shells (sometimes called Mexican hats) that use suction to help the nipples come out.

Some women notice from early on in pregnancy that their breasts occasionally secrete a yellowish discharge. This discharge is perfectly normal, and consists of *colostrum*, which your baby will feed off in the first few days of life. You can find out more about colostrum and nipple shapes in Chapter 14.

Sciatica

Some women experience pain extending from their lower back to their buttocks and down one leg or the other. This pain or, less commonly, numbness is known as *sciatica*, because it is caused by pressure on the sciatic nerve, a major nerve that branches from your back, through your pelvis, to your hips, and down your legs. You can relieve mild cases of sciatica with bed rest (shift from side to side to find the most comfortable position), warm baths, or heating pads applied to the painful areas. If you develop a severe case of sciatica, you may need to ask your GP for referral to a physiotherapist.

Shortness of breath

You may find that as pregnancy proceeds, you become increasingly short of breath. The hormone progesterone affects your central breathing centre and may cause these feelings of breathlessness. Furthermore, as your enlarging uterus presses upward on your diaphragm, your lungs have less room to expand normally.

When Joanne was pregnant with her second child, she used to be so short of breath that the only books she could read to her daughter were ones with very short sentences. *The Cat in the Hat* had to sit on the shelf until after she delivered!

In most cases, shortness of breath is perfectly normal. If you're worried that your shortness of breath is more serious, read the sections on deep vein thrombosis and pulmonary embolus in Chapter 17.

Stretch marks

Stretch marks are an almost inevitable part of pregnancy. Some women do manage to avoid stretch marks, whilst others probably have a genetic predisposition for them.

Stretch marks can vary in colour from brown to pinkish-red, but tend to fade to silvery-grey or white several months after delivery. No cream or ointment is completely effective in preventing stretch marks. Many people think that rubbing vitamin E oil on the belly helps prevent stretch marks or helps them fade faster, but the effectiveness of vitamin E has never been proven scientifically. Your best bet is to avoid excessive weight gain and to exercise regularly, to keep your tummy muscles toned.

Swelling

Swelling (also called *oedema*) of the hands and legs is very common in the third trimester. Oedema most often occurs after you've been on your feet for a while, but it can happen throughout the day. Swelling tends to be even more common in warm weather.

Contrary to popular wisdom, no evidence indicates that lowering your salt intake or drinking a lot of water prevents swelling or makes it go away.

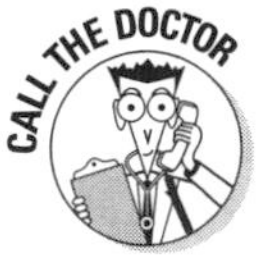

Although swelling is a normal symptom of pregnancy, it can occasionally be a sign of pre-eclampsia (see Chapter 16). If you notice a sudden increase in the amount of swelling, or a sudden large weight gain – 5 pounds (about 2.3 kilograms) or more in a week – or if the swelling is associated with significant headaches or right-sided abdominal pain, call your practitioner immediately.

For ordinary swelling, try the following:

- Keep your legs up whenever you can.
- Stay in a cool environment.
- Wear support tights that aren't restricting around your knees.
- When you're in bed, don't lie flat on your back; try to lie on your side.

Urinary stress incontinence

Leaking a little urine when you cough, laugh, or sneeze isn't unusual when you're pregnant. This kind of *urinary stress incontinence* occurs because your growing uterus is putting pressure on your bladder. Relaxation of the pelvic floor muscles increases the problem during the late second and third trimesters. And sometimes the baby may give the bladder a swift kick and cause it to leak urine. *Pelvic floor exercises* – in which you repeatedly contract the pelvic floor muscles as if you're trying very hard not to pee – can prevent or markedly reduce the problem. (See Chapter 13.) Some women continue to experience a little stress incontinence even after delivery, but it usually goes away after about 6 to 12 months.

Pelvic floor exercises don't just help with stress incontinence – a recent study in the *British Medical Journal* confirms that women who do regular pelvic floor exercises during pregnancy are less likely to need a forceps delivery (see Chapter 11).

Varicose veins

You may notice that a small road map has suddenly appeared on your lower legs (and sometimes the vulvar area). These marks are dilated veins, referred to as *varicose veins*, caused by the pressure of the uterus on major blood vessels. Pregnancy also causes the muscle tissue inside your veins to relax and your blood volume to increase, and both of these can add to the problem. Women with light skin or with a family history of varicose veins are particularly susceptible. Very often, the bluish-purple veins fade after delivery, but sometimes they don't disappear completely. Varicose veins are usually painless, but occasionally they may be associated with discomfort, achiness, or pain.

In rare instances, a blood clot develops in the superficial veins of the legs. This condition, called *superficial thrombophlebitis*, isn't a serious problem; it's often successfully treated with rest, leg elevation, warm compresses, and special stockings. A clot that forms in the deep veins of the leg is more serious (see Chapter 17 for a discussion of *deep vein thrombosis*).

You can't prevent varicose veins – you can't fight heredity – but you can reduce their number and severity by following these tips:

- Avoid standing for prolonged periods of time.
- Avoid wearing clothes that are very tight around one part of your leg, like socks with tight elastic.

- If you have to stand or sit still, move your legs around from time to time to stimulate circulation.
- Keep your legs up whenever you can.
- Wear support tights – you may be able to get these on prescription from your GP if your varicose veins are causing you a lot of aching.

Thinking about Labour

Toward the end of your third trimester, you're likely to think more about delivery and anticipate what that's going to be like. Many of our patients want to know the time of the onset of labour and whether they can do anything to influence this timing or bring it on sooner. In this section, we give some answers to these rather complicated questions.

Writing a birth plan

Practitioners are very keen for you to be involved in how your labour is managed. A list of your own labour ideas is called a *birth plan*. The exact content of your birth plan depends entirely on your priorities; however, issues you might want to raise could include:

- Will I – and my partner – be kept informed of labour progress at all times?
- Can I have the same midwife with me throughout labour?
- Will all staff introduce themselves to me when I see them for the first time?
- Will my midwife respect my wish to have a natural delivery without pain relief, if that's what I want and all is progressing smoothly?
- What facilities for TENS machines, epidural, or other kinds of pain relief are available (see Chapter 10 for more details on the alternatives)?
- Does the hospital have facilities for a water birth? Can I book these facilities in advance?
- Can my baby be delivered straight onto my tummy if all goes smoothly?
- Can my partner cut the umbilical cord?
- Will I be encouraged to breast-feed immediately?

Your baby's and your physical wellbeing are your practitioner's primary concern. If your baby shows signs of being in distress, your practitioner may recommend an intervention that you wouldn't ideally have wanted. However, knowing that you've made it clear in your birth plan that you want to be kept informed at all times, or consulted if there is more than one feasible option, can help you to feel much less anxious.

Writing a birth plan is the ideal opportunity for you and your partner to discuss at your leisure the part she wants you to play in your baby's delivery – and your views on the subject. Do tell your partner if there are any roles you feel strongly about playing or not playing. However, remember that *she's* the one going through all the hard work, so try to be as supportive as you can.

Timing labour

'When am I going to have this baby?' We hear this question all the time as the due date approaches and wish we had a foolproof way of knowing, but not even a crystal ball works. Sometimes a woman whose cervix is long and closed goes into labour within 12 hours of an internal examination, although other women can walk around for weeks with a cervix dilated to 3 centimetres (1.2 inches). Some signs that something may happen include loss of the *mucous plug* (not really a plug but thick mucous produced in the cervix), *bloody show* (an unfortunately named and blood-tinged mucous discharge), increasing frequency of Braxton-Hicks contractions, and diarrhoea. But nothing is a sure sign of labour. Loss of the mucous plug or bloody show may occur hours, days, or weeks before labour, or in some cases, not at all. This unpredictability may add to your anxiety, but it also makes the whole process more exciting.

Women have tried all kinds of tricks (Chinese food, enemas, and raspberry tea, to name a few) to induce labour on their own, but nothing – short of medical induction – really has been proven to work. Sex might help if you have enough energy (see Chapter 20)!

Vigorously rubbing or massaging the nipples can cause contractions, but it shouldn't be performed at home because it can lead to hyperstimulation of the uterus (that is, too-frequent contractions), which isn't healthy for you or your baby. It's not a sure thing, in any case, because as soon as you stop the nipple stimulation, the contractions usually also stop.

Using perineal massage

In the past few years, *perineal massage* has generated a great deal of interest. This process involves using an oil or cream on the *perineum* (the area between the vagina and the rectum) and massaging the area in preparation for childbirth, and reduces your chance of needing an episiotomy (see Chapter 11). Although trials haven't shown a clear benefit, there's no harm in trying it – you might even ask your partner to help.

Hitting the Home Stretch: Antenatal Visits in the Third Trimester

The National Institute of Clinical Excellence (NICE) recommends that during your first pregnancy, you have routine third trimester checks at 28, 31, 34, 36, 38, 40, and 41 weeks; however, some practitioners may see you every two weeks (depending on the care pattern in your part of the country). Most of these visits involve the usual measurements (see Chapter 6): blood pressure, urine, foetal heart rate, and fundal height. At 28 or 30 weeks you will also have a blood test to check again for anaemia (see Chapter 6). These checks are also an excellent time to discuss any concerns or queries that you might have about the final stages of your pregnancy, labour, or delivery.

If you haven't delivered by your due date, your practitioner will see you again at 41 weeks for a check-up, and to discuss induction of labour (see Chapter 10). By 41 weeks the placenta may not be able to support your baby as well, and your baby is more likely to run into unexpected – and potentially serious – problems. So while no women (well, very few) would actually choose to be induced, doing so may well be the safest way to ensure you go home with a healthy bundle of joy.

Preparation for Parenthood Classes

All hospitals offer preparation for parenthood classes. Sometimes called childbirth classes or antenatal classes, these sessions prepare you for much more than delivery. You can find out about pregnancy, labour, pain relief, and childbirth, as well as antenatal exercises, relaxation techniques, and tips on caring for your baby. These classes are free, and are usually held weekly for 8–10 weeks in your third trimester.

JUST FOR DADS

Preparation for parenthood classes are aimed at dads too, so you won't be the only man there. These classes are a great opportunity for you to find out what you can expect, and give you and your partner ideas about how you can help her through labour.

At preparation for parenthood classes, you should be offered a chance to tour the labour ward – if the offer isn't made, ask at the hospital.

Some women prefer to attend private classes, and you can ask your GP or midwife for more details about local private classes. The classes run by the National Childbirth Trust (NCT) are popular and widely available. NCT classes need to be booked well in advance and you will have to pay for them. Many mothers find that they feel more comfortable with the greater emphasis of NCT classes on natural/drug-free childbirth than hospital classes offer. You can find out about the NCT by contacting them by post at The National Childbirth Trust, Alexandra House, Oldham Terrace, Acton, London W3 6NH; phone: 0870 7703236; e-mail: `enquiries@national-childbirth-trust.co.uk`; Web site: `www.nctpregnancyandbabycare.com`.

One of the many benefits of preparation for parenthood classes is that these sessions are a great way to meet other parents-to-be from your area. Many NCT groups still have regular reunions of their members ten years on!

Recognising Causes for Concern

During the final weeks and months of pregnancy, you see your practitioner more often than before. Still, certain questions and problems may arise between visits. Everything starts to heat up during the later stages of the third trimester, with both the baby and your body preparing for delivery. Here are some of the key things that may lead you to call your doctor.

Bleeding

If you experience any significant bleeding, let your practitioner know immediately. Some third-trimester bleeding is harmless to you and your baby, but sometimes it can have serious implications – so always get any bleeding checked out. Possible causes of third-trimester bleeding include:

- Preterm labour
- Inflammation or irritation of the cervix or the harmless rupture of a superficial blood vessel on the cervix, either of which can occur after sex
- Placenta previa (see Chapter 16) or a low-lying placenta
- Placental separation or abruption (see Chapter 16)
- Bloody show (see Chapter 10). This show is usually less than the amount of blood you would see during a normal menstrual period, and it's often mixed with mucous

Breech presentation

A baby is in a so-called *breech* position when its buttocks or legs are down, closest to the cervix. Breech presentation happens in 2 to 4 per cent of all singleton deliveries.

A woman's risk of having a breech baby decreases the further along she goes in her pregnancy. About 1 in 4 women find their baby in the breech position at their 22-week check. As pregnancy progresses the baby will usually move into a head-down position so that by 30 weeks the chance of the baby being in a breech position is 1 in 12, reducing to 1 in 20 by 34 weeks, and about 1 in 35 by 40 weeks.

If your baby is still in breech position by about 36 weeks, the hospital doctor will discuss your options – including a 'wait and see' approach, trying to turn the baby to a head-down position from the outside, or assessing your pelvic size and your baby's head size to see whether elective caesarean section is necessary. You can find out more about breech positions and caesarean section in Chapter 16.

Decreased amniotic fluid volume

The medical term for decreased amniotic fluid volume is *oligohydramnios*, and is usually found from an ultrasound scan. No obvious reason may exist for decreased amniotic fluid volume to occur, although it can be linked with intrauterine growth restriction (we describe more in the 'Foetal growth problems' section later in this chapter), preterm rupture of the membranes, or other conditions. Usually, a mild decrease in amniotic fluid isn't a major cause for concern; your practitioner begins to monitor you more closely to make sure that no problem arises. See Chapter 16 for more details about problems with amniotic fluid.

Decreased foetal movement

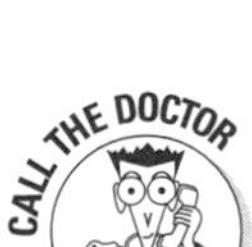

If you're not feeling the amount of foetal movement that you've been accustomed to, let your practitioner, or the labour ward, know. Foetal movement is one of the most important things to pay attention to as you near your due date (see the section 'Movin' and shakin': Foetal movements' earlier in this chapter).

Foetal growth problems

You may find out at a routine antenatal visit that your practitioner thinks that the measurements of your uterus are either too big or too small. This finding isn't a cause for immediate alarm. Your practitioner may suggest that you have an ultrasound examination to get a better idea of how big the baby is. Ultrasound is used to measure parts of the baby – the size of the head, the abdomen's circumference, and the thighbone's length. Your practitioner then plugs these measurements into a mathematical formula that gives the estimated foetal weight (EFW). That estimate is then entered on a curve plotting the baby's age in weeks against weight (see Figure 8-4), which represents the average growth of thousands of foetuses at each gestational age.

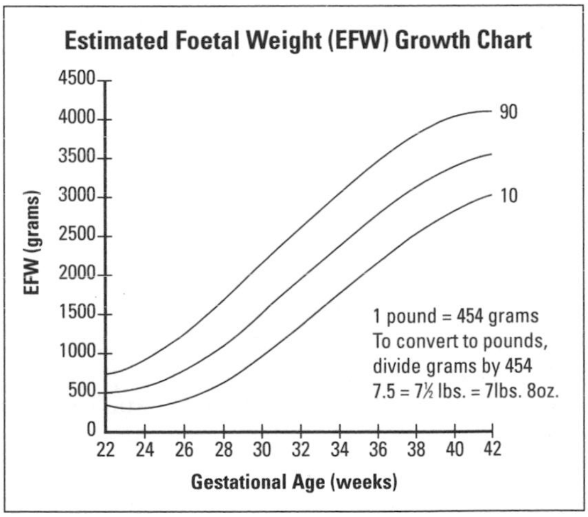

Figure 8-4: Average foetal weights at different points during pregnancy.

Your practitioner can check to see where your baby's weight falls on the curve and thus tell which percentile the baby is in. If the baby's weight is anywhere between the 10th and the 90th percentiles, the weight is considered normal. Remember, not every baby is at the 50th percentile, so the 20th percentile is still normal and no reason to worry.

Keep in mind that, although ultrasound is an excellent tool for assessing foetal growth, it isn't perfect. Judging the baby's weight by an ultrasound examination isn't the same as putting the baby on a scale. Weight estimates can vary by as much as 10 to 20 per cent in the third trimester due to variations in body composition. So if your baby is outside the normal range, don't worry.

If your baby measures very large (*macrosomia*), your practitioner may suggest that you have another glucose screen to check for gestational diabetes (see Chapter 16). If your baby is especially small (*intrauterine growth restriction*), your doctor may suggest that you be followed more closely – that you undergo Cardiotocograph tests (CTGs) and repeat ultrasound examinations to keep an eye on foetal growth. We go into problems with foetal growth and how to manage them in greater detail in Chapter 16.

Leaking amniotic fluid

If you notice that your underwear is wet, several explanations are possible. It may be a little urine, vaginal discharge, the release of the mucous plug in the cervix, or actual leakage of amniotic fluid (also known as *rupture of the membranes*). Often, you can tell what it is by examining the fluid. Mucous discharge tends to be thick and globby, while vaginal discharge is whitish and smooth. Urine has a characteristic smell and doesn't flow continuously without your effort. Amniotic fluid, on the other hand, is normally clear and watery and often is lost in spurts. Sometimes you have a big gush of water when membranes rupture, but if the membrane has only a small hole, the leakage may be scant.

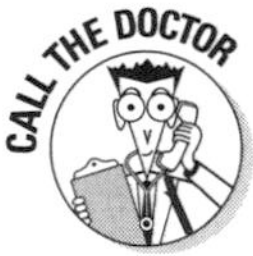

If you leak what you think may be amniotic fluid, call your practitioner right away. If you aren't preterm and the amniotic fluid is clear, leaking fluid isn't an emergency; however, most practitioners want you to let them know so that they can tell you what to do. If the fluid is bloody or greenish-brown, let your practitioner know immediately. Greenish fluid means that the baby has had a bowel movement (meconium) inside the uterus. Most of the time, such an event doesn't indicate a problem, but sometimes it means that the baby is being stressed. Your practitioner makes sure that the baby is okay by monitoring the baby's heartbeat (probably by performing a Cardiotocograph test).

Pre-eclampsia

Pre-eclampsia is a condition unique to pregnancy. Pre-eclampsia combines high blood pressure, swelling of your legs, hands (and sometimes face), and protein in your urine. This condition isn't uncommon; it occurs in 1 in 15 of all pregnancies, and can range from being very mild to being a serious medical condition. If you develop signs or symptoms of pre-eclampsia, you'll need to be monitored more frequently and may need extra tests. Chapter 16 provides you with the signs and symptoms of pre-eclampsia.

Preterm labour

Preterm labour is defined as labour before 37 weeks, which includes both contractions and changes in your cervix. Of course, you won't know if your cervix is changing unless you have an internal examination – which is why any regular, persistent, and uncomfortable (or painful) contractions should always prompt you to contact the labour ward or your practitioner. Getting checked out early increases your chance of being diagnosed early, which in turn improves your chances of successful treatment. Medications aimed at arresting premature labour work best if the cervix is dilated less than 3 centimetres (1.2 inches). If labour occurs after 35 weeks, your practitioner probably won't try to stop your contractions except in rare circumstances (such as poorly controlled diabetes).

CALL THE DOCTOR

If you find that you're having regular, uncomfortable, persistent contractions (more than five or six in an hour) and you're not yet 35 to 36 weeks pregnant, call your practitioner. Also, if you think your membranes have ruptured (your water has broken) or if you're having any bleeding, call your practitioner immediately. See Chapter 16 for more detailed coverage of preterm labour.

When the baby is late

At your first antenatal check, you'll be given a *due date* (the anticipated birth date for your baby) and you may spend the rest of your pregnancy aiming towards that 'D Day'. But if you want to stay sane, don't rely on delivering on that exact day – only about 1 in 20 women do.

TECHNICAL STUFF

Your due date is given because that's the number of weeks into pregnancy on which more women deliver than any other. The further away from your due date, the less likely you are to deliver – about 4 out of 5 women deliver between 37 and 42 weeks. If you haven't delivered by 40 weeks, your practitioner will raise the question of induction – you can find out more in Chapter 10.

TIP

Sitting at home biting your nails and waiting to go into labour is bad enough – but friends phoning every five minutes to check whether 'it' has happened yet can test you patience to the very limits! You may want to think about leaving your answerphone on with a 'Don't call us, we'll call you' message – or getting your partner to remind all your friends and family (tactfully) of the level of stress that well-meant enquiries can bring.

Getting Ready to Head to the Hospital

You're so close to delivery now that it's a good idea to make sure you're ready to walk out of the door and head for the hospital. You probably won't want to stop to pack a suitcase at the last minute, nor will you have time to stop off at the shops for a baby car seat. Getting these must-do items off your pre-delivery checklist now will free you up to concentrate on the important things, like that 437th daily trip to the loo.

Packing your suitcase

Many women find it comforting to know that their bag is packed for the trip to the hospital or birthing centre. Having your bag ready allows you to concentrate on watching for signs of labour and helps keep you from worrying about being prepared. Excitingly, of course, you're going to be packing for two!

REMEMBER

Some women put off packing their labour bag until the last minute, assuming that once they go into labour, they'll have time to pack before the contractions become too frequent. Sarah was one of these, and discovered the hard way that things don't always go according to plan. She ruptured her membranes before she had a single contraction, then promptly went into fully-fledged labour. Not only did Sarah still need to pack her bag, she had to crawl into the loft to get her suitcase – not to be recommended.

TIP

What you pack for the hospital depends on the sort of labour you want. If you want to deliver to the sound of soothing womb music or breaking waves, for example, don't forget to pack tapes and a personal stereo! You might want to include items from the following list.

- For you:
    - Two loose nighties (front opening, for breast-feeding)
    - Slippers and socks
    - Hairbrush, toothbrush, and toiletries
    - Nursing bras and breast pads (ask for them at any pharmacy)
    - Old undies – the baggier the better – and sanitary towels
    - Clothes to go home in
    - Hot water bottle (great for relieving pain in labour, but the hospital won't provide one)

  - Water spray to cool your face
  - Camera (and film)
  - Snacks and a drink (for during and after labour)
  - Change for the hospital's phones and parking meters
  - Your address book
  - Birth announcement cards, stamps, and a pen
- For baby:
  - Nappies
  - 3 vests (with snap fastenings at the bottom)
  - 3 babygrows
  - 2 cardigans
  - Shawl or cot blanket
  - Socks, hat, and mittens (depending on the time of year)
  - A car seat (see the section 'Choosing – and using – a car seat')

Choosing – and using – a car seat

REMEMBER

Taking your baby home from hospital in a car means you'll need to get a car seat sorted out before you go into labour. The law in the UK states the following:

- All children under 3 years must be carried in an appropriate child restraint.
- All car seats and safety restraints must comply with the safety standard ECE R44/03 (all new car seats for sale in the UK comply with this standard).
- All car seats and safety restraints must be fitted according to manufacturers' instructions (practise beforehand – otherwise getting out of the hospital car park to take your baby home might take much longer than you anticipated).

Some areas of the UK have car seat loan schemes for use when you take your baby home from hospital. If you think this option may be useful, have a word with your midwife or health visitor.

We recommend that you always buy a new car seat (or borrow one from the hospital if you can, and if you're not going to need one in future) – your baby's safety is just too important to take chances. In any larger store (baby or department) the assistant will be able to advise you on a suitable car seat. You'll need to check that the seat you choose

- is suitable for infants from birth
- has a five-point safety harness with straps that adjust from the front
- offers plenty of head and neck support

Other considerations include:

- Can the seat be fitted on top of your pram or pushchair (yes, they do exist)?
- Is the cover easy to clean?
- Can the seat convert from a static car seat to a rocking chair when you're at home?

TIP

If you want to cover your baby, buckle the harness first, and then put a blanket over him – a blanket under the harness, or even a bulky clothing garment like a snowsuit, may make the harness too loose.

REMEMBER

If your car has airbags, never put your baby's car seat on the front seat, even if the seat is backward facing. Airbags pose a real threat of suffocation to your baby if they inflate when your baby is in their path.

Chapter 9

Understanding Antenatal Testing

In This Chapter

- Screening and invasive testing for foetal abnormalities
- Understanding ultrasound
- Looking at other antenatal tests and procedures

Some of the biggest advances in antenatal care in the last few decades have been in the area of screening your unborn baby's health. 'Passing' your home pregnancy test is just the beginning – during pregnancy you'll undergo several different tests to make sure that both you and your baby are healthy.

Two main sets of tests for foetal abnormalities (such as Down's syndrome and spina bifida, detailed later in this chapter) exist:

- **Non-invasive tests (known as *screening*).** These tests involve a blood test or an ultrasound scan. Non-invasive tests carry no risks, but only tell you whether you are at high or low risk of having an affected baby.
- **Invasive tests.** These tests, such as amniocentesis and chorionic villus sampling (you can find out what these are by reading on), are carried out on your womb, or the fluid or structures inside, and give you a definitive answer, but they both carry a small risk to your baby.

Every pregnant woman in the UK should be offered one of the screening tests discussed in this chapter. If you're not offered a screening test, it's important to ask why not. If you have any particular risk factors, or if your screening test suggests that you are at high risk of having a baby affected by a medical condition such as *Down's syndrome* (a chromosome abnormality), you will be offered an invasive test.

Non-Invasive (Screening) Tests

Non-invasive, or screening, tests are carried out routinely as part of your health care during pregnancy.

Screening tests carry no physical risk to you or your baby and the majority of women who have these tests prove to have a low risk of having an affected baby. You may be tempted to have a test just to reassure yourself, but remember, these tests don't tell you for certain if you have an affected baby – just how high your risk is. If your results show that you're at high risk (usually a risk of more than 1 in 250), you'll be offered an amniocentesis (see the section on 'Invasive Tests for Foetal Abnormalities' later in this chapter for more about this). Such tests carry a small risk to your baby, so if you're not sure you could go through with an invasive test, think carefully before having the tests discussed in this section.

Screening for alpha-foetoprotein

AFP stands for *alpha-foetoprotein,* a protein made by the foetus that also circulates in the mother's bloodstream. This screening test looks at the levels of AFP circulating in your bloodstream, which closely reflects the amount of AFP your baby is producing. Doctors use a simple blood test to check the level of AFP, usually between 15 and 18 weeks into your pregnancy. The test result is affected by weight, race, and pre-existing diabetes, so it is adjusted for these factors.

AFP can usually indicate whether a pregnancy is at risk for certain complications and may indicate:

- Underestimation of the foetus's age (how far along you are in your pregnancy)
- The presence of twins – or more
- Bleeding that may have occurred earlier in the pregnancy (for more on this see Chapter 6)
- Neural tube defects (spina bifida, anencephaly, and other defects causing abnormalities in the nervous system such as paralysis, extra fluid in the brain, or mental retardation)
- Abdominal wall defects (protrusion of the foetus's abdominal contents through a defect in the abdominal wall)
- Rhesus disease (see Chapter 16) or other conditions associated with *foetal oedema* (abnormal fluid collection in the foetus)

- Increased risk for low birth-weight, pre-eclampsia, or other complications (see Chapter 16)
- *Congenital nephrosis* (a rare foetal kidney condition)
- Foetal death or foetal abnormalities

Screening for Down's syndrome

Down's syndrome – the most common chromosomal abnormality in babies – can be tested for using the same sample of blood that's used for the AFP. This screening test also helps to identify women at risk of having babies with other chromosomal abnormalities, like *Trisomy 18* or *Trisomy 13* (an extra copy of either the number 18 or 13 chromosome).

Rolling out the red carpet for a Down's syndrome first-trimester test

Chorionic villus sampling (CVS) and early amniocentesis are the only tests that can give definitive information about foetal chromosomes during the first trimester. But researchers have been trying to develop non-invasive, risk-free screening tests that can help determine if a foetus is at increased risk for certain problems, primarily Down's syndrome. Using a combination of a special ultrasound measurement, called *nuchal translucency*, and certain blood tests, researchers believe that 80 to 90 per cent of affected foetuses may be detected through screening. These first-trimester screening tests are usually performed between the approximate gestational ages of 10 weeks and 4 days to 13 weeks and 6 days. Here's how the tests work:

- **Nuchal translucency:** This test uses ultrasound to measure a special area behind the foetus's neck. Only physicians specially trained in the procedure should conduct a nuchal translucency test. When measurements of nuchal translucency are combined with blood screening tests, the accuracy of these tests is probably increased.
- **Serum screening:** Tests that check the levels of PAPP-A, a substance produced by the placenta, and hCG, a hormone in the mother's blood, may help screen for Down's syndrome in the first trimester. When PAPP-A, hCG, and nuchal translucency are used together to check for foetal abnormalities, the procedure is known as the combined test. This test isn't available throughout the UK on the NHS (although you can ask your GP about getting one done privately), because most hospitals have a system in place already for screening for Down's syndrome and the two tests have a fairly similar accuracy rate. The main advantage of the first-trimester test is that if you do have a high-risk result, you can have an invasive test to get an absolute answer earlier.

You'll be offered a screening test to assess your risk of having a baby with Down's syndrome. You should be offered blood or ultrasound testing regardless of your age, although, as you get older, the chance of having a baby affected by Down's syndrome steadily increases.

Your practitioner performs the Down's syndrome screening test by measuring two, three, or four substances in the blood (called the double, triple, and quadruple tests, respectively):

- AFP
- hCG (human chorionic gonadotropin)
- uE3 (a form of oestrogen)
- Inhibin A (a substance secreted by the placenta)

If your results suggest that you're at high risk of having an affected baby, you'll be offered an amniocentesis (see 'Invasive Tests for Foetal Abnormalities' later in this chapter). If you're over 37 you can ask automatically for an amniocentesis.

Screening with ultrasound scans

An ultrasound scan is an incredibly useful, non-invasive tool that allows you and your doctor to see the baby inside your uterus. A device called a *transducer* emits sound waves. The sound waves are reflected off the foetus and converted into an image that appears on a monitor. (Some examples of ultrasound photos are provided in Chapter 22.) You can see almost all the structures in the foetus's body, and you can see the foetus moving around and performing all its normal activities – kicking, waving, and so on. The best time to view the baby's anatomy is around 18 to 22 weeks, but detecting a foetal heartbeat should be possible as early as 6 weeks.

An ultrasound examination doesn't hurt. A doctor or ultrasonographer spreads gel or lotion over your abdomen, and then moves the transducer around through the gel. A full bladder isn't necessary because the amniotic fluid surrounding the foetus provides the liquid needed to transmit the sound waves to create a clear or detailed picture. Picture quality varies, depending on maternal fat, scar tissue, and the foetus's position.

Ultrasound is like a check-up for the foetus and can provide information about the following:

- Number of babies present
- Gestational age

- Rate of foetal growth
- Foetal position, movement, and breathing exercises (the foetus moves its chest and abdomen as if it were breathing air)
- Foetal heart rate
- Amount of amniotic fluid
- Location of placenta
- Foetal anatomy, including the identification of some birth defects

A detailed ultrasound can examine these structures:

- Arms and legs
- Bladder
- Brain and skull
- Face
- Genitalia
- Heart, chest cavity, and diaphragm
- Kidneys
- Spine
- Stomach, abdominal cavity, and abdominal wall

Many women like the idea of having an early ultrasound scan to see their baby for the first time. If all is going smoothly, however, you're unlikely to be offered an ultrasound scan until you're at least 12–14 weeks pregnant. Most areas routinely offer two scans – one at about 12–14 weeks (the best time to check the accuracy of your due date) and one at 18–20 weeks (the best time to check the baby's anatomy). However, if any aspect of your pregnancy is not going according to plan, you may be offered other scans to check on the baby's progress.

Understanding screening accuracy

You can become incredibly confused trying to work out which is best of the apparently endless permutations for screening tests you're offered to screen for foetal abnormalities. The National Institute of Clinical Excellence (NICE) has, fortunately, done most of the hard work for you.

NICE has issued guidelines on which tests offer a detection rate above 60 per cent (in other words, if 100 women carrying foetuses with Down's syndrome had the test, the condition would be diagnosed in at least 60 of them) and a *false negative rate* (high-risk results which turn out to be normal) of under 5 per cent. Table 9-1 shows some of these tests.

Table 9-1 NICE Recommended Screening Tests

11–14 weeks	Nuchal translucency testing
	The combined test (nuchal translucency, hCG, PAPP-A)
14–20 weeks	The triple test (hCG, AFP and uE3)
	The quadruple test (hCG, AFP, uE3 and inhibin A)
	The integrated test (nuchal translucency, PAPP-A + hCG, AFB, uE3, inhibin A)
	The serum integrated test (PAPP-A+hCG, AFB, uE3, inhibin A)

Source: www.NICE.org.uk

NICE also highlights a number of even more accurate tests, with a detection rate of over 75 per cent and a false positive rate of under 3 per cent. After April 2007, only these most accurate screenings will be in use. Table 9-2 outlines some of the screenings.

Table 9-2 NICE Recommended Screening Tests from April 2007

11–14 weeks	The combined test (nuchal translucency, hCG, PAPP-A)
14–20 weeks	The quadruple test (hCG, AFP, uE3, and inhibin A)
	The integrated test (nuchal translucency, PAPP-A + hCG, AFB, uE3, inhibin A)
	The serum integrated test (PAPP-A+hCG, AFB, uE3, inhibin A)

Source: www.NICE.org.uk

Invasive Tests for Foetal Abnormalities

Two main forms of invasive test for foetal abnormality are in use in the UK:

- Amniocentesis
- Chorionic villus sampling (CVS)

Both these invasive tests require considerable skill, so are carried out by an obstetrician or maternal-foetal medicine specialist (see Chapter 2) under ultrasound control. Invasive tests give you a definitive answer as to whether your baby is affected by the foetal abnormality being tested for.

All invasive tests carry a small risk of complications – the most dangerous being miscarriage. CVS and amniocentesis are equally accurate, and carry similar levels of risk of miscarriage. CVS has the advantage that it can be carried out earlier than amniocentesis (at between 9 and 11 weeks into your pregnancy). However, this timing means that you can't have screening tests (as explained in the section 'Non-Invasive (Screening) Tests', earlier in this chapter) beforehand to check if you're at high risk of having a baby with a foetal abnormality, because the screening tests don't give an accurate result before about 11 weeks into your pregnancy. Many women, therefore, prefer to have a screening test, and then invasive testing in the form of an amniocentesis only if they turn out to be at high risk.

Invasive tests involve testing the developing baby's chromosomes. Chromosomes carry the genetic information that determines what a person is like. Certain abnormalities in chromosome number or structure can lead to problems in the baby. For example, *Down's syndrome*, one of the more common chromosomal abnormalities associated with severe mental retardation, may occur if the foetus has an extra copy of chromosome 21 (people normally have 46 chromosomes).

Amniocentesis, chorionic villus sampling (CVS), and other tests detect such abnormalities in chromosome number and structure by yielding an enlarged picture of the individual chromosomes called a *karyotype*. Additionally, a couple with a known family or ethnic group risk for carrying a child with a genetic disease (cystic fibrosis, for example) have the same material tested for such diseases.

Amniocentesis

Used to check for genetic abnormalities, amniocentesis will usually be carried out between 15 and 20 weeks. If you need an invasive test earlier than this, you usually get invited to have a chorionic villus sampling, or CVS, instead (see the section 'Chorionic Villus Sampling' later in this chapter for more details). You can read more about when amniocentesis is used in the 'Reasons for having an amniocentesis' section.

A genetic *amniocentesis* primarily tests to make sure that 23 chromosome pairs are present and that their structure is normal. The amniocentesis doesn't routinely test for all possible genetic diseases or birth defects. The amniotic fluid cells must be incubated before your doctor can read the results of a genetic amniocentesis, so results usually arrive in one to two weeks.

During the amniocentesis procedure, you lie flat on your back and an ultrasound image is taken to locate the foetus and the amniotic sac. Your doctor, or an ultrasound technician, then inserts a thin needle through your abdomen and uterus into the amniotic sac (see Figure 9-1). After the examiner has withdrawn enough amniotic fluid to test (usually about 15 to 20 cc, or 1 to 2 tablespoons), the needle is removed. The amniotic fluid can then be tested in a variety of ways.

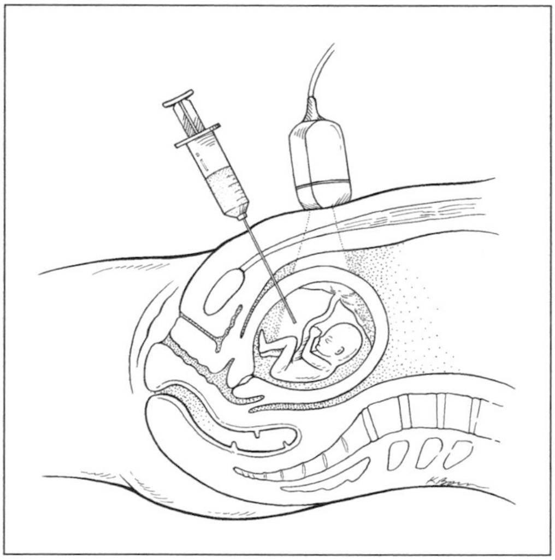

Figure 9-1: An amniocentesis procedure.

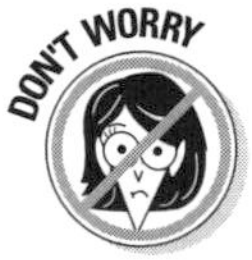

Amniocentesis typically lasts no longer than one to two minutes, but this may seem like an eternity to an anxious woman. The procedure is mildly uncomfortable but not terribly painful. Many women feel a slight, brief cramping sensation as the needle goes into the uterus and then a weird pulling sensation as the fluid is withdrawn through the needle. Having an amniocentesis performed isn't altogether pain-free, but most women report that it isn't as bad as they expected. Afterwards, your doctor may advise that you rest and avoid strenuous activity and sex for a couple of days.

Reasons for having an amniocentesis

Your practitioner may recommend a genetic amniocentesis for the following conditions or situations:

- Your age is 37 or more at your due date.
- You had an elevated AFP (see the section 'Screening for alpha-foetoprotein' earlier in this chapter).
- You had abnormal results from the Down's syndrome screening (see Screening for Down's syndrome' earlier in this chapter).
- Your ultrasound scan was abnormal, indicating, for example, poor foetal growth or suspected structural abnormalities.
- You had a previous child or previous pregnancy with a chromosomal abnormality.
- You're at risk of having a baby with a certain genetic disease.

Your practitioner may perform amniocentesis for other reasons, including:

- **Preterm labour:** An infection within the amniotic fluid may be a cause of preterm labour. To check for such infection your practitioner sends the fluid to a lab for tests. If an infection is present, your doctor may want to deliver your baby immediately to minimise harm to you and the baby.
- **Rhesus sensitisation:** Patients with Rhesus sensitisation are sometimes monitored with a test known as *delta OD-450*, in which the amniotic fluid is examined for evidence of broken-down foetal red blood cells. See Chapter 17 for more on Rhesus sensitisation.
- **Lung maturity studies:** Certain tests on the amniotic fluid can determine if the foetus's lungs are mature enough for the baby to be delivered.

Risks and side effects of amniocentesis

Amniocentesis carries a risk of miscarriage. If a non-invasive screening shows a high-risk result (see the section on 'Non-Invasive (Screening) Tests' earlier in this chapter), you'll have to decide whether to proceed with an amniocentesis – even though your chances of having an unaffected baby may be over 99 per cent. The following symptoms or problems can occur after an amniocentesis, but remember, not all patients have these:

- **Cramping:** Some women experience cramping for several hours after the procedure. The best treatment for this cramping is rest.
- **Spotting**: *Spotting*, which is light vaginal bleeding, may last one to two days.

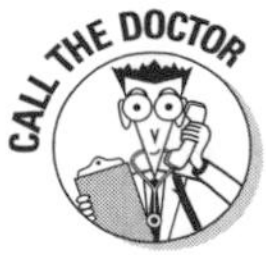

- **Amniotic fluid leak:** A leakage of 1 to 2 teaspoons of fluid through the vagina occurs in 1 to 2 per cent of patients. In the great majority of these cases, the membrane seals over within 48 hours. Leakage stops and the pregnancy continues normally. However, if you experience a large amount of leakage, or persistent leakage, call your doctor.

- **Foetal injury:** Injury to the foetus is extremely rare because of ultrasound guidance.
- **Miscarriage:** Although amniocentesis is considered very safe, it's still invasive, and is associated with an increased risk of miscarriage of about ½ per cent.

An amniocentesis performed later in the pregnancy – later than 20 weeks – doesn't carry the same risk of miscarriage that an early amniocentesis does. Later amniocentesis carries only a very small risk of infection, rupture of membranes (breaking the water), or onset of labour.

Chorionic villus sampling

Chorionic villi are tiny, budlike pieces of tissue that make up the placenta. Because chorionic villi develop from cells arising out of the fertilised egg, they have the same chromosomes and genetic make-up as the developing foetus. By checking a sample of chorionic villi, your doctor can see whether or not the chromosomes are normal in number and structure, determine the foetal sex, and test for some specific diseases (if the foetus is at risk for these diseases).

Your doctor performs a chorionic villus sampling (CVS) by withdrawing placental tissue (containing chorionic villi) either through a hollow needle inserted through the abdomen (*transabdominal CVS*) or through a flexible catheter inserted through the cervix (*transcervical CVS*, see Figure 9-2), depending on where the placenta is located within the uterus and the uterus's general shape and position. Your doctor uses ultrasound equipment as a guide as she performs the procedure. She then examines the tissue under a microscope, and the cells are cultured in a laboratory.

Like amniocentesis, CVS raises the risk of miscarriage slightly – about ½ to 1 per cent. Neither CVS method is more risky than the other. The person performing the test should have plenty of experience doing the procedure; experience helps reduce the risk of miscarriage.

CVS results are typically available in seven to ten days. The main advantage that CVS has over amniocentesis is that it can provide information earlier in the pregnancy. This time factor may be important to some women who feel that termination is an option if severe abnormalities are present.

Unlike amniocentesis, CVS can't measure AFP (refer to the section 'Non-Invasive (Screening) Tests' for more information about AFP). However, your practitioner can take this measurement from maternal blood drawn at 15 to 18 weeks into the pregnancy.

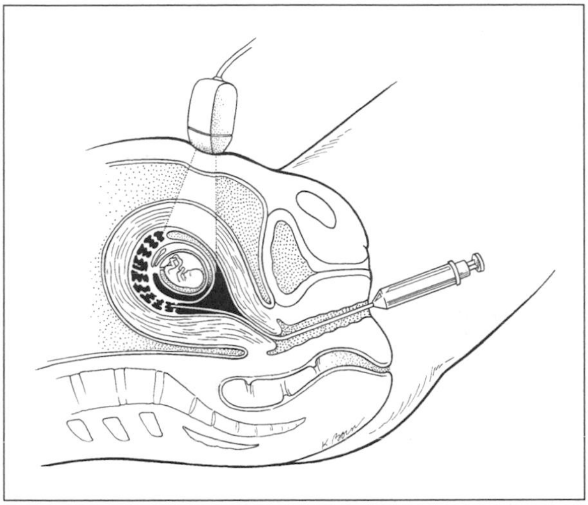

Figure 9-2: In trans-cervical CVS, your doctor uses a flexible catheter inserted into the cervix to withdraw a tiny amount of placental tissue, using ultrasound as a guide.

REMEMBER

If you undergo CVS or amniocentesis and are Rhesus negative, you should receive an injection of Anti-D following the procedure to prevent you from developing Rhesus disease (see Chapter 16).

Other Antenatal Tests and Procedures

Most of the tests in this section are rarely done – the tests are necessary only if you have a specific problem, and are usually done in medical centres that specialise in foetal medicine. These tests may sound scary, but we include them just to let you know what might be available if you develop a problem.

Foetal echocardiogram

A *foetal echocardiogram* is an ultrasound focused on the foetal heart. A maternal-foetal medicine specialist, a paediatric cardiologist, or a radiologist usually performs this procedure. You may need a *foetal echocardiogram* if you have a history of diabetes or a family history of congenital heart disease, or if an ultrasound shows any signs of a heart abnormality. Your practitioner may recommend a foetal echocardiogram if she sees *any* structural problem on ultrasound, because heart abnormalities are often associated with other birth defects.

Doppler studies

Ultrasound can be used to perform Doppler studies of foetal and umbilical blood flow. These studies are a way of assessing blood flow to various organ systems and also within the placenta. A Doppler study is sometimes used as a test of wellbeing in foetuses with IUGR (intrauterine growth restriction). See Chapter 16 for more on IUGR.

Cardiotocography

If you have any concerns during your third trimester, your practitioner is likely to send you to the labour ward for monitoring with a Cardiotocograph (CTG).

CTG testing measures the foetal heart rate, foetal movement, and uterine activity by a special monitoring machine. Your practitioner hooks you up to the device, which picks up uterine contractions and the baby's heart rate and generates a tracing of both. The CTG is similar to the device used during labour to monitor the foetal heart rate and contractions. You also receive a button to press each time you feel a foetal movement. The monitoring goes on for about 20 to 40 minutes. The doctor then looks at the tracing for signs of *accelerations*, or increases, in the foetal heart rate. If accelerations are present, and occur often enough, the test is considered *reactive*, and the foetus is thought to be healthy and should continue to be so for three to seven days. (The foetus is healthy in more than 99 per cent of cases.) If the accelerations aren't adequate (that is, the test is *non-reactive*), you still have no cause for alarm. In 80 per cent of cases, the foetus is fine, but further evaluation is needed.

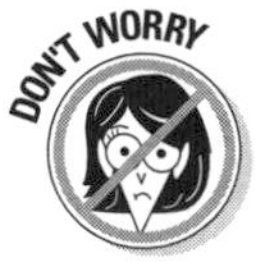

If your practitioner recommends that you have a CTG, it's almost always just a precaution. CTGs are perfectly safe, non-invasive tests of your baby's wellbeing, and provide extremely useful reassurance that all's progressing smoothly.

Doppler velocimetry

A doctor performs a Doppler velocimetry test only in certain situations such as the occurrence of certain foetal problems (like intrauterine growth restriction – see Chapter 16), or if you have high blood pressure. In this test, your doctor performs a special type of ultrasound examination and then assesses the blood flow through the umbilical cord.

Foetal blood sampling

This test lets your doctor obtain blood for rapid chromosomal diagnosis when time is critical. Your doctor may perform this test in order to diagnose foetal infections, to detect evidence of foetal anaemia, or to diagnose and treat a condition called *non-immune hydrops* (where fluid accumulates abnormally in the foetus).

For foetal blood sampling – also known as *PUBS* (*percutaneous umbilical blood sampling*) or *cordocentesis* – a maternal-foetal medicine specialist withdraws foetal blood from the umbilical cord, under ultrasound guidance. The procedure is similar to an amniocentesis except that the doctor directs the needle into the umbilical cord rather than into the amniotic fluid. The risk of foetal loss is about 1 per cent, but other risks include infection, or rupture of the membranes.

Some foetuses develop anaemia, which can be treated *in utero* (within the womb) with a blood transfusion directly into the umbilical cord. Conditions that may lead to anaemia include certain infections (such as parvovirus), genetic diseases, or certain blood group incompatibilities (see Chapter 16).

Part III

The Big Event: Labour, Delivery, and Recovery

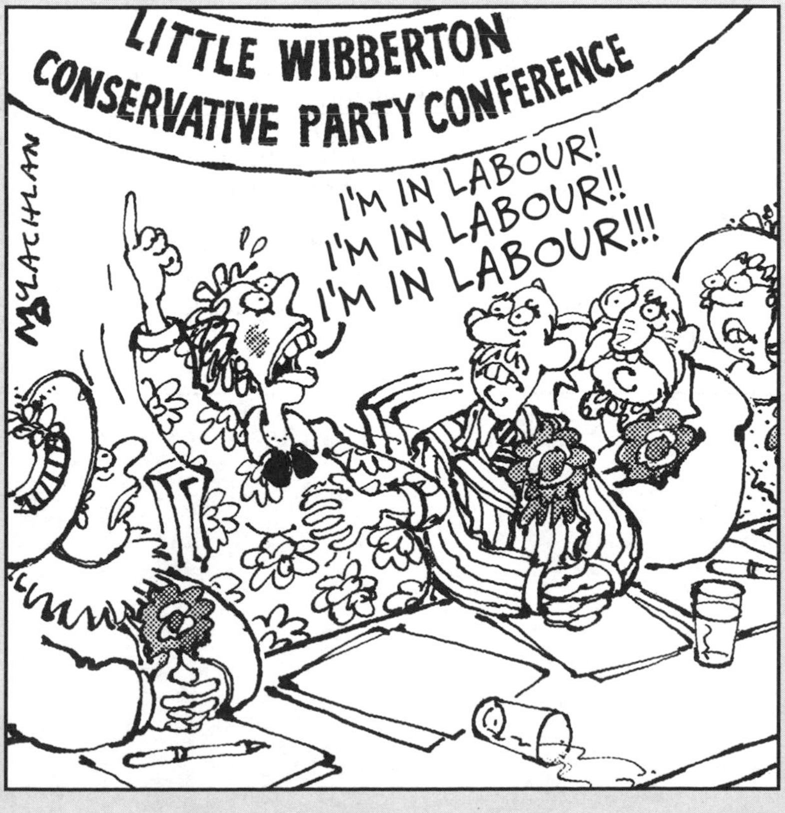
LITTLE WIBBERTON
CONSERVATIVE PARTY CONFERENCE
I'M IN LABOUR!
I'M IN LABOUR!!
I'M IN LABOUR!!!
McLACHLAN

In this part . . .

And now the moment you've all been waiting for. . . . Like pregnancy itself, childbirth can go more smoothly if you know what's going to happen. Practitioners in the UK are very focussed on involving you in the decision-making for your labour, including choices about pain relief options. This part aims to give you the information you need to take a fully informed role in your labour. We also describe what you can expect once your baby is born, and some of the details that may help you in caring for your newborn, as well as the changes you can expect your own body to go through after delivery. We've made this part fairly comprehensive, so you can be prepared for every eventuality – even though for most women, labour and delivery go smoothly.

Chapter 10

I Think I'm in Labour!

In This Chapter

- Working out if you're in labour
- Being admitted to the hospital or birthing centre
- Keeping an eye on the baby's vital signs during labour
- Inducing labour in special circumstances
- Looking at the three stages of labour
- Managing the pain of childbirth
- Considering home and water births

Despite the incredible advances that have been made in science and medicine, no one really knows what causes labour to begin. Labour may be triggered by a combination of stimuli generated by the mother, the baby, and the placenta. Or labour may begin because of rising levels of steroid-like substances in the mother or other biochemical substances produced by the baby. Because we don't know exactly how labour starts, we also can't pinpoint exactly when it will occur.

Being unsure whether or not you're really in labour is fairly common. Even a woman expecting her third or fourth child doesn't always know when she's genuinely in labour. This chapter helps you better identify your own labour (but you still may find yourself calling your practitioner several times or even making many trips to the hospital or birthing centre, only to find out that what you think is labour really isn't).

Knowing When Labour Is Real – and When It Isn't

You may experience some of the early symptoms of labour before labour actually begins. Rather than indicating that you're in labour, these symptoms suggest that labour may occur in the next few days or weeks. Some women experience these labour-like symptoms for days or weeks, and others experience them only for several hours. Going into labour isn't usually as dramatic as it's portrayed in sitcoms or soaps. Women very rarely lack the time they need to get to the hospital before they deliver.

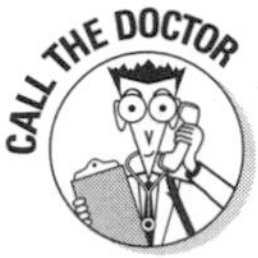

If you think you're in active labour, don't run to the hospital immediately. Instead, telephone the labour ward, or your practitioner, first.

Noticing changes before labour begins

As you near the end of your pregnancy, you may recognise certain changes as your body prepares for the big event. You may notice all these symptoms, or you may not notice any of them. Sometimes the changes begin weeks before labour begins, and sometimes they begin only days before.

- **Bloody show:** No, the bloody show isn't the latest Hollywood slasher movie. As changes in your cervix take place, you may expel from your vagina some mucous discharge mixed with blood. The blood comes from small, broken capillaries in your cervix.
- **Diarrhoea:** Usually a few days before labour, your body releases *prostaglandins*, which are substances that help the uterus contract and may cause diarrhoea.
- **Dropping and engagement:** Especially in women who are giving birth for the first time, the foetus often drops into the pelvis several weeks before labour (see Chapter 8). You may feel increased pressure on your vagina and sharp pains radiating to your vagina. You also may notice that your whole uterus is lower in your belly and that you're suddenly more comfortable and can breathe more easily. You may also feel the need to go to the loo more often, as your baby's head pushes against your bladder.
- **Increase in Braxton-Hicks contractions:** You may notice an increase in the frequency and strength of *Braxton-Hicks contractions* (see Chapter 8). These contractions may become somewhat uncomfortable, even if they don't grow any stronger or more frequent. Some women experience strong Braxton-Hicks contractions for weeks before labour begins.
- **Mucous discharge:** You may secrete a thick mucous discharge known as the *mucous plug*. During your pregnancy this substance plugs your cervix, protecting your uterus from infection. As your cervix starts to thin out (*efface*) and dilate in preparation for delivery, the plug may wash out.

Expectant mothers ask . . .

Q: 'I've never had a contraction, so how do I know what one feels like?'

A: A *contraction* occurs when your uterus's muscle tightens and pushes the baby toward the cervix. Usually, contractions are uncomfortable and, therefore, unmistakable. But many women worry that they won't know that they're having contractions. You can tell whether you're experiencing contractions by using a quick and easy trick. With your fingertips, touch your cheek and then your forehead. Finally, touch the top part of your abdomen, through which you can feel the top part of your uterus (the *fundus*). A relaxed uterus feels soft, like your cheek, and a contracting uterus feels hard, like your forehead. You can also try this exercise if you think you may be in pre-term labour (see Chapter 16 for more information).

Telling false labour from true labour

Distinguishing true labour from false labour isn't always easy. But a few general characteristics can help you determine whether the symptoms you're experiencing mean you're in labour.

In general, you're in false labour if your contractions

- Are irregular and don't increase in frequency
- Disappear when you change position, walk, or rest
- Are not particularly uncomfortable
- Occur only in your lower abdomen
- Don't become increasingly uncomfortable

You're more likely to be in actual labour if your contractions

- Grow steadily more frequent, intense, and uncomfortable
- Last about 40 to 60 seconds
- Don't go away when you change position, walk, or rest
- Occur along with leakage of fluid (due to rupture of the membranes)
- Make normal talking difficult or impossible
- Stretch across your upper abdomen or are mainly in your back, radiating to your front

Sometimes the only way you can know for sure whether you're in labour is by seeing your practitioner or going to the hospital. When you arrive at the hospital, a doctor, or midwife, performs a pelvic examination to determine whether you're in labour. The practitioner may also hook you up to a monitor to see how often you're contracting and to check how the foetal heart responds. Sometimes you find out straight away whether you're truly in labour. But the practitioner may need to keep you under observation for several hours to see whether the situation is changing.

Deciding when to call the labour ward or your practitioner

If you think you're in labour, call the labour ward or, if you have a named midwife or doctor, call them. Don't be embarrassed if he tells you that you're probably *not* in labour (it happens to many women). If your contractions are occurring every 5 to 10 minutes and they're uncomfortable, definitely call. If you're less than 37 weeks and feeling persistent contractions, don't sit for hours counting their frequency – call the labour ward or your practitioner immediately.

Call the labour ward or your practitioner if any of the following apply to you:

- Your contractions are coming closer together, and they're becoming increasingly uncomfortable.
- You have ruptured membranes. Having your water break may appear as a small amount of watery fluid leaking out, or it may be a big gush. If the fluid is green, brown, or red, let the labour ward or your practitioner know straight away.
- *Meconium* (your baby's first bowel movement) usually happens after the baby is born, but 2–20 per cent of babies pass meconium during labour, most commonly if they're born past their due date. Passing meconium doesn't necessarily indicate that anything is wrong, but it can occasionally be associated with foetal stress.
- You have bright red heavy bleeding (more than a heavy menstrual period) or are passing clots, in which case you should go to the hospital immediately (after calling the labour ward or your practitioner).
- You're not feeling an adequate amount of foetal movement (see Chapter 8 for more information).
- You have constant, severe abdominal pain with no relief between contractions.
- You feel a foetal part or umbilical cord in your vagina. Go to the hospital immediately.

Checking for labour with an internal examination

When a practitioner is trying to determine whether you're in labour, he performs an internal examination to look for several things:

- **Dilation:** Your cervix is closed for most of your pregnancy but may gradually start to dilate during the last couple of weeks, especially if you've had a baby before. After active labour begins, the rate of cervical dilation speeds up, and the cervix dilates to 10 centimetres (about 4 inches) by the end of the first stage of labour. Often, you're considered to be in active labour when your cervix is about 4 centimetres (1½ inches) dilated or 100 per cent effaced.
- **Effacement:** Effacement is a thinning out or shortening of the cervix, which happens during labour. Your cervix goes from being thick (uneffaced) to 100 per cent effaced. See Figure 10-1.
- **Position:** When labour begins, the baby typically starts out facing to the left or right side. As labour progresses, he rotates until the head assumes a face-down position so that the baby comes out looking at the floor. Occasionally, the baby rotates to the opposite position and comes out face-up, looking at the ceiling – commonly termed OP (occipito-posterior), but don't be surprised to hear this described as the 'face-to-pubes' position.

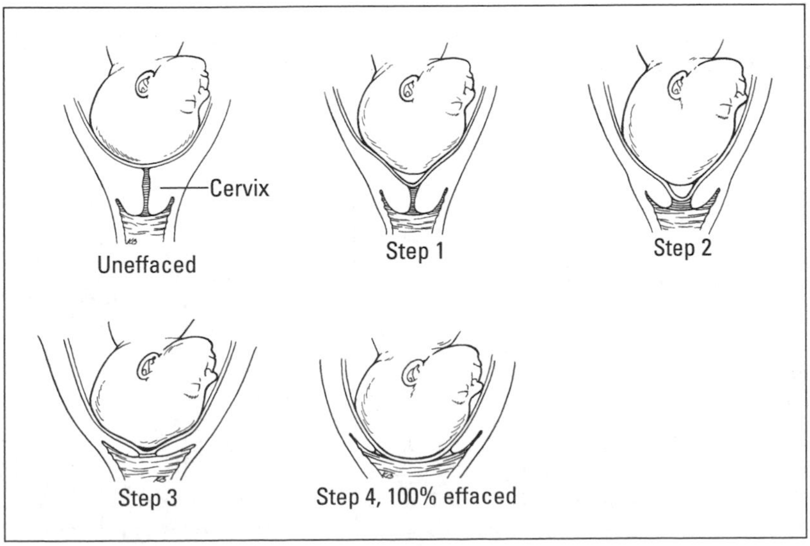

Figure 10-1: During cervical effacement, the cervix progresses from an uneffaced state to 100 per cent effaced and partially dilated.

Getting Admitted to the Hospital

Whether you're in labour, being induced, or having an elective caesarean delivery, you need to be admitted to your hospital's delivery wing. When you phone the hospital, the labour ward may ask you to come straight up to be monitored, or tell you to go to one of the hospital wards first for an assessment.

Although each hospital or birthing centre has its own system, getting settled in usually follows this routine when you arrive at the ward:

- A midwife asks you to change into a gown.
- A midwife asks you questions about your pregnancy, your general health, your obstetric history, and when you last ate. If you think your waters have broken or you're leaking fluid, let the midwife know.
- A midwife or doctor performs an internal examination to see how far your labour has progressed.
- Your contractions and the foetal heart rate are monitored using a foetal monitor. The foetal monitor has two attachments, one to monitor the baby's heart rate and one to monitor your contractions. The foetal monitor generates a *foetal heart tracing*, which is a paper record of how the baby's heart rate rises and falls in relation to your contractions (see Figure 10-2).
- A midwife or doctor may take a blood sample and put an IV (*intravenous*) line in your arm (for delivering fluids and, possibly, medications).

TIP

You may want to hand over any valuables you have with you to your partner or other family member (or simply leave them at home).

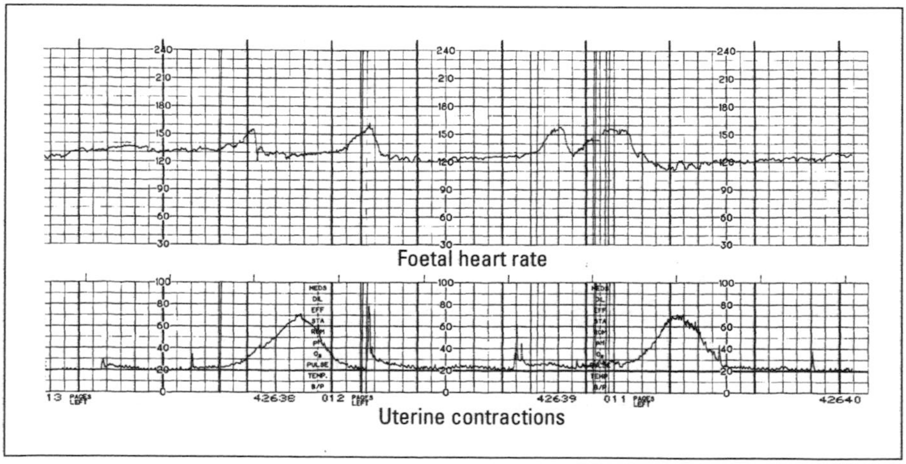

Figure 10-2: The foetal heart rate and uterine contractions.

Monitoring Your Baby

While you're in labour, your practitioner may keep an eye on your baby in a number of different ways to make sure that he is tolerating the whole process well. Most hospitals, and most practitioners, have their own ways of deciding when to place foetal monitors and which ones to place. Although some low-risk patients may require only intermittent monitoring, other patients are better off with continuous monitoring. Sometimes knowing whether continuous monitoring makes sense isn't possible until you're in labour and your practitioner can see how the baby is responding.

Foetal heart monitoring

Labour puts stress on both you and the baby. Foetal heart monitoring provides a way to make sure that the baby is handling the stress. In some hospitals, all patients in labour are routinely monitored; in others, patients who are at low risk for complications may be monitored only intermittently. Monitoring can be done through several techniques.

External monitoring

External foetal monitoring is usually called CTG (refer to Chapter 9 for more about CTG). Electronic foetal heart monitoring uses either two belts or a wide elastic band placed around the abdomen. A device attached to the belt, or under the band, uses an ultrasound-Doppler technique to pick up the foetal heartbeat. A second device uses a gauge to pick up the contractions. An external contraction monitor can show the frequency and duration of contractions, but it can't provide very accurate information about how strong they are. An external foetal heart monitor gives information about the foetus's response to contractions and records *long-term variability* – that is, periodic changes in heart rate (which are a good sign).

You may hear your practitioner use the following terms to describe the foetal heartbeat:

- **Normal:** About 120 to 160 beats per minute.
- **Bradycardia:** A decrease in the foetal heart rate, to below 120 beats per minute, which lasts for more than two minutes.
- **Tachycardia:** An increase in the foetal heart rate to above 160 beats per minute for more than two minutes.
- **Accelerations:** Brief increases above baseline in the foetal heart rate, often after a foetal movement. Accelerations are a reassuring sign.

- **Decelerations:** These are intermittent decreases below the baseline foetal heart rate. The significance of decelerations depends on their frequency, how far the heart rate drops, and when they occur in relation to contractions. Decelerations are classified as early, variable, or late, according to when they occur in relation to contractions.

Internal monitoring

Most women are only monitored externally, but internal monitoring is performed if the baby's progress needs to be very closely observed. To place an internal foetal monitor (also called an internal scalp electrode), the membranes (waters) must be ruptured and the cervix dilated to at least 1 or 2 centimetres (⅓ to ¾ inch). During an internal examination, the monitor is passed through the cervix via a flexible plastic tube. This procedure is no more uncomfortable than a pelvic examination. The tiny electrode is then attached to the baby's scalp. The process is quite safe and is only rarely associated with a local infection or a slight rash on the baby's head.

Other tests of foetal health

If the information from the foetal monitor raises concerns or is ambiguous, your practitioner can perform other tests to help determine how to proceed with your labour.

If your practitioner is concerned about how well the baby is tolerating labour, he may want to perform a *scalp pH test*. The pH is a measure of the degree of acidity in the baby's blood. Stressed babies have more acidic blood. This test is possible only if the membranes are ruptured and the cervix is dilated at least 1 to 2 centimetres (⅓ to ¾ inch) – and if the hospital where you're labouring has a pH testing machine.

When conducting a scalp pH test, a plastic cone is inserted into the vagina so that a tiny portion of the foetal scalp becomes visible. The scalp is gently wiped with a swab and then pricked with a small blade (similar to the way you may have a finger-prick blood test taken in a doctor's surgery), and a tiny sample of foetal blood is collected into a glass tube. The blood sample is put into a pH machine to find out how well the baby is tolerating labour.

Nudging Things Along: Labour Induction

To *induce* labour means to cause labour to begin before it starts on its own. An induction is *medically indicated* (becomes a medical necessity) when the risks of continuing the pregnancy are greater – for the mother or the baby – than the risks of early delivery.

Problems with the mother's health that may warrant induction include

- Pre-eclampsia (see Chapter 16 for more information)
- The presence of certain diseases, such as diabetes or cholestasis (see Chapter 16), which may improve after delivery
- An infection in the amniotic fluid, such as chorioamnionitis
- Foetal death

Potential risks to the baby's health that may warrant induction include

- The continuation of the pregnancy well past the due date – the rate of foetal death increases significantly after a mother passes her 41st to 42nd week
- Ruptured membranes before the start of labour, a situation that may place the baby at risk of developing an infection
- Intrauterine growth retardation (see Chapter 16)
- Suspected *macrosomia* – a foetus weighing 4 kilograms (9 pounds) or more
- Rhesus incompatibility, with complications (see Chapter 16)
- Decreased amniotic fluid (*oligohydramnios*)
- Meconium aspiration – the baby breathes in meconium (an early foetal bowel movement)
- Tests of foetal wellbeing indicating that the foetus may not be thriving in the uterus

In the UK, induction for non-medical reasons – for convenience, or because you're under the care of a particular consultant who's only available at certain times – is very much the exception.

If you haven't gone into labour by 41 weeks, you should be offered a *membrane sweep*, which means that your practitioner carries out a vaginal examination to encourage your cervix to produce hormones that may trigger labour. If you choose not to have a membrane sweep, or the one you have does not start labour, you should be offered an admission date to induce labour.

REMEMBER

You have a right to refuse induction of labour when you are past your due date, but doing so does increase the risks to your baby – we certainly wouldn't recommend this course of action.

Inducing labour

The way in which labour is induced depends on the condition of the cervix. If your cervix isn't favourable, or *ripe* (thinned out, soft, and dilated), your practitioner may use various medications and techniques to ripen it. Occasionally, this technique alone may put you straight into labour.

The most common agent used for cervical ripening is a type of *prostaglandin* (a substance that helps soften cervical tissue and cause contractions), administered either as a gel or a tablet. A midwife or doctor places the prostaglandin into the vagina, which may cause mild contractions. Another less common option used to ripen the cervix is a medication called misopristol, which is administered in the same way. If your cervix isn't yet ripe, you can't place it on the windowsill for a couple of days like granny did with tomatoes or bananas. If you need induction, you're likely to be admitted to hospital in the evening and given prostaglandin to ripen the cervix at bedtime. Then your practitioner can administer *oxytocin* (a synthetic hormone similar to one that your body naturally releases during labour) to induce labour in the morning.

If your cervix is already ripe, you're likely to be admitted in the morning, and labour is induced either by administering oxytocin intravenously or by rupturing your membranes (often called *breaking your water*). The doctor performs an *amniotomy*, or rupturing of the membranes, with a small plastic hook during an internal examination. This procedure usually isn't painful. After the amniotomy, doses of oxytocin are administered by an intravenous infusion, to induce labour. You begin with very little medication, and the level of medication increases at regular intervals until you have adequate contractions. Sometimes labour starts within a few hours after the induction is started but may take much longer. Occasionally, induction may take as long as two days to really get things going.

A common misconception is that oxytocin makes labour more painful – it doesn't. Oxytocin is similar to the hormone that your body naturally releases during labour, and it is administered in about the same doses that your body would produce to cause normal labour.

Augmenting labour

Doctors can also use oxytocin to augment labour that is already happening. If your contractions are inadequate, or if labour is taking an unusually long time, your practitioner may use oxytocin to help move things along. Again, the contractions produced as a result of this augmentation are no stronger and no more painful than contractions that occur during a spontaneous labour.

Getting the Big Picture: Stages and Characteristics of Labour

Each woman's labour is, in some ways, unique. One individual woman's experience may even vary from pregnancy to pregnancy. Anyone who delivers babies knows all too well that labour can always surprise you. As doctors, we may expect a woman to deliver quickly and find that her labour takes a long time, and those women who we think will take forever sometimes deliver very rapidly. Still, in the vast majority of pregnant women, labour progresses in a predictable pattern.

Your practitioner can track your progress through labour by performing internal examinations every few hours. How easily you progress through labour is measured by how quickly your cervix dilates and how smoothly the foetus moves down through the pelvis and birth canal.

Doctors become concerned over the progress of labour if it's too slow or if the cervix stops dilating and the foetus doesn't descend. They have a shorthand system for describing the variables that determine how easily a woman makes her way through labour: the three Ps (passenger, pelvis, and power). The baby's size and position (the passenger), the pelvis's size, and the contractions' strength (the power) are all important factors. Your practitioner must pay attention to all these factors, because if labour doesn't progress normally, it may be a sign that the baby would be better off delivered with assistance – with forceps or vacuum, or by caesarean delivery.

If you're going through your first delivery, the entire labour process is likely to last between 12 and 14 hours. For deliveries after the first one, labour is usually shorter (about 8 hours). Labour is divided into three stages, described in the following sections.

The first stage

The first stage of labour occurs from the onset of true labour to full dilation of the cervix. This stage is by far the longest (taking an average of 11 hours for a first child and 7 hours for subsequent births), and is divided into three phases: the early (latent) phase, the active phase, and the transition phase. Each phase has its own unique characteristics.

Early or latent phase

During the early phase of the first stage of labour, contractions occur every 5 to 20 minutes in the beginning, and then increase in frequency until they're less than 5 minutes apart. The contractions last between 30 and 45 seconds at first, but as the first phase continues, they work up to 60 to 90 seconds in length. During the early phase, your cervix gradually dilates to 3 to 4 centimetres (1 to 1½ inches) and becomes 100 per cent effaced.

The entire early phase of the first stage of labour lasts an average of 6 to 7 hours in a first birth and 4 to 5 hours for subsequent births. But the length of labour is unpredictable, because knowing when labour actually begins is difficult to pinpoint.

In the beginning of the early phase, your contractions may feel like period pains, with or without back pain. Your membranes may rupture, and you may have a bloody show (see the section 'Noticing changes before labour begins' earlier in this chapter). Early on in this phase, you may be most comfortable at home. If you're hungry, eat a light meal (soup, juice, or toast, for example), but not a very heavy one – in case you later need anaesthetic to deal with labour complications. You may want to time your contractions, but you don't need to be obsessive about it.

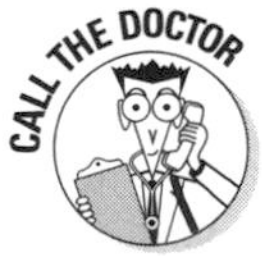

If you start to become more uncomfortable, the contractions occur with more frequency or intensity, or your membranes rupture (your water breaks), call the labour ward or your practitioner.

Many women find that walking around makes them more comfortable and distracts them from the pain during the early part of labour, others prefer to rest in bed – do whatever works for you.

Active phase

Labour's active phase is usually shorter and more predictable than the early phase. For a first child, it usually lasts 5 hours, on average. For subsequent babies, it lasts about 4 hours. Contractions occur in this phase every 3 to 5 minutes, and they last about 45 to 60 seconds. Your cervix dilates from 4 to 8 or 9 centimetres (1½ to 3½ inches).

You may feel increasing discomfort or pain during this phase, and you may have a backache as well. Some women experience more pain in the back than in the front, a condition known as back labour. This may be a sign that the baby is facing toward your front rather than toward your spine.

By this time, you're probably already in the hospital or birthing centre. Some patients prefer to rest in bed; others would rather walk around. Do whatever makes you comfortable, unless your practitioner asks that you stay in bed to be monitored closely. Now is the time to use the breathing and relaxation techniques you may have practised in childbirth classes.

If you need pain relief, let your practitioner know (for more information on pain relief, see the section 'Handling labour pain' later in this chapter). Your partner may help ease your pain by massaging your back.

Transition phase

Many practitioners consider the transition period as part of the active phase, but we prefer to label it separately. During the transition phase, contractions occur every 2 to 3 minutes and last about 60 seconds. The contractions during this phase are very intense. Your cervix dilates from 8 or 9 to 10 centimetres (3½ to 4 inches).

In addition to very intense contractions, you may notice an increase in bloody show and increased pressure, especially on your rectum, as the baby's head descends. During this last phase of the first stage of labour, you may feel as if you need to have a bowel movement. Don't worry; this sensation is a good sign and indicates that the foetus is heading in the right direction.

You may start to get frustrated or want to give up at this point – but remember, it's almost over.

If you feel the urge to push, let your practitioner know. You may be fully dilated, but try not to push until your practitioner tells you to do so. Pushing before you're fully dilated can slow the labour process or tear your cervix.

Practise breathing exercises and relaxation techniques, if they work for you. When you want pain medication or an epidural anaesthetic, let your practitioner know.

Potential problems during labour's first stage

Most women experience labour's first stage without any problems. But if a problem arises, the following sections prepare you with the information you need so that you handle it with a clear and focused mind.

Power problems

If your uterus isn't contracting often enough, your contractions may not do their job properly. This condition can stop your labour from getting going, or slow down the dilation of your cervix.

Rupturing your membranes will often help the contractions to get going effectively. If rupturing your membranes doesn't do the trick, your practitioner may recommend an intravenous infusion of oxytocin, as mentioned in the section 'Inducing labour' earlier in this chapter.

Further problems may result in you needing a caesarean section. Whether this happens will depend on several things, the most important being whether the baby is showing signs of being distressed, and how you are coping with the labour.

Passenger and pelvis problems

For your first baby, your cervix should dilate at a *minimum* rate of 1.2 centimetres (½ inch) an hour, and your baby's head should descend about 1 centimetre (⅓ inch) an hour. If you have delivered previously, the cervix should dilate at least 1.5 centimetres (½ inch) an hour, and your baby's head should descend about 2 centimetres (¾ inch) an hour. If your cervix dilates too slowly or if the baby's head doesn't descend at a normal rate, the possibility of cephalo-pelvic disproportion (also known as passenger problems) will be considered.

Cephalo-pelvic disproportion can occur because your baby's head is too big (unlikely unless he's a real whopper, over about 4 kilograms or 9 pounds), or simply in the wrong position. Your baby's head is not a perfect sphere, and is much wider in some directions than others; when your baby's head is bent forward, with his chin on his chest, this is the easiest position for getting him out. If your baby is lying with his back towards yours, his position is described as being *posterior* or *occipito-posterior*. This position stops his head from bending forwards normally. Fortunately, the baby's whole body may turn during labour so that he comes out in a normal position. If the baby doesn't turn, getting him out will be much harder work, and you are quite likely to need a forceps delivery or even a caesarean section.

Your baby's passage is determined not just by his size but also by the shape of your pelvis – in the same way that your baby's head is not a perfect sphere, your pelvis is narrower in some directions than others. Fortunately, as before, your baby's head and upper body often turn during labour to a more favourable position.

REMEMBER

If you've had a normal vaginal delivery in the past, your chances of having a normal delivery this time round are increased. If this is your first pregnancy and your baby's head has engaged before you go into labour, you have a good chance of avoiding passenger or pelvis problems.

The second stage

Labour's second stage begins when you're fully dilated (at 10 centimetres or 4 inches) and ends with your baby's delivery. This part is the pushing stage and takes about one hour for a first child and 30 to 40 minutes for subsequent births. The second stage may be longer if you have an epidural. We describe the second stage in detail in Chapter 11.

The third stage

The third stage occurs from the time of delivery of the baby to delivery of the placenta and usually lasts less than 20 minutes for all deliveries. We go into more detail about this stage in Chapter 11.

Handling Labour Pain

During labour's first stage, pain is caused by contractions of the uterus and dilation of the cervix. The pain may feel like severe menstrual cramps at first. But in labour's second stage, the stretching of the birth canal as the baby passes through it adds a different kind of pain – often a feeling of great pressure on the lower pelvis or rectum. But none of this pain needs to be excruciating, thanks to well-practised breathing and relaxation exercises and, in many cases, modern anaesthetic. If this is your first labour, you won't know exactly what the pain is like, or how you're going to react to it, until you're actually there. Just remember that this is *your* labour, and if ever a woman had the prerogative to change her mind, it's now. So if you discover that natural labour isn't the exhilarating experience you had always imagined, you have every right to ask for any pain relief going – and if it's smoother and less scary than you thought, feel free to stick to breathing techniques. Sometimes, your practitioner may decide that intervention is necessary for the wellbeing of the baby, but all the staff involved in your labour will do their best to let you be in charge, or will at least discuss or explain what they're planning and why.

You and your partner may have had long discussions about how you would help her with her breathing, mop her sweating brow, and whisper sweet nothings between contractions. You may also have decided on a natural labour with no drug intervention. If your partner suddenly changes her mind and wants every drug going, you won't improve the situation by reminding her that, as she told you last week, epidurals are for wimps. Go with the flow – the baby may belong to both of you, but the pain is hers to deal with.

Techniques for managing pain are explained in antenatal or preparation for parenthood classes (refer to Chapter 8 for more details on these classes).

The following sections explain some of the options offered to you to reduce labour pain.

Breathing exercises

Whether you choose other pain relief or not, you can still use breathing exercises, which can be remarkably effective at reducing pain during contractions, especially in the earlier part of labour. Breathing exercises are particularly useful if you remind yourself that breathing through each contraction is bringing you closer to delivery. Do practise beforehand, though – it's amazing how complicated breathing can seem in the middle of a contraction!

TENS

TENS (which stands for transcutaneous electrical nerve stimulation) involves stimulating your spinal nerves by way of a weak electric current passed through pads attached to your lower back and connected to a hand-held machine. This stimulation helps to block out the pain of labour. You adjust the current yourself, so are completely in control. TENS is completely safe for you and your baby, but the pain blocking does take a while to build up. Some hospitals have machines you can borrow, but you should check with your midwife. If no TENS machines are available your midwife should be able to tell you where you can hire one.

Gas and air

Every hospital or birthing centre has an Entonox machine, which lets you breathe in a mixture of 50 per cent nitrous oxide (a strong painkilling gas) and 50 per cent oxygen. This gas and air machine takes about 20 seconds to start working, reaching a peak effect within about 45–60 seconds. If you start to breathe by using this machine at the start of a contraction, and breathe deeply but at a normal rate, the pain relief should take effect by the time the contraction becomes really uncomfortable.

Although the Entonox machine helps, it doesn't completely get rid of the pain, and the gas and air mixture can make you feel light-headed. That fuzzy feeling makes gas and air, on the whole, unsuitable for the second stage of labour, when you need all your concentration to push effectively.

Pethidine and meptid

Pethidine is a powerful sedative drug, usually injected into your muscle and effective within about 15 minutes of the injection. Pethidine shouldn't slow labour down, but if administered late in your labour (if your baby is born within three hours of the last pethidine dose), the drug can affect your baby's breathing just after delivery. If breathing difficulties do occur, your baby may need to be given an antidote to reverse the effects of the pethidine. Meptid gives the same sedative benefits as pethidine, but without the complications.

Epidural

Because most of the pain of labour is concentrated in your uterus, vagina, and rectum, concentrating pain relief on these regions is the sensible thing to do. *Epidural anaesthetic* is the most common kind of region-specific pain relief used in the UK.

An epidural is given by a tiny, flexible, plastic catheter inserted through a needle into your lower back and threaded into the space above the membrane covering the spinal cord. Before putting the needle in, the anaesthetist numbs your skin with a local anaesthetic. While the needle is going in, you may feel a brief tingling sensation in your legs, but the process isn't really painful for most women. Once the catheter is in place, medication can be sent through it to numb the nerves coming from the lower part of the spine – nerves that go to the uterus, vagina, and perineum.

The catheter (not the needle) stays in place throughout labour in case you need a top-up dose of the anaesthetic to get you through the rest of labour and delivery. A major advantage of epidural anaesthetic is that it provides only a small dose of pain medication.

The nerves that control sensation are more sensitive than those that control movement, allowing you some movement in your legs after an epidural. However, because your sensory nerves run very close to your motor nerves, large doses of anaesthetic can temporarily affect your ability to move your legs during labour.

Sometimes the epidural takes away the sensation you feel when your bladder is full, so you may need a *urinary catheter* (a rubber tube passed into your bladder via your urethra – the tube your urine normally passes down when you pee) to empty your bladder. The *mobile* or *walking epidural* is a variation. The mobile epidural involves injecting a larger amount of more diluted local anaesthetic. This epidural is not available at every hospital, and is sometimes less effective than the more common anaesthetic – but the epidural does let you move around during labour, and means you should be able to avoid a urinary catheter.

Epidurals are extremely effective – providing total pain relief in over 90 per cent of women. Epidurals don't have any effect at all on your baby, but can reduce the strength of contractions and prolong your labour, and may increase your chance of needing a forceps delivery. However, epidurals don't increase your chance of needing a caesarean section.

Although complications of epidurals are rare, you do need to be aware of some situations that can occur. The risk of your blood pressure falling suddenly is up to 1 in 20, but can be reduced by giving you fluids through a drip. In about 1 in 100 cases, the epidural may not be effective because the needle is pushed through the membrane surrounding the spinal cord. In about 1 in 1000 cases, giving the local anaesthetic once this membrane has been breached can cause temporary paralysis of your legs and a nasty headache.

General anaesthetic

When you have *general anaesthetic*, you're made fully unconscious by an anaesthetist using a variety of medications. General anaesthetic causes you to sleep through your baby's delivery. Doctors almost never use this technique for labour, and it is only rarely used for caesarean deliveries because it's associated with a higher risk of complications. But if, in a caesarean delivery, you have a clotting problem that rules out placing a needle into your spinal column, or if the caesarean is an emergency and there isn't enough time to place an epidural, general anaesthetic should be used.

Considering Alternative Birthing Methods

Increasing numbers of women are expressing interest in non-traditional or alternative birthing methods, and more and more possibilities are available. The following options certainly aren't for everyone, but knowing what's available can be helpful.

Delivering without drugs – natural childbirth

Natural childbirth works on the idea that pain, fear, and tension are linked. If you know what to expect and feel in control, you will be less scared, which in turn will help you feel less tense.

Natural childbirth puts the emphasis on you choosing what positions are comfortable, how mobile you want to be, and what techniques you want to use to be as comfortable as possible. Natural childbirth can be practised in a hospital setting, birthing centre, or at home.

The National Childbirth Trust can be particularly helpful if you're interested in natural childbirth. Contact the NCT by post at The National Childbirth Trust, Alexandra House, Oldham Terrace, Acton, London W3 6NH; by phone: 0870 7703236; by e-mail: enquiries@national-childbirth-trust.co.uk; or visit their Web site: www.nctpregnancyandbabycare.com.

Giving birth at home

Home births are still relatively uncommon in the UK, although for some women, a home birth provides an ideal environment to deliver their baby. A midwife usually attends a home birth, and an obstetric team from the hospital should be on call in case problems arise. Home births are certainly more appropriate for women who are at very low risk for complications. The data on the safety of home births is conflicting: Although some studies demonstrate that home births are associated with greater risks for both the mother and baby, others show that home births are at least as safe as hospital births for healthy, low-risk women.

REMEMBER

Delivering a baby is illegal for anyone other than a midwife or doctor, except in an emergency. If a home birth is for you, make sure that you've made the necessary plans with your practitioner.

Immersing yourself in a water birth

Water births refer to spending much of labour immersed in water, with the option of even delivering the baby in the water. Water births usually take place in a birthing centre, with the help of a midwife, although some hospitals may provide birthing pools or baths. Although some professionals in the medical community feel that a water birth is a safe procedure, others have concerns about its safety.

Chapter 11

Special Delivery: Bringing Your Baby into the World

In This Chapter

- Pushing to the finish in a vaginal delivery
- Helping things along with forceps or vacuum extractors
- Preparing for a caesarean delivery
- Looking at the first few moments after delivery

When you reach the end of the second stage of labour, you're very close to the point of delivery. Now is the time you've been waiting for. You can prepare yourself for delivery by taking childbirth classes and by reading this book, for example. And remember that your practitioner and her assistants in the delivery room guide you through the process – accept and rely on their help. Trust in yourself and let this natural process move along one step at a time.

Babies are delivered in one of three ways: through the birth canal by your pushing, through the birth canal with a little assistance (by using forceps or a *ventouse* – a vacuum cup which helps pull your baby out), or by caesarean delivery. The method that's right for you depends on many different factors, including your medical history, the baby's condition, and the size of your pelvis relative to your baby's size.

Having a Vaginal Delivery

Most expectant mothers spend a great deal of time during the 40 weeks of pregnancy thinking ahead to the actual delivery. If you're having a baby for the first time, birth may seem pretty scary. Even if you have had a child before, worrying a bit until you see your beautiful baby is normal. A little knowledge goes a long way, though, and being informed and prepared for all possibilities is always helpful.

The most common method of delivery is, of course, a vaginal delivery (Figure 11-1 gives you an overview of the process). You'll probably experience what doctors call a *spontaneous vaginal delivery,* which means that it occurs as a result of your pushing efforts and proceeds without needing a great deal of intervention. If you do need a little help, forceps or a vacuum extractor may be used. A delivery requiring the use of one of these tools to help pull the baby out is called an *operative vaginal delivery*. We cover both types of delivery in this chapter.

During the first stage of labour, your cervix dilates and your membranes (usually) rupture. When your cervix is fully *dilated* (open to 10 centimetres – or 4 inches), you reach the end of the first stage of labour and are ready to enter the second stage, in which you push your baby through the birth canal (vagina) and actually deliver it. At the end of the first stage, you may feel an overwhelming sensation of pressure on your rectum. You may feel as if you need to have a bowel movement. This sensation is likely to be greatest during contractions and is caused by your baby's head descending in the birth canal and putting pressure on neighbouring internal organs.

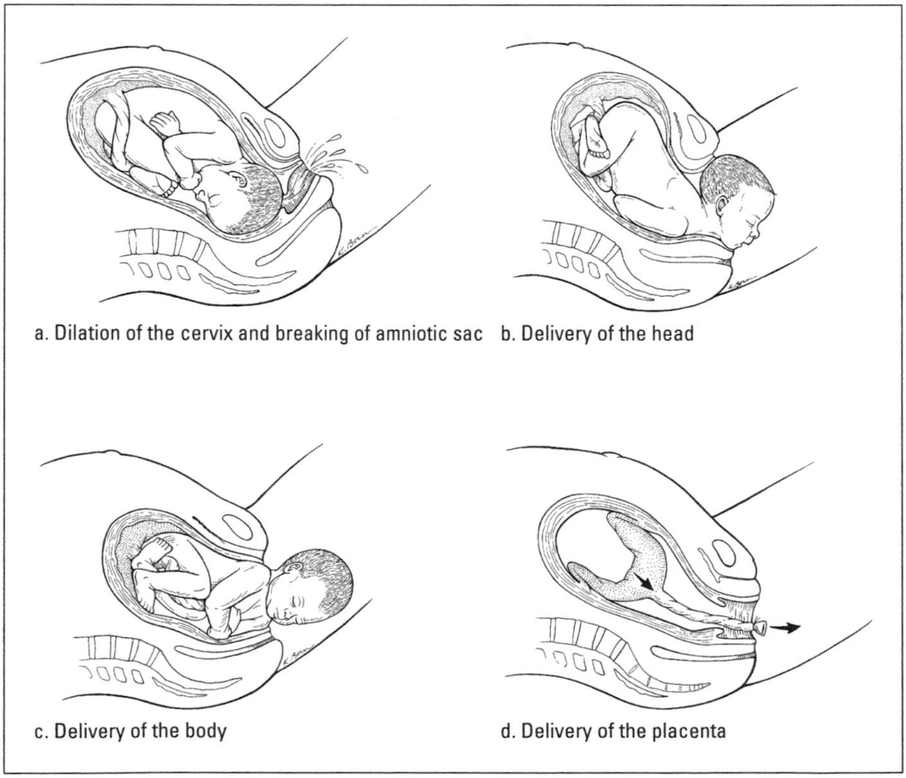

Figure 11-1: An overview of the delivery process.

If you have an *epidural* (a type of regional anaesthetic used to take away the pain of labour – see Chapter 10), you may not feel this pressure, or the feeling may be less intense. If you do feel this pressure, let your practitioner know, because it's probably a sign that your cervix is getting close to being fully dilated and it may be time for you to push. Your practitioner performs an internal examination to confirm that your cervix is fully dilated – and if it is, she tells you to start pushing.

Whether your doctor or midwife is actually coaching you during pushing varies from hospital to hospital and from practitioner to practitioner. The important factor is that someone is with you to help you through this stage of labour.

Occasionally, you may be fully dilated when the foetal head is still relatively high up in the pelvis. In this case, your practitioner may want you to wait until the contractions make the head descend more before you start to push.

Pushing the baby out

Pushing can take less than half-an-hour, but usually lasts from about half-an-hour to two hours. Pushing often takes less time if you've had a baby before. The time taken to push your baby out also depends on the baby's size and position and whether you've had an epidural (refer to Chapter 10). Pushing the baby out is known as the second stage of labour.

You have several possible positions in which to push (see Figure 11-2). The *lithotomy position* is the most common, in which you lean back and pull your flexed knees to your chest. At the same time, you bend your neck and try to touch your chin to your chest. The idea is to get your body to form a C shape. The position isn't the most flattering, but it does help to align the uterus and pelvis in a position that makes delivery relatively easy.

Other positions that may work are the squatting or knee-chest variations. The advantage of squatting is that you have gravity working with you. A disadvantage is that you may be too tired to hold the position for very long, and any monitoring equipment, or an intravenous line you may have connected to you, can be cumbersome. The knee-chest position is one in which you push while on all fours. This position is sometimes helpful if the baby's head is rotated in the birth canal in such a way that makes pushing the baby out in the lithotomy or squatting positions difficult. The knee-chest position may be awkward for some women and difficult to stay in for very long. Finding the one position that feels and works best for you may take a bit of experimentation.

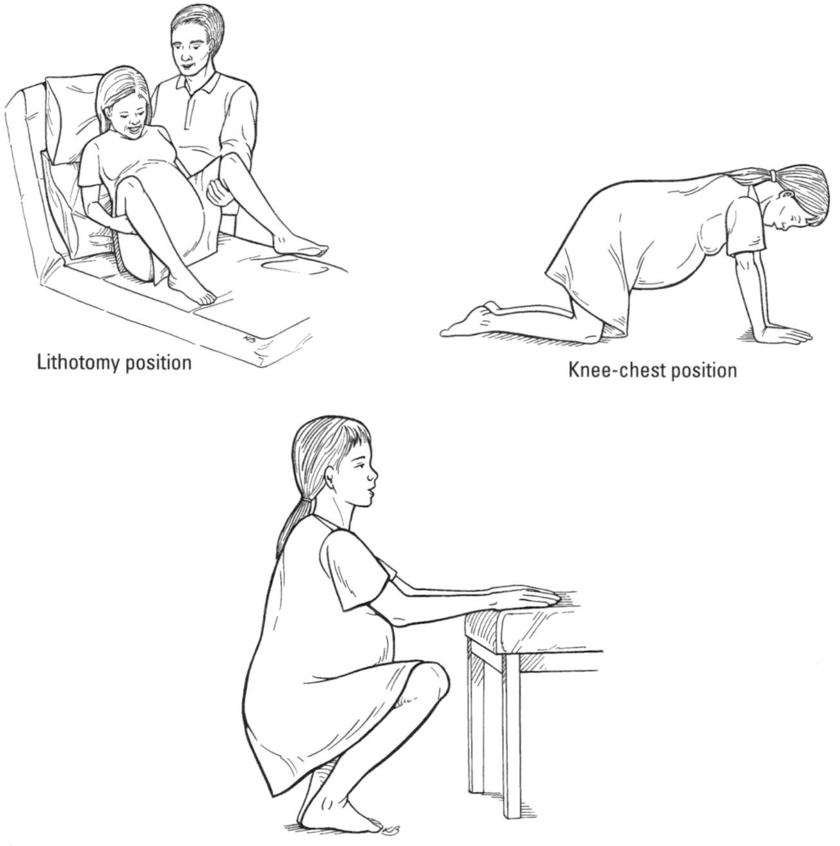

Figure 11-2: Positions you can assume in childbirth.

TIP

If you find that you're not making progress, try changing positions.

When you start to feel a contraction, your practitioner probably tells you to take a deep, cleansing breath. After that, you inhale deeply again, hold in the air, and push like mad. Focus the push toward your rectum and *perineum* (the area between the vagina and the rectum), trying not to tense up the muscles of your vagina or rectum. Push like you're having a bowel movement. Don't worry or be embarrassed if you pass a stool while you're pushing (if it happens, a midwife quickly cleans the perineum). Passing a stool is the rule rather than the exception, and all the people helping to take care of you have seen it many times before – in fact, it's a sign that you're pushing correctly, so congratulate yourself. Trying to hold a stool in only impedes your efforts to push the baby out.

To watch or not to watch

Some partners want to see everything that's happening during childbirth; others feel uncomfortable even being in the delivery room. Likewise, some women want their partners to witness everything, and others prefer that their partners do not see them in this situation.

Communicate your feelings about being watched to your partner so that you can make each other feel as comfortable as possible. The last thing you need is for you or your partner to be embarrassed during a time that should be one of joy and happiness.

Hold each push for about ten seconds. Many midwives count to ten or ask your birth partner to count to ten to help you judge the time. After the count of ten, quickly release the breath you have been holding, take in another deep breath, and push again for another ten seconds, exactly as before. You probably push about three times with each contraction, depending on the length of the contraction.

Be warned: Labour is very hard work for your partner. Whatever you do, don't try, as Sarah's husband did, to break the monotony. He had the job of counting to ten for each push, and about 90 minutes in, started counting in Russian instead, just for a change. Sarah did not find this funny, and neither did he after she told him exactly what she thought of his attempt to be clever. Remember, all the focus should be on your partner at this crucial time.

Between contractions, try your best to relax and rest so that you can get ready for the next one. You may like your birth partner to give you some ice cubes or pat your forehead with a damp, cool cloth.

After your baby gets far enough down the birth canal, the top of the head becomes visible during your pushing efforts. When the top, or crown, of your baby's head stays visible between pushes, it's called *crowning*. After the contraction, the baby's head may again disappear back up into the birth canal. This retraction is normal. With each push, the baby comes down a little farther and recedes a little less afterward.

Getting an episiotomy

Just before it's born, the baby's head distends the *perineum* (the area between the vagina and the rectum) and stretches the skin around the vagina. As the baby's head comes through the vagina's opening, it may tear the tissues in the back, or *posterior*, part of the vaginal opening, sometimes even to the point that the tear extends into the anus and rectum (your back passage). To minimise tearing of the surrounding skin and perineal muscles, your practitioner may make an *episiotomy* – a cut in the posterior part of the vaginal opening large enough to allow the baby's head to come through with minimal tearing or to provide extra room for delivery. The decision to make an episiotomy is usually made by your practitioner moments before you deliver (see the nearby sidebar 'Expectant mothers ask . . .' for more details). Although an episiotomy decreases the likelihood of a severe tear, it doesn't guarantee that you won't get one (that is, the cut made for the episiotomy may tear open even further as the baby's head is delivered). Episiotomies are more common in women having their first baby, because the perineum stretches more easily after a previous birth.

Just before your baby's head is born, your practitioner will tell you to stop pushing and to pant in short breaths. This can be hard to do, not to mention incredibly frustrating when you're so close. However, this action helps your practitioner to deliver the baby's head as slowly as possible, reducing the chance of your tearing.

Most tears or lacerations that occur during delivery are in the perineum or are extensions of an episiotomy. Occasionally, especially when the baby is exceptionally large or you have an operative vaginal delivery, lacerations can occur in other areas, such as the cervix, on the vagina's walls, the labia, or the tissue around the urethra. Your practitioner examines the birth canal carefully after delivery and sews up any lacerations that need to be repaired. These lacerations usually heal very quickly and almost never cause long-term problems.

Handling prolonged second-stage labour

If you're having your first child and you remain in the second stage of labour for more than two hours (or three hours if you have an epidural), the labour is considered prolonged. If you're having your second or subsequent child, a second stage nearing one hour (or two hours if you have an epidural) is also considered prolonged.

A prolonged second stage may be due to inadequate contractions or to *cephalo-pelvic disproportion* (see Chapter 10). Sometimes, the baby's head is in a position that blocks further descent. You may be advised to try changing your position to push more effectively. Sometimes forceps do the trick (see 'Assisting Nature: Operative Vaginal Delivery', later in this chapter) if the baby's head is low enough in the birth canal. If all else fails, your doctor may recommend a caesarean delivery (see later in this chapter for more on caesareans).

Expectant mothers ask . . .

Q: 'Do I really need an episiotomy?'

A: The answer to this question depends on many factors, including the point of view of your practitioner. The real problem is that it's very hard to predict if, or how much, your perineum will tear if you don't have an episiotomy. Many practitioners believe that repairing a controlled cut in the perineum is easier than repairing any uncontrolled tear through the skin and perineal muscles that may occur without an episiotomy. Also, almost all episiotomies are *mediolateral*– angled away from your anus. This should mean that if the tear does extend, it's less likely to reach the muscles of your anus. A tear that reaches your anus is called a third-degree tear, and can sometimes cause significant problems with incontinence of faeces (or poo).

The big moment: Delivering your baby

When the crown of the baby's head remains visible between contractions, your practitioner helps get you into position to deliver. As you're pushing, your perineum is getting more and more stretched out.

With each push, the baby's head descends farther and farther until finally it comes out of the birth canal. After the baby's head delivers, your practitioner tells you to stop pushing, just as she did before the baby's head came out (see 'Getting an episiotomy' earlier in this chapter).

Your practitioner checks at this point to see whether the *umbilical cord* (the cord connecting your baby's tummy button to your placenta) is wrapped around the baby's neck. Entanglement, as this is called, is quite common and almost always no need to worry. Your practitioner simply removes the loop from around the baby's neck before delivering the rest of her.

Finally, your practitioner instructs you to push again to deliver the baby's body. Because the head is typically the widest part, delivery of the body is usually easier. The first part of the baby to emerge after the head is, of course, the shoulder. During the delivery of your baby's first shoulder, you're offered an injection of oxytocin or syntometrine, helping the placenta's delivery and reducing blood loss.

Occasionally, though, the baby's shoulders may be stuck behind the mother's pubic bone, which makes delivery of the rest of the baby more difficult. This situation is known as *shoulder dystocia.* If you have this problem, your practitioner can perform various manoeuvres designed to dislodge the shoulders and deliver the baby. These methods include

- Applying pressure directly above your pubic bone to push away the entrapped shoulder
- Flexing your knees back to allow more room for delivery
- Rotating the baby's shoulders manually
- Delivering the posterior arm of the baby first

Although shoulder dystocia can occur in women with no risk factors, certain characteristics make this condition more likely:

- Very large babies
- Gestational diabetes
- Prolonged labour
- History of large babies or babies with shoulder dystocia

Delivering the placenta

After the baby is born, the third stage of delivery begins – the delivery of the placenta, also known as the *afterbirth* (refer to Figure 11-1). This stage lasts only about 5 to 15 minutes. You still have contractions, but they're much less intense. These contractions help separate the placenta from the uterus's wall. After this separation occurs and the placenta reaches the vagina's opening, your practitioner may ask you to give one more gentle push. Many women, exhilarated by and exhausted from the delivery, pay little attention to this part of the process and later on don't even remember it.

Repairing your perineum

After the placenta is out, your practitioner inspects your cervix, vagina, and perineum for tears or damage and then repairs (with stitches) the episiotomy or any tears. (If you didn't have an epidural and you have sensation in your perineum, your practitioner will use a local anaesthetic to numb the area before repairing it.)

After the practitioner finishes with the repairs, she cleans your perineal area, removes your legs out of the leg supports if you had any, and gives you warm blankets. You may also continue to feel mild contractions; these contractions are normal and actually help to minimise bleeding.

Assisting Nature: Operative Vaginal Delivery

If the baby's head is low enough in the birth canal and your practitioner feels that the baby needs to be delivered immediately or that you can't deliver the baby vaginally without some added help, she may recommend the use of forceps or a ventouse (suction cup) to assist the delivery. Using either of these instruments is called an *operative vaginal delivery*, and an obstetrician carries out such deliveries (refer to Chapter 2 to find out more about obstetricians). A forceps or ventouse delivery may be appropriate when

- You've pushed for a long time, and you're too tired to continue pushing hard enough to deliver.
- You've pushed for some time, and your practitioner thinks you won't deliver vaginally unless you have this type of help.
- The baby's heart rate pattern indicates a need to deliver the baby quickly.
- The baby's position is making it very difficult for you to push it out on your own.

Figure 11-3 shows *forceps,* two curved, spatula-like instruments that are placed on the sides of the baby's head to help guide it through the outer part of the birth canal. The ventouse is placed on the top of the baby's head, to which suction is applied to allow your practitioner to pull the baby gently through the birth canal.

Both techniques are safe for you and the baby if the baby is far enough down in the birth canal and the instruments are used appropriately. In fact, these techniques can often help women avoid caesarean delivery (but not always – see the next section). The decision to use forceps or ventouse often depends upon your practitioner's judgement and experience and the baby's position.

If you haven't had an epidural, you may need extra local anaesthetic for a forceps or vacuum delivery, and most doctors perform an episiotomy to make extra room. After the forceps or ventouse is applied, the doctor asks you to continue to push until the head emerges. The forceps or ventouse is then removed, and the rest of the baby is delivered with your pushing.

If forceps are used, very often the baby is born with marks on her head where the forceps were applied. If this happens to your baby, don't worry – it's quite typical, and the marks disappear within a few days. A ventouse may cause the baby to be born with a round, raised area on the top of the head where the extractor was applied. This mark, too, goes away in a few days.

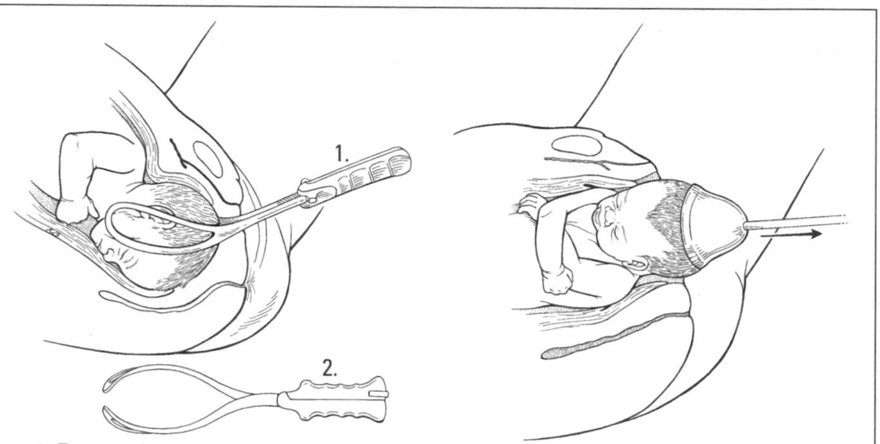

Figure 11-3: Two ways to help the process of a vaginal delivery along: (a) using forceps or (b) a ventouse to help guide the baby through the birth canal.

Having a Caesarean Delivery

Many patients wonder whether they'll need a caesarean. Sometimes your doctor knows the answer before labour even begins – if you have placenta praevia (see Chapter 16), for example, or if the baby is in a *transverse lie* (the baby is lying sideways within the uterus rather than head-down). But most of the time, neither you nor your doctor can know whether you'll need a caesarean until you see how your labour progresses and how your baby tolerates labour.

REMEMBER

Because a caesarean is a surgical procedure, it is always performed under sterile conditions, in an operating theatre, and by an obstetrician.

Before the caesarean section operation begins, an anaesthetist puts an *intravenous line* (a plastic tube inserted into your vein, allowing drugs and fluids to be put into your system) in your arm. A *catheter* (a tube passed up the tube you pee through into your bladder) is put into your bladder, your belly is cleaned with an antiseptic solution, and sterile sheets are placed over your belly. One of the sheets is lifted up to create a screen so that you and your partner don't have to watch the procedure. (Although childbirth is usually an experience shared by both parents, a caesarean delivery is still a surgical operation. Most doctors feel that the procedure isn't something that expectant parents should watch, because it involves scalpels, bleeding, and exposure of internal body tissue that's normally not seen, which is disturbing to many people.)

Many hospitals allow your partner to stay in the operating room during a caesarean delivery, but this decision depends on the nature of the delivery and on hospital policy. If the caesarean is an emergency, the doctors and nurses are moving quickly to ensure the safety of both the mother and the baby, which may make it necessary for the partner to wait elsewhere.

The exact place on the woman's abdomen where the incision is made depends on the reason she's having the caesarean. Most often, the incision is low, just above the pubic bone, in a transverse direction, parallel to (and just below) the top of your bikini-line, which is why it's called a *bikini-line incision*. Much less frequently, the incision is vertical, along the midline of the abdomen.

After the doctor makes the skin incision, she separates the abdominal muscles and opens the inner lining of the abdominal cavity, also called the *peritoneal cavity*, to expose the uterus. She then makes an incision in the uterus itself, through which the infant and placenta are delivered. The incision in the uterus can also be either transverse (most common) or vertical (sometimes called a *classical incision*), depending again on the reason for the caesarean and previous abdominal surgery. After delivery, the uterus and abdominal wall are closed with *sutures* (stitches), layer by layer. A caesarean delivery takes 30 to 90 minutes to perform.

Understanding anaesthetics

The most common forms of anaesthetic used for caesarean deliveries are epidural and spinal. (Refer to Chapter 10 for more information on anaesthetic.) Both kinds of anaesthetic numb you from mid-chest to toes but also allow you to remain awake so that you can experience your child's birth. You may feel some tugging and pulling during the operation, but you don't feel pain. Sometimes the anaesthetist injects a slow-release pain medication into the epidural or spinal catheter before removing it in order to prevent, or greatly minimise, pain *after* the operation.

If the baby has to be delivered in an emergency and there's no time to place an epidural or spinal anaesthetic, a general anaesthetic may be needed. You're then asleep during the caesarean and totally unaware of the procedure. Also, general anaesthetic may be needed in some cases because of complications in pregnancy that make it unwise to place epidurals or spinals.

Looking at reasons for caesarean delivery

The reasons your doctor may perform a caesarean delivery are many (see the list later in this section), but all are about delivering your baby in the safest, healthiest way possible while also maintaining your wellbeing. A caesarean delivery can be either planned ahead of labour (*elective*), unplanned during labour (when the doctor determines that delivering the baby vaginally isn't safe), or done as an emergency (if the mother's or the baby's health is in immediate danger).

If your practitioner feels that you need a caesarean delivery, she'll discuss with you why it is needed. If your caesarean is elective or if it's done because your labour isn't progressing normally, you and your partner have time to ask questions. If your baby is in a breech position, you and your practitioner may consider together the pros and cons of having either an elective caesarean delivery or a vaginal breech delivery (see Chapter 16). Both deliveries carry some risks, and often your practitioner asks you which risks are most acceptable to you. If the decision to perform a caesarean is due to a last-minute emergency, the discussion between you and your doctor may happen quickly, while you're being wheeled to the operating theatre.

If things seem hurried or rushed when you're on your way to the operating theatre for an emergency caesarean, don't panic. Doctors and midwives are trained to handle these kinds of emergencies.

The doctor may suggest that you have a caesarean delivery for one of many different reasons, of which these are the most common:

- The baby is in an abnormal position (breech or transverse; see Chapter 15).
- Placenta praevia (see Chapter 16).
- You've had extensive prior surgery on the uterus, including previous caesarean deliveries or removal of uterine fibroids. (See Chapter 15 for more information on vaginal births after caesarean delivery.)
- Delivery of triplets or more.

Reasons for unplanned but non-emergency caesarean delivery:

- The baby is too large in relation to the woman's pelvis to be delivered safely through the vagina – a condition known as *cephalo-pelvic disproportion* (CPD) – or the position of the baby's head makes vaginal delivery unlikely.
- Signs indicate that the baby isn't tolerating labour.
- Maternal medical conditions preclude safe vaginal delivery, such as severe cardiac disease.
- Normal labour comes to a standstill.

Reasons for emergency caesarean delivery:

- Bleeding is excessive.
- The baby's umbilical cord pushes through the cervix when the membranes rupture.
- Prolonged slowing of the baby's heart rate, or other signs of severe distress.

Other than the fact that the baby and placenta are delivered through an incision in the uterus rather than through the vagina, for the baby, a caesarean delivery makes little difference. A baby delivered by a caesarean before labour usually doesn't have a conehead, but she may if you're in labour for a long time before having the caesarean. (For more on coneheads, see Chapter 12.)

Women who have laboured for a long time only to find that they need a caesarean delivery are sometimes, understandably, disappointed. This reaction is natural. If it happens to you, keep in mind that what is ultimately most important is your safety and your baby's safety. Having a caesarean delivery doesn't mean that you are, in any way, a failure or that you didn't try hard enough. Practitioners stick to basic guidelines when monitoring progress through labour, and those guidelines are all about giving you and your baby the best chance for a normal, healthy outcome.

All surgical procedures involve risks, and caesarean delivery is no exception. Fortunately, problems following caesarean aren't common. The main risks of caesarean delivery are

- Excessive bleeding, rarely to the point of needing a blood transfusion
- Development of an infection in the uterus, bladder, or skin incision
- Injury to the bladder, bowel, or adjacent organs
- Development of blood clots in the legs or pelvis after the operation

Recovering from a caesarean delivery

After the surgery is finished, you're taken to a recovery area, where you stay for a few hours, until the hospital staff can make sure that your condition is stable. Often, you can see and hold your baby during this time.

The recovery time from a caesarean delivery is usually longer than from a vaginal delivery because the procedure is a surgical one. Typically, you stay in the hospital for two to four days – sometimes longer, if complications arise. Check out Chapter 13 for details about recovering from a caesarean delivery.

Congratulations! You Did It!

After their babies are born, women may experience any and every kind of emotion. The spectrum of feelings is truly infinite. Most of the time, you're completely overcome with joy when your long-awaited baby finally is born. You may be incredibly relieved to see that your baby appears healthy and obviously okay. If your baby requires extra medical attention for some reason and you can't hold her immediately, you may be upset or, at the very least, disappointed. Just remember that very soon you'll have her to hold and enjoy for the rest of your life. Some women feel too scared or overwhelmed to care for their baby straight away. Don't feel guilty about any such feelings – they, and most others, are completely normal. Just take one moment at a time – you've come through a phenomenal event.

Shaking after delivery

Almost immediately after delivery, most women start to shake uncontrollably. Your partner may think that you're cold and offer you a blanket. Blankets do help some women, but you aren't shivering because you're cold. The cause of this phenomenon is unclear, but it's nearly universal – even among women who have caesarean deliveries. Some women feel nervous about holding their babies because they're shaking so much. If you feel this way, let your partner or your midwife hold your baby until you feel up to it.

DON'T WORRY

Don't be concerned at all about uncontrollable shaking after delivery – it usually goes away within a few hours.

Understanding postpartum bleeding

After delivery – either vaginal or caesarean – your uterus begins to contract in order to squeeze the blood vessels closed and thus slow down bleeding. If the uterus doesn't contract normally, excessive bleeding may occur. This condition is known as *uterine atony* and it can happen when you have multiple babies (twins or more), if you have some infection in the uterus, or if some placental tissue remains inside the uterus after the placenta is delivered. In some cases, excessive bleeding happens for no apparent cause. If excessive bleeding happens to you, your practitioner may first massage your uterus to get it to contract. If massage doesn't solve the problem, you may be given more oxytocin (see 'Delivering the placenta' earlier in this chapter). If you have some placental material remaining in your uterus, it may need to be removed by reaching inside the uterus or by a *D&C* (dilation and curettage), which involves scraping the uterus's lining with an instrument. Generally, the bleeding stops without a problem, however, if it doesn't stop with these medications and procedures, your doctor will discuss other forms of treatment with you.

Hearing your baby's first cry

Shortly after delivery, your baby takes its first breath and begins to cry. This crying is what expands your baby's lungs and helps clear secretions. In contrast to stereotype, most practitioners don't spank a baby after it's born, but instead use some other method to stimulate crying and breathing – rubbing the baby's back vigorously, for example, or tapping the bottom of the feet. Don't be surprised if your baby doesn't cry the very second after it's born. Often, several seconds, if not minutes, pass before the baby starts making that lovely sound.

Cutting the cord

If there are no immediate concerns about your baby, she is lifted onto your tummy as soon as she is delivered so that you can look at her. While she's on your tummy, her umbilical cord is clamped and cut. Once this is done, your baby's condition is checked.

If any question marks exist over your baby's condition straight after birth, her cord will be clamped and cut immediately, and she will be taken to a resuscitation table with a warming lamp in the delivery room. This is just a precaution, and your baby is very likely to be returned to you within a few minutes.

Checking your baby's condition

All babies are evaluated by the Apgar score, named after Dr Virginia Apgar, who devised it in 1952. This score is a useful way of quickly assessing the baby's initial condition to see if she needs special medical attention. Five factors are measured: heart rate, respiratory effort, muscle tone, presence of reflexes, and colour, each of which can be given a score of 0, 1, or 2, with 2 being the highest score. The Apgar scores are calculated at both one and five minutes. An Apgar score of 6 or above is perfectly fine. Because some of the characteristics are partially dependent on the infant's gestational age, premature babies frequently get lower scores. Factors such as maternal sedation can also affect a baby's score.

Many new parents anxiously await the results of their child's Apgar score. In fact, an Apgar score taken one minute after the baby is born indicates if the baby needs some resuscitative measures but is not useful in predicting long-term health. An Apgar score taken five minutes later can indicate if resuscitative measures have been effective. Occasionally, a very low five-minute Apgar score may reflect decreased oxygenation to the baby, but it correlates poorly with future health. The purpose of the Apgar score is merely to help the hospital staff identify babies who may need a little extra attention in the very early newborn period – it is certainly no indication of whether your baby will get into Oxford or Cambridge.

Chapter 12

Hello, World! Your Newborn

In This Chapter

- Making first impressions
- Adjusting to the first days of life in the hospital
- Taking care of your baby at home
- Making your baby 'legal'
- Knowing when to call the doctor

For 40 weeks, you and your baby have been in one body, and if you're like most women, you've focused on staying healthy to help your baby grow and on preparing to deliver him safely. Now suddenly, your baby is out in the world, and you finally get to take your first real look at him. In this chapter, we give you an idea of what to expect when you first meet your little darling and how to manage those first days at home.

Looking at Your Bundle of Joy – Goo, Blotches, and All

Immediately after delivery, your practitioner puts your baby on your belly or hands him over to a midwife for some judicious cleansing and towelling off before putting him in your arms.

In the first moments after your baby is born, you may be overwhelmed by feelings of love. The shock and relief of it all may also daze you. You also think that your baby is the most beautiful thing you've ever seen – then again, maybe you don't. Contrary to the fairy tales you see on TV soaps and in magazines everywhere, babies don't always come out clean and smelling like a spring shower. Your baby is far more likely to be covered with some of your blood, amniotic fluid, and white goo known as *vernix*. His skin may be blotchy, and your baby may even have suffered a few bruises during delivery. None of these aesthetic glitches last for long, and they won't have any ill effect on your baby.

Feeling a little hesitant at first, or even overwhelmed at the sight of your new baby isn't uncommon. Often it takes a few days before you establish a true connection or bond with your baby. If you're feeling a little detached, don't worry. As reality sets in and you get to know your baby, you feel much better. Of course, it goes without saying that many women are just overwhelmed with love from the first moment.

You notice many other features about your new baby's appearance – from his little stump of an umbilical cord to the amazingly long fingernails and toenails. And you observe his first behaviours – from the initial cry to the way he startles at loud noises. In this section, we go over many of the characteristics you're likely to notice in your newborn.

Your baby will be checked out thoroughly by a health care professional within 24 hours of birth, and any abnormalities will be looked for in detail then. If you need any reassurance in the mean time, just ask your midwife or doctor.

Vernix caseosa

No, not a character from the *Asterix* cartoons, but a thick, white, waxy substance that typically covers a newborn baby from head-to-toe. The formal name for this substance is *vernix caseosa*, a phrase with Latin roots meaning cheesy varnish. Vernix is a mixture of cells that have sloughed off from the outer layer of the baby's skin and of debris from the amniotic fluid. If your baby is born prematurely or by caesarean section, it may be more noticeable, and if your baby passed meconium while inside the uterus (see Chapter 8), the vernix may look a little greenish.

Regardless of what it looks like, most of the vernix probably comes off when the midwife dries off your baby. There's no reason to leave the vernix on the baby's skin. Whatever vernix doesn't come off in the drying process is probably absorbed within the first 24 hours.

Caput and moulding

Caput succedaneum – more commonly called *caput* – refers to a circular area of swelling on the baby's head located at the spot that pushed against the cervix's opening during delivery. The exact location of the swelling varies, depending on the position that the baby's head was in. The swollen area can range in size from only a few millimetres in diameter to several centimetres. Caput generally goes kaput within 24 to 48 hours after birth.

Babies who are born headfirst (*vertex*) often go through a process known as *moulding*. This moulding occurs because throughout labour, as the baby descends gradually through the birth canal, it 'fits' its way along. Moulding doesn't cause any harm. The bones and soft tissues in the baby's head are designed to allow this moulding to happen. The result of this moulding is often a baby with a cone-shaped head. By 24 hours after delivery, the moulding usually disappears, and the baby's head appears round and smooth.

Some women, particularly those who have had children before or who had rapid labour, have babies with no moulding. Also, babies born in the breech presentation or by caesarean section may not have moulding.

TIP

Don't forget to let your baby's first visitors know about moulding. Sarah's first baby came out with a head like a rugby ball, but everyone cooed over him anyway. Weeks later she discovered that her brothers-in-law had been madly debating the best way to tell her gently that she'd given birth to an alien and that only blind mother love was preventing her from seeing it.

Sometimes, during the passage through the birth canal, a baby's ears can also fold down into strange positions. The same thing can happen with the baby's nose, so that at first it may appear *asymmetric*, or pushed to one side, but these features are no reason to rush your baby to a plastic surgeon. These minor oddities are temporary and disappear during the first few days.

Black-and-blue marks

DON'T WORRY

Quite often, babies are born with black-and-blue marks on their heads from the labour and delivery process. These marks may happen because the forces of labour put so much pressure on the baby's scalp, or as a result of a forceps or vacuum delivery. A bruise doesn't indicate that anything harmful has occurred; it's merely a reflection of how vigorous the labour process can be. Most black-and-blue marks go away within the first few days of life.

Blotches, patches, and more

Most people think of newborn skin as blemish-free, but babies have all kinds of spots and markings – most of which disappear within a matter of days or weeks. Some of the most common newborn skin conditions include

- **Dry skin:** Some babies, particularly those who are born late, have an outer layer of skin that looks shrivelled like a raisin and peels off easily shortly after birth. You can use lotion or baby oil, if needed, as a moisturiser.
- **Haemangiomas:** A type of reddish spot, known as a *haemangioma*, may not appear until a week or so after delivery. It can be almost any size, large or small, and can occur anywhere on the infant's body. Although the majority go away in early childhood, some persist. You can treat the spots that become bothersome (because of their appearance). Discuss treatment options, if needed, with your GP.
- **Mongolian spots:** Bluish-grey patches of skin on the lower back, buttocks, and thighs are especially common in Asian, Southern European, and Afro-Caribbean infants. These patches are usually called *mongolian spots*. They often disappear in early childhood.
- **Neonatal acne:** Some babies are born with tiny white or red pimples around the nose, lips, and cheeks, and some develop them weeks or months later. These bumps are completely normal and are sometimes called *neonatal acne*, *milk spots*, or *milia*. Don't rush to the GP – the little bumps disappear in time.
- **Red spots:** Reddish discolouration on the skin, whether very deep and dark or light and hardly noticeable, is very common in newborns. Most of these discolourations go away or fade, but some may persist as birthmarks. One type of discolouration in particular, *erythema taxicum*, can be extensive – it looks like a bad allergic rash, and it comes and goes over the baby's first few days of life.
- **Stork bites:** You may notice small ruptured blood vessels around your baby's nose and eyes or on the back of his neck. These marks are commonly known as *stork bites* and *angel kisses*. Stork bites are common in newborns, and they also disappear after a while, although it sometimes takes weeks or months.

Baby hair

Some babies enter the world totally bald, while others come out looking like they need a haircut. The amount of hair present at birth doesn't necessarily predict what the baby's hair will look like later on. Generally, newborn hair thins out and is replaced by new hair. Different babies grow hair at different rates; some have relatively little hair even at a year of age, while others already need a trip to the beauty salon.

Often, a soft, fine layer of dark hair, which can be especially prominent on the forehead, shoulders, and back, covers babies' bodies. This hair is called *lanugo*, and like so many aspects of a newborn's appearance, is quite normal. Lanugo is most common in preterm babies and in infants of mothers who have diabetes. It falls out within several weeks of life.

Extremities

Newborn babies often assume a position similar to the one that they became familiar with inside the uterus, the so-called *foetal position*. You may notice that your baby likes to be curled up a bit, with his arms and legs bent and fingers balled into a fist.

Watch out for those nails, though. Newborn fingernails and toenails may be surprisingly long and sharp. Because babies can easily scratch themselves, keep the nails relatively short (some mothers also dress their babies in little mittens, to prevent accidental scratches). Pick up a pair of baby nail scissors or clippers from your local pharmacy.

A good time to trim fingernails and toenails is when your baby is fast asleep and oblivious to what you're doing.

Eyes and ears

At birth, a baby's vision is quite limited. Newborns can only see objects that are close-up and see things best at a distance of about 7 to 8 inches away (the approximate distance from your baby's eyes to your face when you're breast-feeding, making feeding time a great opportunity to bond). Babies also respond to light and appear to be interested in bright objects.

All newborn babies have dark blue or brown eyes, regardless of what colour eyes the parents have. By the age of four months, baby eye colour changes to the permanent hue. Right after birth, the whites of your baby's eyes may have a bluish tint. This tint is normal and disappears in time.

Often, a newborn's eyes may appear a little swollen or puffy. The whole delivery process causes this puffiness; it's perfectly normal, and it quickly subsides. Babies are fully able to hear from the moment they're born, which is why you may notice that your baby reacts with a startled motion to loud or sudden noises. Newborns also can distinguish various tastes and smells.

Conjunctivitis (an eye infection) in your baby may be caused by chlamydia. If your baby has persistent sticky eyes from birth, make an appointment with your GP to discuss the possibility of chlamydia (see Chapter 17 for details).

Genitalia and breasts

Babies are often born with a swollen or puffy scrotum or labia. The breasts also may appear slightly enlarged. Maternal hormones that cross the placenta cause this swelling. Sometimes, high maternal hormone levels may even cause the baby to secrete whitish or pinkish discharge from the breasts (known as witch's milk) or from the vagina (like a period) in female babies. Like so many newborn characteristics, these secretions are both normal and transient; they go away within a few weeks after birth.

Umbilical cord

The stump of your baby's umbilical cord probably has a little piece of plastic attached to it. After delivery, your practitioner closes the cord with a small plastic clamp and then cuts it. Usually, your practitioner removes this clamp before you take the baby home. Then the umbilical cord stump quickly dries up and shrivels so that it looks like a hard, dark cord. Within one to three weeks, the stump usually falls off. Don't try to pull it off.

To keep the stump clean, you can dip a cotton swab in boiled, cooled water and clean around the base. However, some doctors think this cleaning is unnecessary – unless a lot of gooey stuff is around the base.

Newborn size

In general, newborn babies weigh anywhere from about 6 to 8 pounds (about 2,700 to 3,600 grams) and measure 18 to 22 inches (46 to 56 centimetres) long. The exact size depends on the baby's gestational age (the number of weeks the pregnancy lasted), genetics, and other factors, such as whether the mother had diabetes, whether she smoked, how healthy her diet was during pregnancy, and many other reasons.

You may notice that your baby's head seems disproportionately large compared to his body. This feature is true of all newborns. Your baby can't hold up his head and needs time to develop muscles strong enough to hold it up without assistance. You may also notice soft spots on the back and top of your baby's head. These are *fontanelles*, areas where the baby's skull bones meet. Fontanelles allow for the rapid growth of the baby's brain. The back spot (posterior fontanelle) usually closes within a few months, but the anterior or top fontanelle (the one most typically called the soft spot) usually remains until the baby is 10 months to 1 year old.

Baby begins to breathe

Often, the baby starts to cry spontaneously shortly after delivery, but not every baby cries straight away. A full-throated cry is music to the ears of everyone on the hospital staff because they know that the cry triggers the baby's first breathing efforts. Healthy breathing can begin without a loud cry, however, and some babies give only a little whimper. Some babies have normal respiration even if they don't wail at high decibels.

If your baby is slow to start breathing spontaneously, you may notice the doctor or midwife stimulating him by rubbing his back, by drying him off, or by tapping his feet. Contrary to stereotype, your practitioner is unlikely to turn your baby upside down and give him a little spank on the behind to elicit that first cry.

During pregnancy, a foetus receives oxygen through the placenta. After delivery, the baby takes over respiratory function by using his own lungs. While in the womb, a special fluid bathes your baby's lungs, and this fluid is often pushed out during delivery. Sometimes, however, a baby needs extra time and help – in the form of suctioning or stimuli – to expel all the fluid in the lungs.

DON'T WORRY

You may notice that your baby breathes differently than you do. Most babies breathe 30–40 times a minute. A newborn's respiratory rate can also increase with physical activity. Newborns breathe through their noses rather than their mouths. This great natural adaptation enables them to breathe while breast- or bottle-feeding.

You may also think that your baby's belly looks unusually large and protuberant, but it's just a normal new baby's belly.

Knowing What to Expect in the Hospital

After your practitioner is assured that your baby is fine (usually determined by an Apgar test – see Chapter 11 for details), the hospital staff starts cleaning the baby and helping him make a comfortable transition to life outside the womb. Like butterflies emerging from their cocoons, newborns must adjust to a new state of being in various ways. Suddenly, and for the first time, they can breathe on their own and see the wide world around them.

At the hospital, your baby wears an identification bracelet to identify him as yours. All hospitals also require that the mother wear a bracelet with the baby's ID number on it. Most hospitals also take additional security measures to prevent any mix-ups and to prevent unauthorised individuals from gaining access to the ward.

Preparing baby for life outside the womb

A lot happens in the few hours immediately after your baby is born. He has made a pretty significant change and will have a lot to adjust to. The medical staff take immediate action to give him the best start in life.

Keeping your baby warm and dry

Because body temperature drops rapidly after birth, keeping your new baby warm and dry is important. If newborns become cold, their oxygen requirements increase. For this reason, a midwife dries the baby off, places him in a warmer or warmed cot, and then watches his temperature closely. Often the midwife wraps or swaddles the baby in a blanket and puts a little hat on him to reduce the loss of heat from the head – the site of most heat loss (just as your mother told you).

Boosting vitamin K stores

Vitamin K is important in the body's production of substances that help the blood to clot. This nutrient doesn't pass through the placenta to a baby very easily, however, and newborn livers, because they're immature, produce very little of it. So babies are typically low in this nutrient. Because of a shortage of vitamin K, a few babies develop a disease called *haemorrhagic disease of the newborn*. This disease is rare, but giving the baby vitamin K is an important preventive measure. Depending on the hospital's policy, your baby will receive vitamin K, usually by injection.

Understanding baby's developing digestive system

Most babies wet their nappies six to ten times a day by the time they're one week old. The frequency of bowel movements depends on whether you bottle- or breast-feed. Typically, a breast-fed baby has two or more bowel movements per day, whereas a formula-fed baby has only one or two per day.

Don't be surprised if your baby's first stool looks like thick, sticky, black tar – that's normal. This stool is called *meconium*. Ninety per cent of newborns pass their first stool within the first 24 hours, and almost all the rest do so by 36 hours. Later on, the colour of the stools lightens, and the texture becomes more normal. A formula-fed baby typically has semi-formed, yellow-green stools, whereas a breast-fed baby has looser, more granular, yellowish stools.

Most newborns urinate within the first few hours after birth, but some don't urinate until the second day. The passage of meconium and urine is an important sign that your baby's gastrointestinal and urinary tracts are functioning well.

Considering circumcision

Circumcision is the surgical removal of a male infant's penis foreskin. Some families choose to have this procedure carried out for cultural or religious reasons. Circumcision is now uncommon in the UK because no persuasive evidence exists to show that it offers any benefit to the baby.

Routine circumcision is not available on the NHS. Your GP or doctors at the hospital should be able to tell you how to go about organising a private circumcision, if you want your boy to have one.

Spending time in the neonatal intensive care unit

During the hospital stay after delivery (which often lasts only a few hours, but may be up to a few days), most newborns spend most or all of their time with their mothers. But sometimes newborns need the kind of extra attention they can get only in a *neonatal intensive care unit* (NICU) – sometimes called a *special care baby unit* (SCBU). Within such a unit, you may find a special area for critical care, where one-to-one nursing, sophisticated monitors, breathing machines, and so on are available. You may also find the so-called *transitional care unit*, for babies who aren't yet ready to join their mothers but don't need critical, one-to-one care.

If your paediatrician (you can read more about this specialist in Chapter 2) thinks that your baby needs the care offered by the neonatal intensive care unit, it doesn't automatically mean that something is wrong. Often, doctors place babies in special care units for a short while just for observation – or for any number of reasons. These are some of the most common (this list is far from inclusive):

- The baby was born prematurely.
- The baby does not weigh quite enough to make the birth-weight cut-off established by your particular hospital.
- The baby may need antibiotics – for example, because the mother had a fever during labour or because she had a prolonged rupture of membranes prior to delivery.
- The paediatrician may be concerned because the baby's breathing seems somewhat laboured. This reason is a relatively common one for putting a baby under observation for a short period of time.
- The baby has a fever or a seizure.
- The baby is anaemic.
- The baby is born with certain congenital abnormalities.
- The baby requires surgery.

Checking In: Baby's First Doctor's Visit

As well as the initial check-up your baby gets when first born (see the section 'Knowing What to Expect in the Hospital' earlier in this chapter), another formal examination occurs within a day or so of birth. If you have a home birth or are discharged within a few hours of delivery, your GP may carry out this check. Otherwise, your baby will be checked by one of the doctors or midwives at the hospital. When the doctor (or midwife) examines your baby, he checks the baby's general appearance, listens for heart murmurs, feels the fontanelles (the openings in the baby's skull where the various bones come together), looks at the extremities, checks the hips, and generally makes sure that the baby is in good condition.

A few days after delivery, often during a home visit from the community midwife, the midwife will carry out a variety of routine blood tests by pricking your baby's heel with a needle and taking a drop or two of blood (rather than comedian Tony Hancock's famous 'armful'). Your baby's blood is analysed for thyroid disease, *PKU* (a condition in which a person has trouble metabolising some amino acids, the 'building blocks' of protein), and sometimes other inherited metabolic disorders.

DON'T WORRY

The results of your baby's screening tests probably won't come back for a few days, but don't sit around worrying about them. If any of the results need further action, your midwife or doctor will let you know immediately.

Considering heart rate and circulatory changes

Remember how your practitioner checked the foetal heart rate during antenatal visits (see Chapter 3 for more on these visits)? You may have noticed then how fast the beat was. Before birth, the baby's heart rate is, on average, 120 to 160 beats per minute, and this heart rate pattern continues during the newborn period. Your baby's heart rate also can increase with physical activity and slow down when he sleeps.

One of the checks made on your baby at his first check-up is on his heart. If the practitioner hears any kind of *heart murmur* – an extra or different sound to the usual heart beat – your baby will be referred to a consultant paediatrician, usually for a special ultrasound scan called an echocardiogram. But don't worry – many murmurs go away on their own.

Looking at weight changes

Most newborns lose weight during their first few days of life – usually about 10 per cent of their body weight – which, of course, if you weigh only 7 or 8 pounds (3,200 or 3,600 grams), amounts to less than a pound (454 grams). This phenomenon is completely normal and is usually caused by fluid loss from urine, faeces, and sweat. During the first few days of life, the typical infant takes in very little food or water to replace this weight loss. Preterm babies lose more weight than full-term babies, and it may take them longer to regain their weight. In contrast, babies who are small for their gestational age may gain weight more rapidly. Generally, most newborns regain their birthweight by the tenth day of life, by the age of five months, they're likely to double it and by the end of the first year, they triple it.

Bringing Baby Home

Finally, the day comes when the hospital discharges you, and you can bring your baby home with you. This may be the same day as you give birth, or may even be as long as five days after birth, depending on your doctor's advice.

You must have an infant car seat to carry your baby in. Holding a baby while sitting in either the front or the back seat of a car is illegal. The only legal alternative to a car seat is a carrycot, which has the cover on and is secured with special straps. However, we always recommend a car seat. See Chapter 8 for more on selecting an appropriate car seat.

Sometimes the mother is ready to leave the hospital before her baby, for example when the baby is born prematurely and needs time to grow and mature before leaving the hospital, or has jaundice (you can find out more about jaundice later in this chapter).

Whatever the reason, going home without your new baby can cause you and your partner to feel incredibly disappointed and empty. If this happens to you, keep in mind that your feelings are completely normal. Going home alone after all the time you spent anticipating bringing the baby with you is difficult. Just remember that your baby will come home soon, and then you'll forget all about the first few days of separation. What's most important is that your baby comes home healthy.

Settling Baby in at Home

When the time comes, bringing your baby home is a great privilege and a huge responsibility. Suddenly, you are in charge of your baby's care, without the benefit of the hospital staff. You may have a partner, family members, or even a maternity nurse to help, but ultimately the responsibility is now yours. In this section, we go over many of the ways in which you take care of your newborn – everything except feeding, which we cover in Chapter 14.

Bathing

You don't have to give your baby a bath every day – two or three times a week is enough. Of course, your natural instinct may tell you that a daily bath is an essential, but too much water can actually dry your baby's skin out. In between baths, though, you should *top and tail* your baby every day.

Topping and tailing involves washing your baby's face, neck, hands, and bottom with warm (never hot) water. When you top and tail, take off all your baby's clothes except his nappy and vest (the nappy comes off for bottom washing only, to minimise accidents). You can hold your baby on your knee or lay him on a changing table – either way, it's easier than bathing.

Whether you're topping and tailing or bathing, you'll find the following hints helpful:

- Try to choose a time when your baby is wide awake but contented – more rewarding for both of you and much less like hard work.
- Make sure the room is warm enough (16–20°C is just right . . . you should be comfortable wearing your nightie).

- Use a fresh piece of cotton wool for every eye/ear/body part, to avoid spreading infection.
- Have all your supplies ready before you start:
  - Warm water
  - Two towels (in case of accidents)
  - Cotton wool
  - Mild soap and baby shampoo if you like (washing with no soap is fine, too)
  - A clean nappy
  - Clean clothes

To wash your baby's face, dip a piece of cotton wool in warm water and wipe gently around his eyes, from the nose outwards. Don't use soap on your baby's face.

TIP

Clean around your baby's ears with cotton wool, but don't clean inside them. Never put cotton buds in your baby's ears. Cotton buds can damage the sensitive lining of the ear canal, making the ears more prone to infection. (The same applies to adults, by the way.)

Keeping your little squirmer clean

You may find that bathing your squirming baby can be a little difficult, but following these tips can help you both enjoy bath time:

- Using your elbow, test the water temperature to make sure that it isn't too hot. (Your hand may not be as sensitive to heat.)
- Be sure that your baby's head and body are securely supported during the bath. Remember, your baby can't hold up his own head.
- Before you put your baby in the bath, wash his face as you would when you top and tail (see the section 'Bathing' for more about this cleaning method).
- Wash a baby girl's genitals from front to back to avoid washing any stool forward. For boys, clean underneath the scrotum and wash the foreskin without pulling back strongly on it.
- When you dry your baby, pat rather than rub, and pay special attention to the skin creases.
- If your baby has trouble settling down to sleep at night, you may want to consider a bath before bedtime – he may find it relaxing.

Of course we know that you know this, but never leave your baby unattended in the bath.

Burping

Often babies swallow air when they're feeding, especially if they're bottle-feeding. The accumulation of air inside a baby's stomach may make him feel uncomfortable. The good news is that all the discomfort goes away with one big burp. See Chapter 14 for some techniques that you may find helpful for burping your baby.

TIP

Keep a cloth nappy or towel over your shoulder while burping your baby. Babies often spit up some formula or milk when burping, and the cloth protects your clothes.

Sleeping and sudden infant death syndrome (SIDS)

Every new mother's worst nightmare must be the death of their baby from *sudden infant death syndrome* (SIDS), sometimes known as cot death. The causes of SIDS remain unproven, but taking simple precautions when you put your baby to bed reduces the risks enormously:

- Health care professionals recommend that babies sleep on their backs – not on their stomachs, which has been associated with SIDS. To keep your baby turned on his back, roll up a blanket and use it as a prop that prevents him from rolling over.
- Keep the room at the right temperature – invest in a nursery thermometer to make sure the temperature stays between 16 and 20°C.
- Always put your baby to bed with his feet at the foot of the cot, and keep his head uncovered.
- Don't smoke in your baby's room – as if the increased risk of infant chest infections and asthma weren't enough to deter you.

TIP

Other helpful pointers to consider when dealing with your baby's sleeping habits include:

- Keeping bright pictures or hanging objects around the cot to give your baby something interesting to look at when he is lying awake. But be careful not to place pillows or stuffed toys inside the cot, to minimise any risk of suffocation.
- Playing soft music before a nap may help your baby get into the mood for sleep.

- Rocking your baby to sleep. Be aware, however, that you may end up establishing a pattern that's difficult to reverse.
- Preventing your baby falling asleep with a formula- or milk-filled bottle in his mouth. This habit can lead to dental problems like tooth decay.

TIP

Some babies go through what's known as day-night reversal: They sleep during the day but are wide-awake at night. If this behaviour happens to your baby, you can try to keep him more awake during the daytime by stimulating him with pictures, toys, or activities. The good news is that most babies outgrow this syndrome and suddenly reverse their habits. If your baby's habits become a problem for you, you may want to consult your GP or health visitor.

Crying

Babies cry to express themselves. During the first week of life, some babies hardly cry at all and seem incredibly happy and peaceful, but by the second week, they can turn into the loudest criers in the world. Very often your baby is crying for help, and you can do something – feed him, hold him, change his nappy – to make him stop. Sometimes a baby cries for no apparent reason, and you may just have to let it happen – don't feel like a bad parent for doing so. Babies cry when they

- are hungry
- need a nappy change
- have wind and need to be burped
- are tired
- are uncomfortable – their clothes are too tight, they're too hot, or they don't like the position they're in, for example
- are over-stimulated
- want to be held
- want to suck on something

In most cases, you can use your own common sense to figure out how to calm your crying baby. But you may find it helpful at first to have a list of all the tried-and-tested strategies:

- Entertain the baby with a toy.
- Hold the baby in a warm, supportive, loving manner.

- Let the baby rest and relax in a quiet room (quiet except for the sound of his crying, that is) or put the baby down in his cot to rest.
- Play music (but probably not heavy metal!).
- Put the baby in the infant car seat and set the car seat on top of a running washing machine, holding on to it to make sure that the seat doesn't fall off. Some babies find the gentle shaking motion soothing.
- Rock the baby in a rocking chair or a baby swing, walk the baby (in a pram or pushchair or in your arms), or take him for a ride in the car.

If all else fails, and you're assured that your baby seems not to be suffering any real discomfort, you may need to just let him cry. Then the trick is to find a way not to let it bother you. (*Hint:* Try turning up the radio.)

C is for colic

If your baby cries for more than three hours a day, three days a week, for three consecutive weeks – that's colic. Doctors don't know the exact cause, but some think it may be related to intestinal discomfort. You may be lucky and never have this ugly creature rear its head. Or you may be like many of us who can remember the days of colic as if they were yesterday. Colic often starts at about 4 to 6 weeks and ends by about 12 weeks.

When your baby has colic, he cries and cries, with little that can be done to console him. Often this crying happens around 6 to 10 p.m. If you're working outside the home, and this is the time of day when you finally get to be with your baby, you may think that your baby doesn't like you. Be assured that the timing doesn't hinge on you – it's just that the evening hours are the bewitching hours. Thank goodness, colic almost always goes away by itself – if it doesn't, discuss it with your GP or health visitor.

Newborn jaundice

When your baby is 2 to 5 days old, his skin may take on a yellow-orange tint. This condition is known as *physiological jaundice of the newborn*, and it develops in about one-third of all babies. An increase in the concentration of bilirubin in the baby's blood causes jaundice. *Bilirubin* consists of by-products of haemoglobin from the baby's red blood cells, by-products that are normally disposed of through the liver and kidneys. Raised bilirubin levels may occur because a baby's liver isn't yet fully mature. (Significant jaundice is most common in preterm babies, whose livers are especially immature.)

Feeding the newborn early in life may help to decrease the risk of jaundice by keeping the baby well hydrated and stimulating the digestive tract.

If your newborn baby is jaundiced, your midwife will probably take a blood test. Depending on the result, they may advise you to go back to hospital (rare), take another test the next day (less rare), or reassure you that everything will be fine (most common). As long as your baby is looking less yellow by the day, and has been checked at least once, you're unlikely to have anything to worry about.

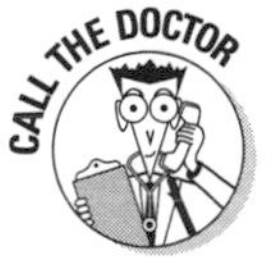

If your baby is still jaundiced when he's more than two weeks old, make an appointment for him with your GP. If, during a period of jaundice, your baby's urine is dark, and his stools are pale, take him to a doctor immediately.

Dummies (For Dummies)

New parents often fall into two schools of thought about dummy use – some can't live without it while others believe it only leads to problems down the road. The biggest advantage of a dummy is that it's often helpful in soothing a crying baby. The downside is that eventually, you need to rid your child of the dummy habit.

Is there any medical benefit or problem associated with the use of dummies? Fortunately, scientific data doesn't show any long-term adverse effects. Some people have been concerned about dummy use and early childhood dental cavities, but a review of the medical literature shows that no such association exists.

Preventing newborn injuries

Knowledge is the best road to prevention, and being aware of the common newborn injuries is the best way to prevent them from happening. The most common injuries to babies are caused by falls from furniture or being dropped, and in older infants (still under a year) falls down stairs or from baby walkers. Your newborn baby may not be able to roll by himself, but it's only a matter of weeks before he can.

From day one, get into the habit of treating your baby as though he can move by himself, and never leave him alone on your bed, on the changing table, or in a baby walker. Always be prepared for the next development stage in your baby's never-ending cycle of mobility.

Shopping for the baby

Newborn fashion is an industry all to itself. Many of the clothes made for babies today are lovely, cute, and adorable – and if you're tempted to buy things by the dozen, you're not alone. But be forewarned: You may end up using not even half the clothes you buy or receive as gifts. Newborns outgrow their clothes at a shocking pace. Also, as you become accustomed to daily life with your new baby, the novelty of sweet little clothes wears off, and your appreciation for practicality takes over.

In addition to clothing, your baby needs a full set of baby-specific household supplies. Here are some suggestions:

- **Toiletries:** Pick up a hairbrush, nail clippers, shampoo, and soap.
- **Linens:** You'll need towels, baby blankets, and cot sheets. Towelling squares are really useful when you burp your baby, or at any time for that matter – babies need no excuse to bring up milk.
- **Furniture:** You'll need a cot eventually, but you may be happy with a carrycot or Moses basket at first, especially if the baby is sleeping in your room. You'll also need a changing table or a changing mat.
- **Changing bag:** These bags come in all shapes and sizes; invest in one with an integral changing mat. A changing bag is invaluable for even the shortest trip away from home – keep it stocked with nappies, wet wipes (for cleaning baby's bottom without the need for water), bottles (if appropriate), a towelling square, and a change or two of clothes.
- **Car seat:** Check out Chapter 8 to find out what to look for.
- **Pram or pushchair:** The selection is almost endless, and you could drive yourself mad working out the pros and cons of them all. Appearance is important, but practicality is even more essential. If you're getting a pushchair and want to use it from birth, you'll need one that lies completely flat – newborn babies shouldn't sit up in pushchairs, as they don't have the muscle strength to control their heads.

REMEMBER

If you're considering buying secondhand baby items, you must check they're safe. The Baby Products Association offers a leaflet, called 'A child's safety is worth every penny', which advises you on what to look for. You can get a copy by calling their leaflet line on 01296 660990.

Registering Your Baby's Birth

Your baby isn't 'official' until you've registered his birth. Go along to your local Register Office in person to register your baby's birth. You can find the details of your local Register Office in the phone book.

In Scotland, you legally have to register your baby's birth within 21 days. In England, Wales, and Northern Ireland, you legally have 42 days to do so.

Be prepared to give the Registrar the following information:

- The sex of your baby
- The date and place of birth of your baby
- Your full name, surname, and date and place of birth
- Your usual address
- Your usual occupation
- The date of your marriage, if you're married

If you're married, either you or your husband can register your child's birth. If you're not married, the mother must do the registering. If you're not married, you don't have to include the father's details on the birth certificate. If you want to include both parents' details and you're not married, both of you will have to attend to register your baby. After all the paperwork is complete, the Registrar will give you:

- A birth certificate (which you'll need if you want to claim child benefit – see Chapter 4 for more on benefits)
- A form to take to your GP so that you can register your baby at his practice

You'll be given a short birth certificate, which is perfectly legal, free-of-charge. If you want a full birth certificate, however (prettier for framing but no more useful for legal purposes), you'll have to pay a fee.

Registering your baby's birth is a legal requirement in the UK.

Recognising Causes for Concern

New parents usually worry and are concerned by any possible signs that something may not be going perfectly with the new baby. If you haven't been around babies much, you may find that your own baby is a little hard to read, especially at first. Babies spit up all the time, and they develop little rashes and other problems. But when should you call the GP? Call your doctor

- If you notice a change in your baby's behaviour – for example, if a baby who usually falls asleep easily suddenly begins to cry a lot, or if a baby who is usually a healthy eater suddenly won't eat at all

- If your baby's breathing becomes laboured or is extremely short, shallow, and rapid
- If your baby has several episodes of diarrhoea or vomiting in a day
- If your baby has fewer than four wet nappies in a day
- If your baby's temperature is higher than 37.8 °C or less than 36.4 °C
- If your baby develops a sudden rash or discolouration of his skin

Chapter 13

Taking Care of Yourself after Delivery

In This Chapter

- Getting better after delivery
- Recovering from caesarean delivery
- Looking at postnatal changes
- Resuming your normal activities

According to the old adage, it takes nine months for a woman to make a baby and nine months for her body to return to normal afterwards. In reality, the time it takes to recover from childbirth varies widely from woman to woman. But most of the changes that your body goes through during pregnancy revert to normal during the *postnatal period* – sometimes called the *puerperium* – which begins immediately after delivery of the placenta and lasts for six to eight weeks.

REMEMBER

You need to make an appointment with your GP for a postnatal check-up about six weeks after you deliver. You can find out more about this appointment in the section 'Checking Your Progress: The First Postnatal Doctor Visit', later in this chapter.

As you go through this period of change, you're likely to have many questions about what you can do to make the postnatal transition as easy as possible. In this chapter, we tell you what life may be like as your body gets back into its old shape, as you begin to have sex again, and as you deal with all the physical and psychological challenges of new motherhood.

Recuperating from Delivery

The average hospital stay after an uncomplicated vaginal delivery is 6 to 36 hours. After a caesarean, you may stay in the hospital for three to four days.

In some hospitals, you spend this recovery period in the same room in which you delivered; in others, you move to a separate postnatal unit. The nurses continue to monitor your vital signs (blood pressure, pulse, temperature, and breathing) and check your uterus's position to make sure that it's firm and well contracted. Nurses (often the same ones taking care of you) also monitor your baby's vital signs. Your nurses can provide you with pain medication that your practitioner has prescribed, if you need it, and help you care for your *episiotomy* (see Chapter 11) or caesarean incision, if you have either one.

Looking and feeling like a new mum

Only in films and on TV do women throw on a sassy pre-pregnancy outfit and leave the hospital looking like they did before they even considered having a baby. Delivery takes a toll, and although most of the changes are fleeting, you'll notice that you look and feel different.

After delivery, your face may be swollen, very red, and possibly splotchy. Some women even have black eyes or broken blood vessels around their eyes and look as though they've just been in a prize fight. All these characteristics are to be expected; the rupture of tiny blood vessels in your face causes them during pushing. Don't be alarmed. You'll look like your old self again in a few days.

You'll also feel like yourself before long, but you're likely to experience *afterpains*, or contractions, persisting sporadically after delivery. These pains are similar to the contractions you experienced during labour and delivery, and they gradually fade away within a few days. You may find the afterpains are more noticeable while you're breast-feeding. If you've given birth before, you may find that the afterpains are much stronger than they were after your first delivery – this is quite normal, and doesn't mean anything's wrong. You may want to talk to your obstetrician or GP about getting painkillers to reduce the discomfort.

Understanding postnatal bleeding

DON'T WORRY

Experiencing vaginal bleeding after delivery is completely normal, even if you had a caesarean delivery. Average blood loss after a vaginal delivery is about half a litre, or one pint. After a caesarean, the average blood loss is twice that – about a litre, or two pints.

The blood coming from your vagina, called *lochia*, may initially appear bright red and contain clots. Over time, the lochia takes on a pinkish and later a brownish colour. The bleeding gradually diminishes in volume, but the flow may persist for three to four weeks after delivery. You may notice that the amount of bleeding increases each time you breast-feed. This increase happens because the hormones that help produce breast milk also cause your uterus to contract, and this contraction squeezes out any blood or lochia in the uterus. Many patients tell us that the bleeding is heavier when they stand up after being in bed for a while. This extra bleeding happens simply because the blood collects in the uterus and vagina while you're lying down, and when you stand up, gravity draws it out – it's perfectly normal.

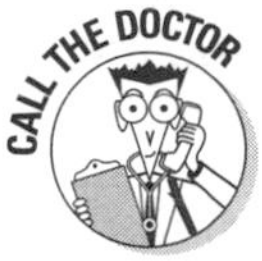

If you have very heavy bleeding with clots that lasts for several weeks after your delivery, let your GP know.

The best way to deal with postnatal bleeding is to use sanitary towels. Pads are available in varying thicknesses to accommodate whatever amount of bleeding you have. Don't use tampons because they may promote infection during the time that your uterus is still recovering. Although the bleeding usually subsides after two weeks, some women experience it for six to eight weeks. Occasionally, fragments of placental tissue stay within the uterus, and this condition can lead to extensive bleeding.

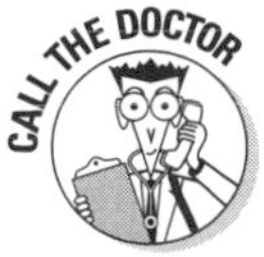

If the bleeding becomes significantly heavier, or starts to smell unusual, let your GP (or midwife, if this happens fewer than 10 days after delivery) know.

Dealing with perineal pain

The amount of pain or soreness you feel in your *perineum* (the area between the vagina and the rectum) depends largely on how difficult your delivery was. If your baby came out easily after only a couple of pushes and you have no episiotomy or lacerations, you probably feel little pain. If you pushed for three hours and delivered a 10-pound budding rugby player, you're more likely to have perineal discomfort. (See tips for handling the pain in the next section.)

The pain you feel has several causes: As the baby comes through the birth canal, it causes stretching and swelling of the surrounding tissues. Also, an episiotomy or tears in the perineum naturally hurt, just as an injury to any other part of your body would. The pain is worse during the first two days after delivery, but then rapidly improves and is usually nearly gone within a week.

Your perineum may be swollen, and if you had an episiotomy, you have stitches closing it up. Sometimes these stitches are visible on the outside, and sometimes they're buried underneath the skin.

Many women are concerned about the stitches used to sew up their episiotomy or lacerations. These sutures aren't meant to be removed – they gradually dissolve over the next one to two weeks. These stitches are strong enough to handle most activities, so don't worry that a sneeze, a difficult bowel movement, or lifting your 10-pound baby will cause them to tear open.

Keeping the perineal area clean to prevent an infection from developing is important. Such an infection is a rare complication, but call your doctor if you notice a foul-smelling discharge or increasing pain and tenderness in the area, especially if you have a fever higher than 38 °C.

Here are the best ways to care for your perineum as it recovers from your delivery:

- Keep the perineal area clean. You may want to use a spray bottle filled with warm water to help clean places that are difficult to reach.
- Some women get relief from pain by taking a *sitz bath*. A sitz bath consists of soaking your bottom in a small amount of warm water. At home, you can sit in a few inches of warm water in the bath. If you have a lot of swelling in the area, putting Epsom salts or sea salts in the water may give you added relief.
- An ice pack applied to the perineum during the first 24 hours after delivery helps minimise swelling and decreases your discomfort.
- Pain relievers such as paracetamol or diclofenac can help ease the pain. These medications aren't a problem if you're breast-feeding.
- Avoid standing for long periods of time, which can make the pain worse.
- After a bowel movement, try not to contaminate the area with the toilet tissue you use to wipe yourself. Clean the area around the anus with a separate toilet tissue, and don't wipe from back to front. If the areas around the anus or the perineum are tender, try to just pat the area dry, instead of wiping. You may find that using baby wipes is really helpful, because they clean the area very well, don't shred, and are gentle on healing tissues.
- Don't insert anything into your vagina (such as a tampon) for the first six weeks.

Relieving the gravitational pressure on your perineum from time to time by getting off your feet and lying down for a short while is important. Finding the time to lie down may be hard given that you're incredibly busy caring for a new baby, but make it a priority. And take heart – usually in a week, and certainly by two weeks, most of your discomfort is gone. If you're extremely uncomfortable, you may want to ask your doctor to prescribe pain medications.

If you had any lacerations that extended near your rectum, you may want to take a stool softener so that bowel movements aren't too painful. At least make sure that you drink extra fluids and consume extra fibre in your diet so that your stool is soft.

Surviving swelling

Immediately after delivery, especially after a vaginal delivery, you may discover that your entire body looks swollen. Don't freak out – it's normal. Many women develop swelling during the last few weeks of pregnancy, and this swelling often persists for a few days into the postnatal period. The intense pushing efforts required to deliver the baby may further cause your face and neck to swell, but this also goes away a few days after delivery. In general, it can take up to two weeks for the swelling to completely go away.

Don't step on the scales the day after you deliver. You may find that you have actually gained weight from all the water you retain during delivery.

Many patients ask, 'Isn't there something you can give me to help relieve the swelling?' Prescribing medication usually isn't necessary because the swelling goes away on its own in a few days, when you're back up and around. Just be patient; you *will* have ankles again.

Coping with your bladder

When you were pregnant, you probably felt like all you did was pee, right? Now, after you've given birth, you may actually find urinating difficult immediately after delivery, or you may feel discomfort when you do urinate. This discomfort is a result of the way the bladder and urethra are compressed when the baby's head and body come through the vagina. The tissues around the opening to the urethra are often swollen after delivery, and this swelling can add to the discomfort.

Some women may need to be *catheterised* (a thin, flexible plastic tube is inserted through the urethra into the bladder) after delivery to help empty the bladder. Urinary problems are sometimes worse in women who have an epidural, because the anaesthetic can hang around in your system for several hours and temporarily make your bladder more difficult to empty. But your bladder regains its normal tone a few hours after delivery, so urinary discomfort is usually a short-lived problem.

If you feel a burning sensation primarily during urination, let your doctor or nurse know, because it may be a sign that you're developing a urinary tract infection.

Some women experience the opposite problem; they find that they don't have good control over their bladder function – that they leak a little urine when they stand up or laugh. This problem is known as *stress incontinence*. Although potentially embarrassing, stress incontinence is nothing serious to worry about. Time usually solves the problem, but in some cases, you may take a number of weeks to get things under control.

Pelvic floor exercises (see 'Doing Pelvic floor exercises' later in this chapter) are great at cutting your chances of developing stress incontinence. Another good strategy is to make a conscious effort to go to the loo at regular intervals to empty your bladder before doing so becomes an emergency.

Battling the haemorrhoid blues

Most of your pushing efforts during delivery are focused toward the rectum, a fact that causes many women to develop *haemorrhoids* (also known as piles) – dilated veins that pop out from the rectum. Unfortunately, having no problems with piles before you go into labour is no guarantee that they won't appear after delivery. If you develop piles during the last part of your pregnancy, they may get worse after delivery. At times, piles can be more uncomfortable than an episiotomy, and they last a little longer. Turn to Chapter 8 for tips on dealing with piles.

The good news is that piles are usually temporary. Postnatal piles typically go away within a few weeks. Sometimes piles don't go away completely, but for the most part they aren't bothersome – they may not trouble you at all for a few months, and then they may be uncomfortable again for a few days, and then get better again.

Using a stool softener – talk to your GP or pharmacist about which ones are suitable – makes bowel movements less painful, and consuming plenty of fibre and fluids helps, too.

Understanding postnatal bowel function

Many women find that they don't have a bowel movement for a few days after delivery. This lack of bowel function may be because you haven't eaten much or because epidurals and some other pain medications sometimes slow down the bowels a little, and your system may take a few days to return to normal.

Avoiding a bowel movement isn't a great idea. You have no reason to be afraid of tearing the stitches. Tearing the sutures is extremely difficult, especially by having a bowel movement.

Continuing to recover at home

By the time you're discharged from the hospital after a vaginal delivery, most of the acute pain is gone. After you get home, however, you can still expect some soreness. The main area of discomfort is around your perineum. No matter how easy your delivery may have been, this part of your body has undergone some real trauma, and it simply needs time to heal.

Try not to let the lingering discomfort associated with having just given birth frustrate you. Keep in mind what an amazing miracle your body has just been through. In addition to dealing with the soreness from delivery, you need to adjust to a new lifestyle – getting up at all hours of the night, changing nappies, and feeding your new baby.

Recovering from a Caesarean Delivery

The hospital stay after a caesarean delivery is generally a few days longer than after a vaginal delivery – usually three to four days in total. If you have a caesarean delivery, you'll be put on a trolley immediately afterward and transported to the recovery room. You may be able to hold your baby in your arms during the trip.

Going to the recovery room

When you're in the recovery room, your midwife and *anaesthetist* (the doctor who deals with local and general anaesthetics) will monitor your vital signs. The midwife periodically checks your abdomen to make sure that the uterus is firm and that the dressing over the incision is dry. Your midwife also checks for signs of excessive bleeding from the uterus. You'll probably have had a catheter in your bladder, and it stays in place for the first night so that you don't have to worry about getting up to go to the loo. You'll also have an intravenous (IV) line in place to receive fluids and any medications your doctor prescribes. If you had an epidural or spinal anaesthetic, your legs may still seem a little numb or heavy. This feeling wears off in a few hours. If you had general anaesthetic (that is, if you were put to sleep), you may feel a little groggy when you get to the recovery room. Just as with a vaginal delivery, you may experience some shaking (see Chapter 11). If you're up to it and if you want to, you can breast-feed your baby while you're in the recovery room (see more about breast-feeding in Chapter 14).

You'll probably have received pain medication in the operating room, and you won't need any more while you're in the recovery room. In some hospitals, if you've had an epidural or spinal anaesthetic, your anaesthetist will inject a long-lasting medication into the catheter that keeps you almost pain-free for about 24 hours. If, however, your pain medication doesn't seem to be working, let your nurse know.

Taking it one step at a time

When your nurse and anaesthetist are confident that your vital signs are stable and that you're recovering normally from the anaesthetic, you'll be discharged from the recovery room – generally about one to three hours after delivery. You'll be transported on a stretcher to the ward, where you'll spend the rest of your recovery time.

The day of delivery

On the day of your caesarean, you should plan on just staying in bed. Thanks to your catheter, you won't need to worry about getting up to go to the loo. If you had your surgery early in the morning, you may feel like getting up later in the evening, even if only to sit in a chair. Just be sure to check with your nurse first to see whether getting up is okay. When you get up the first time, make sure that someone is there to help you.

Although some doctors still prefer that patients not have any food immediately after a caesarean, many doctors now allow women to eat and drink shortly after the surgery. Often, we find that the patient is the best judge of what she should and shouldn't do: If you feel queasy and nauseous, you're better off not eating. But if you feel hungry, drinking liquids and having small amounts of solid food is probably fine.

Like women who have had a vaginal delivery, expect some vaginal bleeding (*lochia*) after a caesarean. The bleeding may be quite heavy during the first few days after your surgery (see 'Understanding postnatal bleeding' earlier in this chapter).

DON'T WORRY

Most women who have a caesarean delivery and have staples in their skin worry that removing the staples will hurt. But don't worry – staple removal is a quick and painless procedure.

The day after

The first day after your surgery, your doctor is likely to encourage you to get out of bed and start to walk around. The first couple of times you get up to walk may be pretty uncomfortable – you may feel pain around the incision in your abdomen – so you may want to ask for a so-called *top up* dose of pain medication 20 minutes or so before getting up.

Make sure someone is with you the first few times you get up to make sure that you don't fall.

Depending on your fluid needs, your doctor may also discontinue your IV line. Most of the time, you're able to drink liquids on the first day, and many doctors also let you eat solid food.

You'll probably have a bandage over your abdominal incision. Sometimes this bandage comes off on day one, but sometimes doctors prefer to leave it on longer.

Understanding post-caesarean pain

You may feel a kind of burning pain at the site of your abdominal skin incision. This pain is worse when you get out of bed or change positions. Eventually, the burning diminishes to a sort of tingling sensation and is much improved within a week or two after surgery.

You may also feel pain from post-delivery uterine contractions – just as women who deliver vaginally do. Pain from contractions diminishes by the second day, although it may recur when you breast-feed, because breast-feeding can trigger more contractions.

You may feel pain in tissues deep beneath your skin. A caesarean isn't a simple slit through the surface of a woman's belly. The incision cuts through several layers of tissue to reach the uterus and each layer must then be repaired. Every one of the repaired incisions can generate pain, which is why you may feel pain deep in your abdomen after a caesarean. This pain usually takes one to two weeks to fade away. Many women tell us that they feel more pain on one side or the other, possibly because the stitches are a little tighter on one side. Whatever the reason, uneven pain is very common and nothing to worry about.

If you have a caesarean delivery after going through labour for hours, you may have perineal pain – from pushing and from any number of internal examinations – on top of everything else. This pain disappears soon after delivery.

Dealing with post-op pain

The amount of pain or discomfort experienced after a caesarean delivery varies from woman to woman, depending on the circumstances of her delivery and on her tolerance for pain. Your doctor can prescribe pain medication, but she will probably specify that the medication shouldn't be given unless you ask for it. (Sometimes this is hospital policy.) So if you want the pain relief, ask for it – before your pain becomes excruciating. Ask for the medication when you anticipate getting out of bed or just before your next dose of medication is due (usually after three or four hours), so that you give your nurse enough time to get it for you.

Getting ready to go home

After surgery, you'll find that each day is noticeably easier and more comfortable than the one before. Over the course of three days, you'll gradually find it easier to get out of bed and walk around. You'll start to eat normally again. You'll also be able to shower – and many women find that first shower a big relief. But please remember that you have just been through not only major surgery but also nine months of pregnancy – and you must recover from both. Some women really do recover quickly and feel like going home after only a couple of days. But many women need more time to feel strong enough to leave the hospital.

The length of your stay may be determined to some extent by how quickly you recover, or by the hospital's policy. Occasionally, you may have to stay in hospital longer because of a post-operative infection or some other complication. But typically, you're ready to go home after about three days.

Here are some indications that you may be ready to go home:

- You tolerate food and liquids without any problem.
- You urinate normally and without difficulty.
- Your bowels are on their way to recovering normal function.
- You have no signs of infection.

Continuing to recover at home

When you're discharged from the hospital after a caesarean delivery, you're well on your way down the road to recovery. However, getting back on your feet after a caesarean delivery takes longer than after a vaginal delivery, so take it easy for the first week or two after you return home.

Taking good care of yourself

Get the help you need from family and friends, if possible. If you can afford it, consider hiring professional help – a maternity nurse – for the first few weeks. (A maternity nurse can be helpful for women who've had vaginal births, too.) Try to keep the household chores you do to a minimum. Avoid running up and down stairs a lot. Devote your energy to taking care of your new baby and taking care of yourself. Pay attention, and your body will clearly let you know how much activity you can handle.

If you've had a caesarean section, many doctors recommend that you don't drive until six weeks after your operation. This restriction is easy to forget with all the other exciting changes going on around you, but a caesarean section is major abdominal surgery.

Most doctors also advise you to postpone any abdominal exercises until after your six-week check-up (see 'Checking Your Progress: The First Postnatal Doctor Visit', later in this chapter), so that the incisions in all the layers of your abdomen have time to heal completely. Most women feel pretty much back to normal by the six-week point; but others need as long as three months to fully recover.

By the time you're home from the hospital, you should be able to eat normally. If you lost a great deal of blood during your surgery, however, you may want to ask your doctor if you should take extra iron supplements.

Noticing changes in your scar

At first, the scar from your caesarean delivery looks reddish or pinkish. In time, the scar may turn a darker shade of purple or brown, depending to some extent on your skin colour. Over the course of a year, the scar will fade and, eventually, assume a very pale colour. If you have dark skin, the scar may be a brownish colour. Most of the time, a caesarean scar is pencil thin or even thinner. A scar from a caesarean delivery may look prominent immediately after the procedure, when the staples are still in place, but after they're removed and the scar has several weeks to heal, you'll observe how it begins to fade into something far less obvious.

Many factors can affect the healing process and thus determine what the scar ultimately looks like. Some women naturally are prone to form a thick type of scar, called a *keloid* – in these cases, doctors really can't do much to change the situation.

You may notice that the area around your incision becomes numb. This numbness occurs because in making the incision, your doctor cut through some of the nerves that transmit sensation in that area. The nerves do grow back, however, and in time the numbness turns into a mild tingling sensation and then returns to normal.

Some women notice a blood-tinged fluid discharge coming from the centre or side of their incision. This drainage sometimes happens when blood and other fluids accumulate under the incision and then seep out. If only a small amount of fluid oozes out and then stops, it's okay.

If you notice persistent blood-tinged or yellowish discharge from your incision, let your doctor know. Occasionally, the incision may open at the point where the drainage occurs – if so, your doctor may want you to take special measures to keep the opening clean so that it heals on its own.

Recognising causes for concern

Most women who have caesarean deliveries recover without any problems. In some cases, however, you may not heal quickly and smoothly. Call your doctor if you notice any of the following:

- If pain from your incision or from your abdomen increases, rather than decreases
- If large amounts of blood or blood-tinged fluid drain from your incision
- If you have a fever higher than 38 °C
- If your incision begins to open up

The Party's Not Over: More Postnatal Changes

Many aspects of postnatal life are the same whether you had a vaginal or a caesarean delivery. Now that you're no longer pregnant, your body begins shifting back to its pre-pregnancy state, and you're in for a number of changes.

Sweating like a . . . new mum

If you're managing to get any sleep at night despite having a new baby in the house, you may find that you wake up drenched in sweat. Even during the daytime, you may notice that you perspire significantly more than usual.

This sweating is very common and is thought to have something to do with fluctuations in hormone levels that occur as your body returns to a non-pregnant state and is very similar to the night sweats and hot flushes that menopausal women get, due to a drop in oestrogen levels. As long as the sweating isn't associated with any fever, it's not a problem and it goes away over the course of the next month or so.

Dealing with breast engorgement

A woman's breasts typically begin to *engorge* – fill with milk – three to five days after she delivers her baby. You may be amazed to see how huge your breasts can really be. If you're breast-feeding, your baby lessens the problem for you as she gets the hang of breast-feeding, figures out how to take in more milk, and establishes a pattern of feeding. (See Chapter 14 for more information about breast-feeding.)

TIP

If you're not breast-feeding, you may find that your breasts stay engorged for 24 to 48 hours (which can be quite painful), and then you begin to feel better. Wearing a tight-fitting supportive bra may make the process a little less uncomfortable. Applying ice packs or bags of frozen peas to your breasts helps the milk to 'dry up', as does taking cold showers. Cold temperature causes the blood vessels in the breasts to constrict, lessening milk production, while warmth causes the blood vessels to dilate, promoting milk production.

Understanding hair loss

One of the stranger aspects of the postnatal return to normality is hair loss. A few weeks or months after delivery, most women notice that they're shedding like crazy. This shedding is normal – it is one of the effects that oestrogen has on your body during pregnancy. This common problem doesn't last long and your hair is usually back to normal by about nine months after delivery.

TECHNICAL STUFF

All hair follicles go through three phases of development: a *resting* phase, a so-called *transitional* phase, and a *shedding* phase. The elevated levels of oestrogen that are present during pregnancy essentially freeze your hair in the resting phase. Within a few months after delivery, all that hair proceeds on to the shedding phase. Suddenly, you notice large amounts of hair sticking in your brush or washing down the drain.

Chasing away the baby blues

The vast majority of women – as many as 80 per cent, studies show – suffer a bout of the blues during the first days and weeks after they deliver. Typically, you begin to feel a little down a few days after the birth, and you may continue to feel vague sadness, uncertainty, disappointment, and emotional discontent for a few weeks. Many women are surprised at the feeling; after all, they've looked forward to motherhood, and they feel sure that they're really thrilled about it.

No one knows for sure *why* women get the postnatal blues, but a few explanations are plausible. First, the shift in hormone levels that comes after delivery can affect mood. Also, when pregnancy ends, a mother must change her whole focus. After focusing on the birth for so many months, she suddenly finds that the big event is over, and she may feel almost a sense of loss. And face it – parenthood brings tremendous anxiety, especially for a first-time mother. Feeling overwhelmed by all the responsibility and all she needs to figure out about caring for a baby isn't unusual for a woman. Add in the physical discomfort – episiotomy repair, breast tenderness, haemorrhoids, fatigue, and the rest – and you begin to wonder how any new mother can avoid feeling a little blue.

REMEMBER

Fortunately, postnatal blues tend to fade away rather quickly, usually by about two to four weeks after the birth. Remember that what you're feeling is extremely common and that it doesn't mean you don't love your child or that you won't be a fabulous parent. Be open about it; let your partner, family members, and friends know how you feel, because you need love and support at this time.

TIP

If you find yourself suffering from the baby blues, remember that you're not the first woman to feel this way. The feeling is as normal as pregnancy itself. And take heart: Those who have already grappled with the problem have found a number of ways to ease the blues. Consider this list of some of the best strategies:

- Lack of sleep compounds the problem of the baby blues. Everything is worse when you're physically fatigued. The amount of stress that you can handle when you've had your rest is much greater than if you haven't slept enough. So try to get more sleep. If the baby is napping, try to lie down and snooze.
- Accept other people's offers of help. In most cases, you don't have to take care of your baby entirely by yourself. You're a great mum, even if you do let Aunt Flo change a nappy or burp the baby.

- Talk about how you feel with other mothers, close family members, and friends. You're likely to find that they felt exactly as you do now. They can empathise with you and offer suggestions for how to cope.
- If possible, try to get some time to yourself. Often, new parents are overwhelmed by the realisation that their time is no longer their own. Get out of the house, if you can. Take a walk, read, watch a film, or get some exercise. Have dinner with your partner or with a friend.
- Pamper yourself with a manicure or pedicure, a trip to the hair salon, or a massage. Often the blues are exacerbated by the fact that your body still isn't back to what it used to be, and doing something that makes you feel beautiful may help.

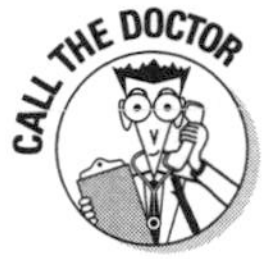

If you have postnatal blues and they don't go away after three or four weeks, if the feeling seems to be getting worse, or if you develop the blues more than two months after your delivery, discuss the situation with your doctor. Your blues may have blossomed into fully-fledged postnatal depression.

Recognising postnatal depression

True *postnatal depression* isn't nearly as common as the blues, but it does affect more women than you may imagine – between 10 and 15 per cent. Postnatal depression usually starts about 2 to 8 weeks after you have your baby, (but sometimes as long as 6 or 12 months after). Symptoms include

- Feeling tired all the time, but having problems sleeping
- Not enjoying life in general or being with your baby
- Lacking interest in caring for your baby
- Bursting into tears for no reason
- Losing your appetite or overeating
- Feeling hopeless
- Feeling guilty
- Finding it hard to cope
- Suffering from anxiety or panic attacks
- Experiencing thoughts of harming the baby or yourself

Postnatal depression goes unnoticed all too often because the symptoms are put down to another cause, or because you feel guilty about feeling depressed when you have a beautiful new baby at home. Postnatal depression is common, it's not your fault, and it's eminently treatable. So if these symptoms sound familiar, it is really important to talk to your GP.

Treatment for postnatal depression includes counselling (group or individual psychotherapy), antidepressant medications, and, rarely, hospitalisation. Your doctor may want to check to see if you have postnatal thyroid disease, which can mask itself as depression or make your depression worse.

For more information on postnatal depression, you can get in touch with the following support groups:

- The Association for Postnatal Illness, 25 Jerdan Place, London SW6 1BE. Tel: 020 7386 0868.
- Meet-a-Mum Association (MAMA), 26 Avenue Road, South Norwood, London SE25 4DX. Tel: 020 8771 5595; Helpline: 020 8768 0123 (Monday–Friday 7–10 p.m.).

Checking Your Progress: The First Postnatal Doctor Visit

Most practitioners ask their patients to come in for a check-up about six weeks after delivery if both the pregnancy and the birth were uncomplicated. If you had a caesarean or some complication, you may be asked to come in earlier.

This check-up is for you, not the baby – although of course you're welcome to take your baby with you. At this postnatal check, your GP chats about your physical recovery, how feeding your baby is going, how you're coping with motherhood, and how you're feeling mentally (all the areas we talk about earlier in this chapter, in fact). Your GP may want to carry out an internal examination and a cervical smear test if you're due for one. Your GP will also chat with you about your contraceptive needs (yes, you've just given birth to the best form of contraception known to man, but there really will be a day when you contemplate having sex again!).

Returning to 'Normal' Life

Your body typically needs six to eight weeks for the changes that you experience during pregnancy to disappear – which means that, after delivery, your body needs some time to get back in shape for your day-to-day activities, let alone for vigorous exercise or sex.

Getting fit all over again

Making exercise a priority after delivery is important for every new mum. Fitness has many important benefits for both your physical and emotional wellbeing – it can help your body recover from the stress of pregnancy, and it helps you feel more even-tempered and better about yourself.

Resume your sports and workouts gradually. Naturally, the amount of exercise you can handle depends on what kind of shape you've been in before and during your pregnancy.

After pregnancy, restoring strength to your abdominal muscles is especially important. In some women, pregnancy causes the abdominal or *rectus* muscles to separate a little, as shown in Figure 13-1. The medical term for this separation is *diastasis*. Doing abdominal exercises to restore these muscles' strength and draw them together is important.

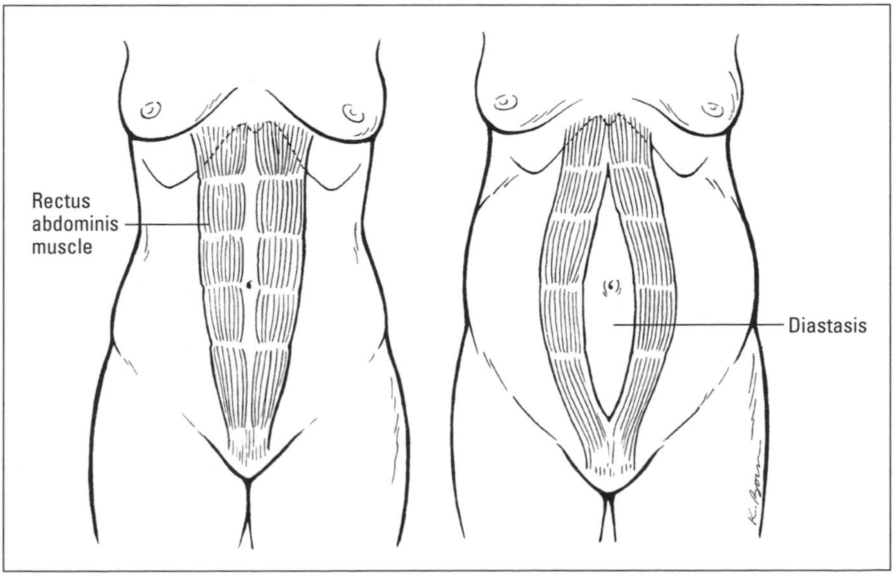

Figure 13-1: After pregnancy, your abdominal muscles may be separated a bit, one side from the other.

Over the course of the two weeks after you deliver, depending on how you feel, you can gradually increase your exercising until you're fully active again. Finding the time for exercise may be a problem, of course, but fitting it into your schedule is worth every effort. Taking care of a newborn can make you feel as though you've just run a marathon, but real exercise is what your body needs. In fact, by improving your overall sense of wellbeing, exercise can make the whole challenge of caring for a new baby much easier.

If you've had a caesarean delivery, don't lift anything in the few weeks after you deliver. You'll need to take extra precautions with other forms of exercise, too. A *physiotherapist* (a health care professional who specialises in exercise) will visit you while you're in hospital to give further advice.

Walking is great exercise for just about everyone (including almost everyone who's had a caesarean delivery). During the first two weeks after delivery, take it slow; but after that, you may find that long or brisk walks are enjoyable for both you and your baby – and a great form of exercise.

Losing the weight

You may feel like jumping on the scales right after delivery to see how much weight you've lost. But take caution – some women do lose a lot of weight quickly after delivery, but some actually gain weight from all the fluid retention. Rest assured that you'll soon weigh less than you did before you delivered, probably about a stone less, but the loss may not register until a week or two after delivery.

Refer to Table 13-1 to see what accounts for the initial weight loss.

Table 13-1	Losing Weight After Birth
Baby	6 to 9 pounds (2.72 to 4.08 kilograms)
Placenta	1 to 2 pounds (0.45 to 0.91 kilograms)
Amniotic fluid	1 to 2 pounds (0.45 to 0.91 kilograms)
Maternal fluids	4 to 8 pounds (1.81 to 3.63 kilograms)
Shrinking uterus	1 pound (0.45 kilogram)

Your uterus continues shrinking for several weeks. Immediately after you deliver, your uterus still extends up to about the level of your navel – about the same point as when you were 20 weeks pregnant. However, because of the excess skin you now have, you probably still look pregnant when you stand up. Don't let your appearance get you down. Your uterus keeps contracting and your skin regains much of its tone until, by about two months after delivery, your belly is down to its pre-pregnancy size.

Most women need two to three months to get back to their normal weight, but, of course, the time varies according to how much weight you gain during pregnancy. A healthy diet and regular exercise help the weight come off.

Try to get as close to your pre-pregnancy weight – or your ideal body weight (see Chapter 5) – as soon as is reasonably possible. You don't have to let a pregnancy turn into a permanent weight gain. If you let each successive pregnancy cause a little more accumulation, your health may suffer in the long run.

Pondering your postnatal diet

Any woman who's just had a baby needs to once again examine her diet. If you're breast-feeding, ensure, as you did when you were pregnant, that you're eating a healthy combination of foods that provide both you and your baby with good nutrition. You also need to make sure you're getting enough fluids. The best approach to weight loss involves exercise, plus a well-balanced diet, low in fat but with a mix of protein, carbohydrates, fruit, and vegetables. (For more information about how to follow a balanced, nutritious diet, see Chapter 5.)

Doing pelvic floor exercises

Pelvic floor exercises are squeezing motions aimed at strengthening the muscles of the pelvic floor that surround the vagina and rectum. These muscles give support to the bladder, rectum, uterus, and vagina. Keeping these muscles strong is key to reducing the adverse effects that pregnancy and delivery can have on this part of your body. If your pelvic floor muscles are very weak, the chances are greater that you will develop *urinary stress incontinence* – a leakage of urine when you cough, sneeze, laugh, or jump – or *prolapse* or *protrusion* of the rectum, vagina, and uterus – in which these organs begin to sag below the pelvic floor.

Pregnancy places extra weight on the pelvic floor muscles, and vaginal delivery stretches and puts added pressure on them – the net result is a general weakening. Some women seem to naturally maintain excellent muscle tone in the pelvic floor after delivery. But other women notice symptoms of weakness – a little urinary incontinence, the feeling that their vagina is loose, or pressure on their pelvic floor from a sagging uterus, vagina, or rectum. The way to strengthen the pelvic floor muscles – to avoid or diminish these symptoms – is to perform pelvic floor exercises.

To perform these exercises, you tighten the muscles around your vagina and rectum. Here's a simple way to find out what it feels like to do the exercises correctly: Sometime when you're urinating, try to stop the flow of urine midstream (sometimes called the emergency stop – but don't try this exercise in a car). Or insert a finger in your vagina and try to tighten the muscles around your finger. If you're doing pelvic floor exercises correctly, your finger feels the squeeze. (Both of these techniques are simply ways of figuring out how to squeeze the muscles, not the way you normally practise the exercise.)

When you're first doing pelvic floor exercises, squeeze the muscles for as many as ten seconds and then release. Squeeze five to ten times per session, and try to do three to four sessions a day. Ultimately, you can build up to the point where you hold each squeeze for 10 seconds and do 25 squeezes per session. Continue to do the exercises four times a day. You can do squeezes while you're sitting, standing, or lying down, and you can do them while you're also doing something else – bathing, cooking, chatting on the phone, watching television, driving your car, or queuing at the supermarket check-out.

Having sex again

If you're like most postnatal women, sex is the last thing on your mind. Many women find that their interest in sex declines considerably during the first weeks and months after pregnancy. But at some point, the fatigue and emotional stress of childbirth ease up, and your thoughts are likely to be more amorous again. For some women (and their lucky partners), the rebound occurs fairly quickly; for others, it may take 6 to 12 months.

The drastic hormonal shifts that occur after delivery directly affect your sex organs. The precipitous drop in oestrogen leads to a loss of lubrication for your vagina, and less engorgement of blood vessels, as well. (Increased blood flow to the vagina is a key aspect of sexual arousal and orgasm.) For these reasons, intercourse after childbirth can be painful and sometimes not all that satisfying. With time, as hormone levels return to their pre-pregnancy norm, the problem tends to correct itself. In the meantime, using a water-based lubricant helps.

The exhaustion and stress of caring for an infant further reduces the desire for sex in some women. Your attention, and your partner's, too, is likely to be focused more on the baby than on the relationship between the parents. Set aside some time for the two of you to be alone together. This time together need not even include sex – just holding, hugging, and expressing feelings for each other.

Most doctors recommend that women refrain from intercourse for four to six weeks after the baby is born in order to give the vagina, uterus, and perineum time to heal and for the bleeding to subside. At your six-week follow-up doctor visit, you can ask your practitioner about various methods of birth control (see the next section).

Choosing contraception

Many people believe that breast-feeding prevents a woman from becoming pregnant. Although breast-feeding *usually* delays the return of ovulation (and, thus, periods), some women who are breast-feeding do ovulate – and do conceive again (see Chapter 14). You may not ovulate the entire time that you breast-feed, or you may start again as early as two months after delivery. And if you don't breast-feed, ovulation begins, on average, ten weeks after delivery, although it has been reported to occur as early as four weeks. If you breast-feed for less than 28 days, your ovulation will usually return at the same time as it does for non-breast-feeding women. So considering your options for birth control before you have sex again is important. Most women have a wide range of birth-control options. But some women have medical conditions that prevent them from using certain methods. Discuss your options with your GP at a postnatal visit.

Chapter 14

Feeding Your Baby

In This Chapter

- Breast or bottle – making the decision that's right for you
- Getting into the breast-feeding routine
- The basics of formula feeding

One of the first big decisions any new parents make is whether to breast-feed their infant or use *formula* (milk, in powder or liquid form, designed for babies) and bottles. Although the majority of parents choose to breast-feed, the decision is by no means an easy one. If you find the decision difficult, take comfort in the fact that both choices are sound and legitimate. In this chapter, we lay out the basic first steps you need, no matter which way you go.

For more tips on feeding your baby, check out *Breastfeeding For Dummies* by Sharon Perkins and Carol Vannais (Wiley).

Deciding between Breast and Bottle

Ask almost anyone – your midwife, your GP, your friends, total strangers – and they will advise you to breast-feed. Bottle-feeding became all the rage in the 1950s, when scientists developed techniques to pasteurise and store cows' milk in formulas appropriate for infant nutrition. Breast-feeding has regained popularity largely because people and organisations (such as the Royal College of Midwives) have recognised its many medical benefits.

The decision whether or not to breast-feed isn't simply a medical one, however: issues of convenience, aesthetics, body image, and even conditions surrounding delivery all play their part. The decision about how to feed the baby is a personal one that every mother must decide for herself. Figuring out how to breast-feed takes an incredible commitment, so don't feel pressured to do so if your heart isn't in it. If you've decided that bottle-feeding is the best decision for you and your baby, don't feel guilty about it.

Sizing up the advantages of breast-feeding

Breast-feeding gives your baby a tailor-made formula for good nutrition, and a whole lot more:

- Human breast milk can strengthen the baby's immune system and help prevent allergies, asthma, and sudden infant death syndrome (SIDS). It can also decrease the number of upper respiratory infections in the baby's first year of life.
- Human breast milk is perfectly designed for your baby's needs, containing all the minerals, vitamins, and other nutrients your baby needs, in exactly the right proportions. Your baby won't need any other source of food for the first 4–6 months of life.
- Mother's milk contains nutrients ideally suited to a baby's digestive system. Cows' milk isn't as easily digested, and your baby can't readily use the nutrients it contains.
- Human milk also contains *antibodies* – substances produced by your body as part of its *immune system* that fight off infection. Antibodies help protect your baby from infection until his own immune system matures.
- Breast-feeding is emotionally rewarding. Many women feel that they develop a special bond with their baby when they breast-feed, and they enjoy the closeness surrounding the whole experience.
- Breast-feeding is convenient. You can't leave home without it. You never have to carry bottles or formula with you.
- Mother's milk is cheaper than formula and bottles.
- You don't have to warm up breast milk; it's always the perfect temperature.
- Breast-feeding provides some form of birth control (though it's not totally reliable – see the section 'Looking at options for contraception' later in this chapter).
- *Lactation* (milk production) causes you to burn extra calories, which may help you lose some of the weight you gained during pregnancy. A breast-fed baby is less likely to get constipated than a bottle-fed baby.

- A breast-fed baby's bowel movements don't have as strong an odour as those babies who formula-feed (and believe us, this odour should not be taken lightly!).
- Breast milk is organic – no additives, no preservatives – and is less likely than cows' milk to cause your baby an allergic reaction.
- Women who breast-feed are likely to reduce their lifetime risk of breast cancer.

TIP

If you're a bottle-feeder your baby can still benefit from a short period of breast-feeding. For example, antibodies, which fight off infection, are especially plentiful in your *colostrum* – the yellowish, watery-looking milk you produce in the first few days after delivery. And breast-feeding for a couple of months will give your baby added protection against infection for several months afterwards.

Checking out the benefits of bottle-feeding

Bottle-feeding also offers plenty of benefits. You may decide to choose this option for any of the following reasons:

- You don't want to breast-feed. If your heart isn't in it, then things aren't going to work out – too much trial-and-error is involved in making breast-feeding work for someone who's not truly committed to succeed.
- You've tried breast-feeding, and your breasts don't produce enough milk to feed your baby (or babies). Lots of women think they can't produce enough milk, but probably about 95 per cent can. In many cases, you'll produce enough milk if you change your breast-feeding technique or patterns.
- Bottle-feeding may better fit your lifestyle. Although many working mothers breast-feed, many feel that juggling the requirements of their job with those of breast-feeding is just too difficult.

  TIP

  Both your baby and you benefit from breast-feeding – even for a short time (refer to the section 'Sizing up the advantages of breast-feeding' earlier in this chapter). If lifestyle is your reason for bottle-feeding, talk to your midwife or health visitor about how to wean your baby off breast-feeding before you return to work, rather than bottle-feeding from the start.
- Bottle-feeding enables others to feed the baby.
- If you have a chronic infection – HIV, for example – bottle-feeding helps ensure that you don't pass the infection to the baby via breast milk.

Women who carry the hepatitis B virus can breast-feed as long as the baby has received the hepatitis B vaccine.

- If you or your baby is very sick after delivery, bottle-feeding may be your only option. Sometimes, a mother can feed with breast milk from a pump, and breast-feed later on, when she or the baby recovers, but this option isn't always possible and often requires the assistance of a breast-feeding specialist.
- If you've had previous surgery on your breasts, bottle-feeding may be your best bet (you may not be able to breast-feed).
- If you take certain medications, bottle-feeding may be best. Some women take medications that can pass through the breast milk and affect the baby adversely. Such drugs include anticancer and anti-leukaemia drugs (such as cyclophosphamide, doxorubacin, methotrexate, and cyclosporin), bromocriptine, lithium, and some migraine treatments (ergotamine, specifically). Ask your GP about any medications you take regularly.

Latching onto Breast-feeding

Pregnancy goes a long way toward preparing your body for breast-feeding. The key pregnancy hormones cause the breasts to enlarge and prepare the glands inside the breasts to lactate. But you can prepare yourself for day-to-day nursing. You can, for example, toughen your nipples a bit – and thus minimise soreness later on – in a few different ways:

- Wear a nursing bra with the flaps down (allowing your clothing to rub against your nipples).
- Roll your nipples between your thumb and forefinger for a minute or so each day.
- Rub your nipples briskly with a flannel after bathing or showering.

Be aware, however, that stimulating your nipples late in your pregnancy can bring on uterine contractions (refer to Chapter 8). When you near the end of your pregnancy, ask your practitioner before doing this kind of stimulation. One way to get around this problem is to avoid the nipple itself and just rub petroleum jelly, or baby oil, over the *areola* (the darker-coloured area around your nipple).

Some women have inverted nipples and worry during pregnancy that their nipples will make breast-feeding difficult. Usually, the problem corrects itself before the baby is born, but a few techniques can help things along:

- Use the thumb and forefinger on one hand to push back the skin around the areola. If this action doesn't bring out the nipple, gently grasp it with your other thumb and forefinger, pull it outward, and hold it for a few minutes. Do this exercise several times a day.

- You can also try wearing special plastic breast cups called Mexican hats (available at most chemists) designed to help draw out the nipple over time.

Start one of these preparation techniques for short sessions during the second trimester and then gradually increase the amount of time you work your nipples or wear the cups until your nipples stay out on their own.

Looking at the mechanics of lactation

The flood of oestrogen and progesterone that your body experiences during pregnancy causes your breasts to grow – sometimes to an astonishing size. This growth starts early, within three to four weeks after conception, which is why the first sign of pregnancy for many women is breast tenderness. As pregnancy progresses, small amounts of serum-like fluid can leak from the nipples. But serious milk production doesn't start until after the baby is born.

During the first days after delivery, the breasts secrete only a yellowish fluid called colostrum, which doesn't contain much milk but is rich in antibodies and protective cells from the mother's bloodstream. Colostrum is gradually replaced by milk.

DON'T WORRY

Don't be alarmed if your baby doesn't seem to get much milk during the first few days. The colostrum is very beneficial on its own. Your baby probably doesn't even have much of an appetite until he is three to four days old – and he is likely to need the first few days to practise sucking movements.

When your baby starts sucking on your breasts, signals are sent to your brain instructing the breasts to start producing milk. About three or four days after delivery, milk production sets in. Milk enters ducts in your breasts, and they become engorged with milk. In the early stages of breast-feeding, you may find that the mere sound of your baby crying or the feel of your baby cuddling next to you can trigger the milk-flow reflex. You may suffer what is known as the wet T-shirt look – but don't worry, it does settle down.

Milk production usually sets in after you've arrived home. When your milk first arrives in your breasts, they can feel rock hard and extremely tender. When your baby starts feeding regularly, this tenderness and hardness settles down.

TIP

Your breasts can become *very* painful when first engorged with milk. Several simple relieving measures may help:

- Squeeze your nipples gently, and massage your breasts towards your nipples (this helps let out some milk and relieves engorgement).

- Wear a well-fitted, supportive nursing bra. Warm or cold *compresses* (you can make one by wrapping a hot or cold wet flannel in a plastic bag) can both provide relief.
- Placing frozen cabbage leaves (put them in your freezer) against your breasts might make you smell like a greengrocer's shop, but can provide rapid relief. We're not joking.

Checking out breast-feeding positions

You can breast-feed in one of three basic positions, as shown in Figure 14-1. Use whichever position works and is comfortable for you and your baby. Most women alternate among the positions.

- **Cradling:** The simplest way is to cradle your baby in your arms with his head next to the bend in your elbow and tilted a bit toward your breast. (See Figure 14-1a.)
- **Lying down:** Lie on your side in bed with the baby next to you. Support the baby with your lower arm or pillows so that his mouth is next to your lower breast, and use your other arm to guide your baby's mouth to the nipple. This position is best for late-night feedings or after a caesarean delivery when sitting up is still uncomfortable. (See Figure 14-1b.)
- **Rugby hold:** Cradle your baby's head in the palm of your hand and support his body with your forearm. Placing a pillow underneath your arm for extra support may help in this position. You can use your free hand to hold your breast close to the baby's mouth. (See Figure 14-1c.)

TIP

Find a comfortable position to breast-feed in – you're going to be there for a while. If you are hunched over, for example, you can strain your back. Both a footstool under your feet and a v-shaped pillow on your lap (for the baby to lie on) will help.

Getting baby to latch on

If you choose to breast-feed, you can get started immediately after delivery, whether you're in the delivery room or the recovery room. Begin as soon as the midwives have checked your baby's health and your baby has settled down a bit from the delivery. Expect to feel a little awkward at first, and try not to get too frustrated.

DON'T WORRY

Many babies don't want to breast-feed immediately. Have patience – you and your baby will eventually get the hang of it. You're both finding out the best way to breast-feed the first few times.

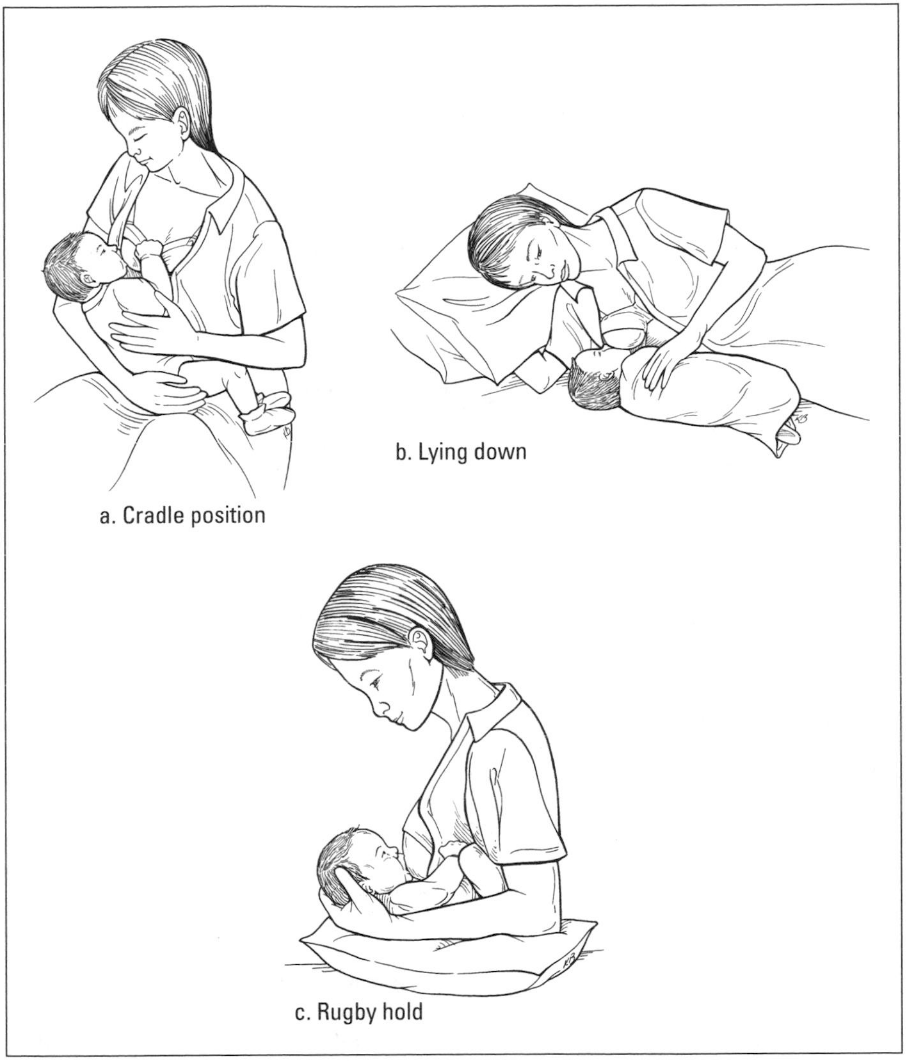

Figure 14-1: The three basic positions for breast-feeding.

Babies are born with a sucking reflex, but many of them don't follow it enthusiastically right from the start. Sometimes babies need some coaxing to latch onto the breast:

1. **Arrange yourself and your baby in one of the basic breast-feeding positions (see the preceding section).**
2. **Gently stroke the baby's lips or cheek with your nipple.**

This action probably causes the baby to open his mouth. If your baby doesn't seem to want to open his mouth, try expressing (gently pressing out) a little milk – colostrum, really – and rubbing some on his lips.

3. **When the baby's mouth is wide open, cradle his head in your hand and bring his mouth to your nipple.**

   Make sure that the entire areola is inside the baby's mouth, because if it isn't, he doesn't get enough milk and you get sore nipples. If your baby is properly latched on, you shouldn't be able to see much of your areola around his mouth.

Orchestrating feedings

After your baby latches on, you know that he is sucking when you see regular, rhythmic movements of the cheeks and chin. Several minutes of sucking may go by before your milk starts flowing. In the beginning, let your baby feed for about five minutes on each breast per nursing session. Over the course of the first three or four days, increase the amount of time on each breast to 10 to 15 minutes. Don't get too hung up about timing the feedings, though; your baby lets you know when he has had enough by not sucking and letting your nipple slip away.

TIP

If your baby stops sucking without letting go of your nipple, insert your finger into the corner of his mouth to break the suction. (If you just pull your breast straight out, you'll end up with sore nipples.)

When switching from one breast to the other, stop to burp your baby by laying him either over your shoulder or your lap and gently patting his back. Figure 14-2 shows you some of the various burping positions. Burp him again when the feeding is finished.

Typically, mothers breast-feed about 8 to 12 times a day (that is, on average, ten times a day). This pattern enables your body to produce an optimal amount of milk, and it allows your baby to get the proper amount of nutrition for healthy growth and development. Try to space the feedings fairly evenly throughout the day; of course, your baby has some influence on the schedule. You don't have to wake your baby for a feeding – unless your GP specifically advises you to do so. You especially don't have to wake your baby at night; if he's willing to sleep through, just count yourself lucky. Nor do you have any reason to withhold a feeding if your baby is hungry – even if only an hour or so has passed since the last feeding. (Also keep in mind that the number of feedings in a day may be less than average if you supplement breast-feeding with some formula feedings.)

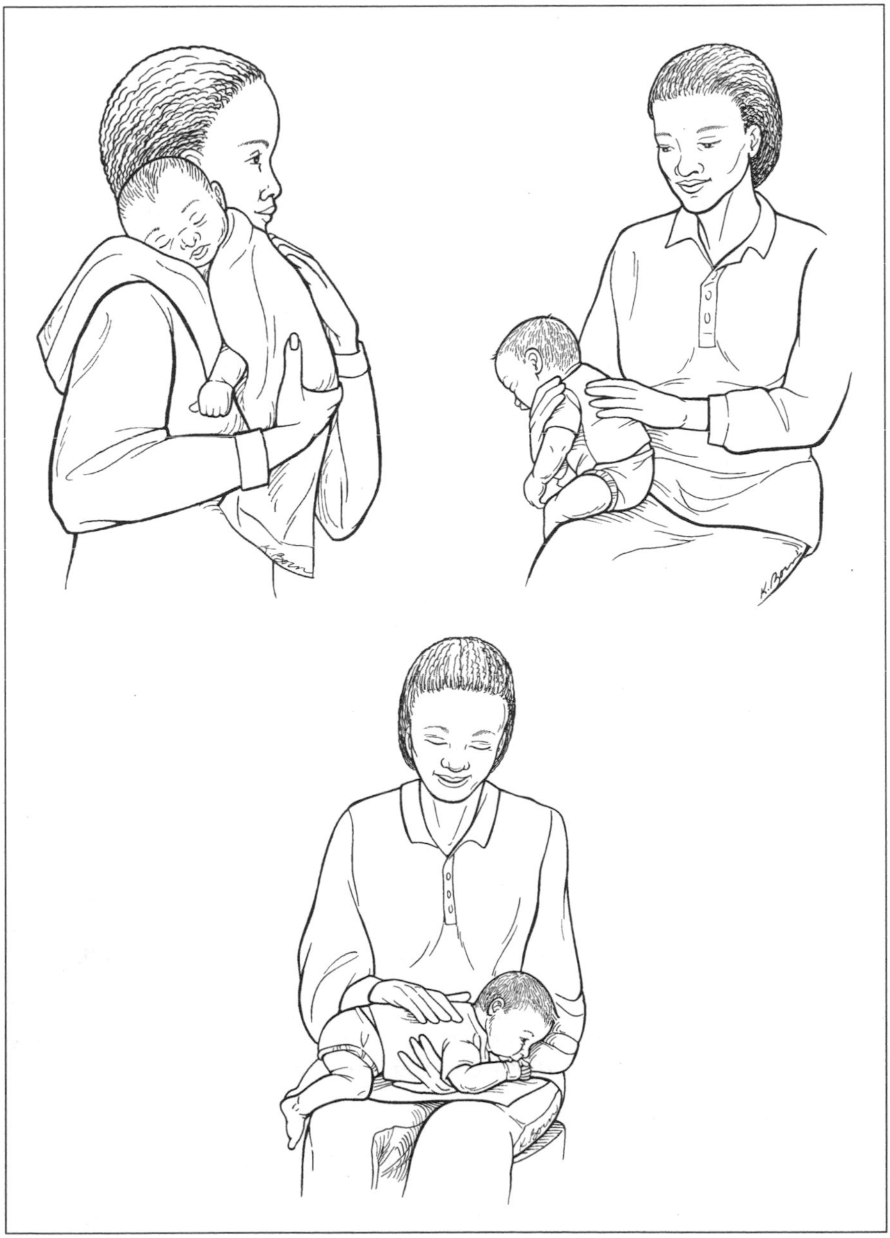

Figure 14-2: You can burp a baby in more than one way. Here are a few of the tried-and-tested positions.

You can tell that your baby is getting enough milk if he

- Feeds ten times a day on average
- Gains weight
- Has six to eight wet nappies a day
- Has two to three yellowish bowel movements (looking like grainy mustard) a day
- Produces urine that's pale yellow (not dark and concentrated)

If your baby isn't meeting these criteria or if you have any concern that your baby isn't getting enough milk, let your health visitor know.

Maintaining your diet

During breast-feeding, as during pregnancy, your nutrition is largely a matter of educated common sense. Your breast milk's quality isn't significantly affected by your diet unless your eating habits are truly inadequate. However, if you don't take in enough calories, your body has a difficult time producing adequate milk. You may also find that your baby reacts a different way to certain foods – for example, he may have more wind if you've eaten particular foods. If you pay attention to how your baby responds to different foods, you can figure out what to avoid.

Breast-feeding women should take in 400 to 600 calories a day more than they would normally eat. The exact amount varies according to how much you weigh and how much fat you gained during pregnancy. Because lactating does burn fat, breast-feeding helps get rid of some of the extra fat stores you may have. But avoid losing weight too fast, or your milk production will suffer. Also, avoid gaining weight while you're breast-feeding.

Unless you were anaemic after delivery (you'll have been advised if you were) you shouldn't need extra vitamins. However, be sure to have plenty of calcium in your diet – Chapter 5 tells you how.

Breast milk is mainly water (87 per cent). To produce plenty of breast milk, you must take in at least 72 extra ounces of fluid per day, which is about nine extra glasses of milk, juice, or water. Don't go overboard, however, because if you drink too many fluids, your milk production may actually decrease.

Keep a cool drink handy when you breast-feed – it can be thirsty work, and breast-feeding's the ideal time to top up your fluid intake.

Looking at options for contraception

Although you're less likely to ovulate while you're breast-feeding, this doesn't guarantee that you won't become pregnant. For a woman who chooses not to breast-feed, it takes an average of 10 weeks after the birth to resume ovulation – that is, to become fertile again. About 10 per cent of women who do breast-feed also begin ovulating again after 10 weeks, and about 50 per cent start up again by 25 weeks – about 6 months – after their babies are born. Clearly, breast-feeding isn't a great form of birth control. Your GP will discuss the options for contraception with you at your six-week check (see Chapter 13 for more on this appointment). But if you do resume sex before this time, using contraception is still essential, even if you're breast-feeding.

The combined oral contraceptive pill can affect the amount of breast milk you produce and it isn't recommended while you're breast-feeding. However, the progesterone-only pill is fine – but remember you need to take this pill within the same three-hour window every day for it to work really effectively.

Determining which medications are safe

Most medications you take get into your breast milk, but usually only in tiny amounts. Paracetamol, for example, is perfectly safe for you to take in standard doses (up to two 500mg tablets four times a day) even if you're breast-feeding. Check with your GP or pharmacist before you use any other medication, even if it isn't a prescription medicine.

Handling common problems

One of the greatest misconceptions about breast-feeding is that it comes easily and naturally to everyone. Breast-feeding takes practice. Problems can range from a little nipple soreness to, in rare cases, infections in the milk ducts.

Sore nipples

Many women experience some temporary nipple soreness during the first few days that they breast-feed. For most women, the pain is usually mild, and it goes away on its own. For some, however, the soreness gets progressively worse and can lead to chapped or cracked nipples and moderate-to-severe pain. If your breasts are heading in this direction, take action before your suffering gets out of hand. The following list outlines some remedies:

- Review your technique to make sure that your baby is positioned correctly. If the baby isn't getting the entire nipple and areola in his mouth, the soreness is likely to continue. Try changing the baby's position slightly with each feeding.

- Increase the number of feedings and feed for less time at each feeding. This way, your baby won't be as hungry and may not suck as hard.
- Definitely continue to feed on the sore breast, even if only for a few minutes to keep the nipple conditioned to nursing. If you let it heal completely, the soreness will only start all over again when you resume feeding from that nipple. We suggest that you feed on the least sore breast first, because that's when your baby's sucking is most vigorous.
- Express a little breast milk manually before you put the baby to the breast. This action helps initiate the milk-flow reflex so that the baby doesn't have to suck as long and as hard in order to obtain a good flow of milk.
- Don't use any irritating chemicals or soaps on your nipples.
- After your baby finishes feeding, don't wipe off your nipples. Let them air-dry for as long as possible. Wiping them with a cloth may cause needless irritation.
- Exposing the nipples to air helps to toughen the skin, so try to walk around the house with your nipples exposed as much as possible. If you wear a nursing bra, leave the flaps open while you're at home. Your nipples toughen from the fabric of your clothes rubbing against them.
- If you're using pads to soak up leakage from your breasts, change them as soon as they get moist, or they may chafe your nipples.
- Try massaging vitamin E ointment, olive oil, or lanolin into sore nipples and then letting them air-dry.
- Apply dry (not moist) and warm (not hot) heat to the nipples several times a day. You can use a hot-water bottle filled with warm water.
- Collect a little breast milk when you finish breast-feeding, and rub it into your nipples.

Clogged ducts

Sometimes some of the milk ducts in the breast become clogged with debris and a small, firm, red lump may form inside the breast. The lump may be tender, but it's usually not associated with a fever or excruciating pain. The best way to treat a clogged breast duct is to try to empty that breast completely after each feed. Start the baby out on that breast when he is most hungry. If the baby doesn't completely empty the breast, use a breast pump on that side until all the milk is drained. Also, applying heat to the lump and massaging it manually is helpful. Most important, keep feeding.

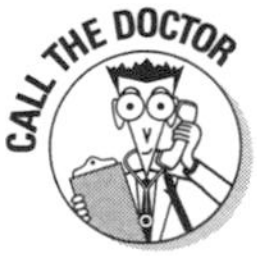

If the lump persists for more than a few days, call your GP to make sure that you're not developing an abscess.

Mastitis (breast infection)

Breast infections (mastitis) occur in about 2 per cent of all breast-feeding women. Bacteria from the baby's mouth usually cause the infections, which are most likely to happen two to four weeks after delivery (but can occur earlier or later than that). Infections are more common in women who are breast-feeding for the first time, who have chapped nipples with cracks or fissures, and who don't empty their breasts completely at feedings.

The symptoms of mastitis include a warm, hard, red breast; high fever (usually over 38 °C); and malaise (similar to having the flu when your whole body aches). The infection in the breast may be diffused, or it may be localised to a particular segment of the breast (known as a lobule). If the infection is localised, the redness may appear as a wedge-shaped area over the infected portion of the breast. If these symptoms develop, make an appointment with your GP as soon as possible – he will probably prescribe antibiotics.

Continue to breast-feed your baby while you have the infection. Mastitis is not harmful to your baby; after all, the bacteria probably came from his mouth. If you stop breast-feeding, the breast becomes engorged, making your discomfort even worse. Paracetamol, ibuprofen, or warm compresses may help relieve the pain from mastitis while the antibiotics take effect (usually about two days). Drink plenty of fluids, and get as much rest as you can to allow your body's natural healing powers to work. Take your medication for the fully prescribed amount of time to help make sure that the infection doesn't recur.

Breast abscess

If mastitis isn't treated aggressively, or if a milk duct remains clogged, a breast abscess can develop. Breast abscesses form in as many as 10 per cent of all cases of mastitis. Symptoms of a breast abscess are extreme pain, heat, and swelling over the area of the abscess, and high fevers (over 38 °C). Sometimes a doctor can treat an abscess with antibiotics, but often the abscess needs to be drained surgically.

If you develop a breast abscess, you can continue to breast-feed on the other side, but you should stop feeding on the side of the abscess until the problem subsides. Check with your doctor before resuming feedings on that side.

Breast-feeding twins

It may seem daunting, but some women with twins successfully breast-feed. Your body can make enough milk for two babies at once, especially if you're persistent and work up your milk production to a high level. Even so, arriving at a system that works for you takes some experimentation. You may breast-feed both babies at once, or each one separately. The advantage to the first alternative is that you don't spend all your time breast-feeding, but the second method is easier. You don't have to deal with one baby finishing first and needing to be burped while the other one is still sucking. (Holding one baby over your shoulder and keeping another one at your breast can be very tricky, no matter how many pillows and props you use.) You may breast-feed one baby, bottle-feed the other, and then alternate at the next feeding. You may breast-feed each baby a little at each feeding and then supplement with the bottle. Or you may breast-feed both babies for most of the day and then supplement with a bottle before bedtime when your milk supply is low.

Women who breast-feed twins need to take in even more extra calories and fluids. You need about 400 to 600 extra calories per day for each baby you are breast-feeding. (Imagine how much you'd have to consume to breast-feed triplets!) Also, you need to increase your fluid intake from 8 to 10 glasses per day to about 10 to 12 glasses per day.

TIP

If you do decide to try breast-feeding twins, count on needing help from other family members and friends. Don't be afraid to ask for it.

Breast-feeding resources

If you'd like to find out more about breast-feeding, plenty of people and organisations are available to give you advice:

- Your midwife (both before and after you leave hospital)
- Your health visitor (who will get in touch shortly after your midwife stops visiting)
- The breast-feeding counsellor at your local hospital
- Friends and family (although beware of conflicting advice from too many sources)
- *Breastfeeding For Dummies* by Sharon Perkins and Carol Vannais (Wiley) – a comprehensive book covering even the smallest details of breast-feeding
- The National Childbirth Trust (Tel: 0870 4448707 8:30 a.m. to 5:00 p.m. Monday to Thursday, 8:30 a.m. to 4:00 p.m. Fridays, for details of your nearest branch), Web site www.nctpregnancyandbabycare.com/nct-online.
- La Leche League (Great Britain), PO Box 29, West Bridgford, Nottingham NG2 7NP. Tel: 0845 1202918, Web site www.laleche.org.uk.
- Association of Breastfeeding Mothers, PO Box 207, Bridgwater, Somerset TA6 7YT. Tel: 0207 8131481 (for recorded information), Web site www.abm.me.uk.
- The Breastfeeding Network, PO Box 11126, Paisley PA2 8YB. Helpline: 0870 9008787, Tel: 0141 8842472, Web site www.breastfeedingnetwork.co.uk.

Bottle-feeding for Beginners

Suppose you've decided to forego breast-feeding in favour of formula. Or you've been breast-feeding for a while, and you want to switch. In this section, we go over what you need to know to get your baby started on bottles.

Stopping milk production

If you do decide to formula feed, you need to stop the process of milk production in your breasts. Milk production is triggered by warmth and breast stimulation. To stop the production of milk, create the opposite environment. Here are some suggestions:

- Wear a tight-fitting bra.
- Apply ice packs to your breasts when they become engorged (usually around the third or fourth day after your baby is born).
- Keep ice packs inside your bra, or use small packages of frozen vegetables, like peas or corn, which you can easily fold to fit within a bra. (We don't recommend going out in public this way, though.)
- Place cold cabbage leaves inside your bra. Cabbage works chemically to reduce the production of milk.
- Let cold water run over your breasts during a shower.

If you're going to breast-feed for a short period of time (6–12 weeks), consider giving your baby one bottle of formula per day while nursing to help make the transition easier. If you're breast-feeding for longer than 6–12 weeks, substituting more and more bottle-feeds for breast-feeds (say, one more daily feed every week) will help your milk tail off naturally.

Engorged breasts can be very uncomfortable. If you're in a great deal of discomfort, you may want to ask your doctor about pain medication. Fortunately, the engorgement usually lasts only 36–48 hours.

Choosing the best bottles and nipples

You won't have any trouble finding a wide choice of bottles and nipples. Some babies definitely demonstrate a preference for one type of bottle or nipple over another. You may have to experiment to discover the tools that work best for you and your baby. One-hundred gram (four-ounce) bottles are good for the first few weeks or months. Later, when your baby drinks a larger amount, you can switch to the larger 200-gram (eight-ounce) bottles.

- Some bottles are actually plastic holders in which you insert little transparent plastic bags that hold the milk or formula. The advantage of this type is that you can throw away the empty milk bag, and you don't have to worry about sterilising the plastic container. Also, because the plastic bag is designed to collapse, less air gets into the bag and into the baby's stomach.
- Some bottles are angled, which also helps to reduce the amount of air taken in by the baby, leading to less wind.
- Nipples come in a wide variety. Newborn nipples have a smaller hole, and the size of the hole increases with the age of the baby (nipples generally come in newborn, 3- and 6-month sizes, and then larger ones for older babies). Orthodontic nipples are designed for a more natural fit. Some nipples are made out of latex, and others of silicone, which are clear and have less odour. Your baby may demonstrate a strong preference for one type over another or may not notice much of a difference.

TIP

Your health visitor is extremely experienced in all the details of bottle-feeding. If bottle-feeding's causing problems, or you want advice on how to start, have a chat with your health visitor.

Feeding your baby from a bottle

You may have decided from day one that breast-feeding is not for you. You may have breast-fed for a few weeks, but have decided to bottle-feed when you go back to work. Or you may just want to give yourself the occasional break by letting dad take the odd night-shift feed.

Whatever your reasons for bottle-feeding, it's worth thinking about the practicalities in advance.

Using a few simple tips makes bottle-feeding much easier:

- The varieties of bottle sterilisers on the market are seemingly endless – ask friends, or your health visitor, about their experiences with the different types.
- Don't save and reuse leftover formula milk, and don't leave prepared milk out of the fridge for long periods – it's more prone to growing bacteria.
- If you want to prepare several bottles in advance, prepare the bottles and water (adding the formula at the last minute) or make up and store the formula in the fridge until you need it.
- Warm bottles with a bottle warmer, a microwave, or in a mug of hot water. Be careful if you use a microwave – it may not warm the milk evenly, so shake the bottle well, then squirt some milk onto the inside of your wrist to check the temperature before you give it to your baby.

Most formula milk comes in powder form, but you can get ready-mixed bottles, too. These are more expensive, but can be useful if you're out and about.

Lots of mothers worry that their baby's tummy upset or rash is due to an allergy to formula milk. In fact, an allergy isn't common, so do talk to your GP or health visitor before you switch to a soya-based or goats' milk variety.

CAUTION

Doctors generally recommend against propping up a baby's bottle by laying it on a pillow next to the baby's mouth, because propping implies that the baby is being left unattended. Also, lying a baby flat on his back with the bottle propped creates more potential for choking. Propping a bottle may also promote tooth decay.

The most common position for bottle-feeding your baby is to hold the baby cradled in one arm, close to your body. Put a pillow on your lap, which eases the strain on your arms and neck. Most parents find it easier to always hold the baby in the same arm and in the same direction. Here are some other tips for bottle-feeding mums:

- Don't swaddle the baby too much or keep him too warm during feeding. The baby may get so comfortable that he falls asleep instead of feeding.
- Change the baby's nappy in the middle of a feed. This may help to keep him awake, so that he can finish the rest of the bottle.
- If your baby has trouble finding the nipple to put in his mouth, stroke his cheek and he will turn in that direction.
- To check to see whether the baby is hungry, put the tip of your finger (a clean finger) into his mouth to see if he starts to suck.
- Keep the bottle tilted in such a way as to completely fill the nipple with the formula, thereby minimising the amount of air your baby gets.

TIP

Burp your baby at least once midway through a feeding and again at the end of a feeding. (Refer to Figure 14-2 for various burping positions.) Babies often take in air along with the milk or formula they drink, and burping helps them to get rid of it – it makes them more comfortable and able to eat more.

Dealing with Baby's Developing Digestive System

Your baby has a brand-new digestive system, and one that requires considerable breaking-in. Long story short: Babies are sick. A lot. Whether they're breast-fed or bottle-fed, newborn babies are likely to vomit as often as two times per day. Baby vomit is called *posset.* Try these suggestions for dealing with this messy phenomenon:

TIP

- Keep a cloth over your shoulder when burping or holding your baby so that you don't have to constantly change, or ruin, your clothes.
- Keep a small bib on your baby during and after feeding so that you don't have to constantly change, or ruin, all the baby's clothes.
- Burp your baby after each feeding. Refer to Figure 14-2 to see some of the most common positions.
- If you're bottle-feeding, stop partway through the bottle to burp the baby, rather than allowing him to drink the entire bottle in one go.
- Don't play with the baby too much after feeding. Jiggling the baby or moving him around a lot can lead to more sicking up.
- After feeding, keep the baby upright (the first two burping positions shown in Figure 14-2 are ideal) for up to half-an-hour. The exact length of time will vary between babies, but you'll soon get an idea of how long is long enough by trial and error.

DON'T WORRY

Possetting is natural, but does seem to produce an awful lot of mess! Many mothers worry that their babies don't keep enough down to feed them adequately. As long as your baby is putting on weight, is opening his bowels regularly, and passing water regularly, he's almost certainly keeping enough milk in his system for his needs.

CALL THE DOCTOR

Two potentially serious conditions that do need treatment can start off with vomiting. Fortunately, these conditions usually give off other clues:

- *Reflux disease* is caused by acid from the stomach refluxing back into the *oesophagus* (gullet). Symptoms include vomiting several times a day, pain when vomiting, irritability, inconsolable crying, gagging, choking, or refusal to feed. If you think your baby is affected, make an appointment with your GP – reflux disease is often easily treatable with medicine, feed-thickeners, or simply propping your baby up during and after feeding.
- *Pyloric stenosis* is where the outflow from the baby's stomach to the rest of the gut becomes swollen and blocked. Pyloric stenosis usually develops in the first month of life. Symptoms include projectile vomiting (the kind that sends your baby's milk out of his mouth to the other side of the room), inconsolable crying, acting hungry straight after feeding, failure to gain weight, failure to pass water or stools adequately, or a lump in the tummy when feeding. If you have any concerns about this condition, take your baby to your GP immediately.

Part IV
Special Concerns

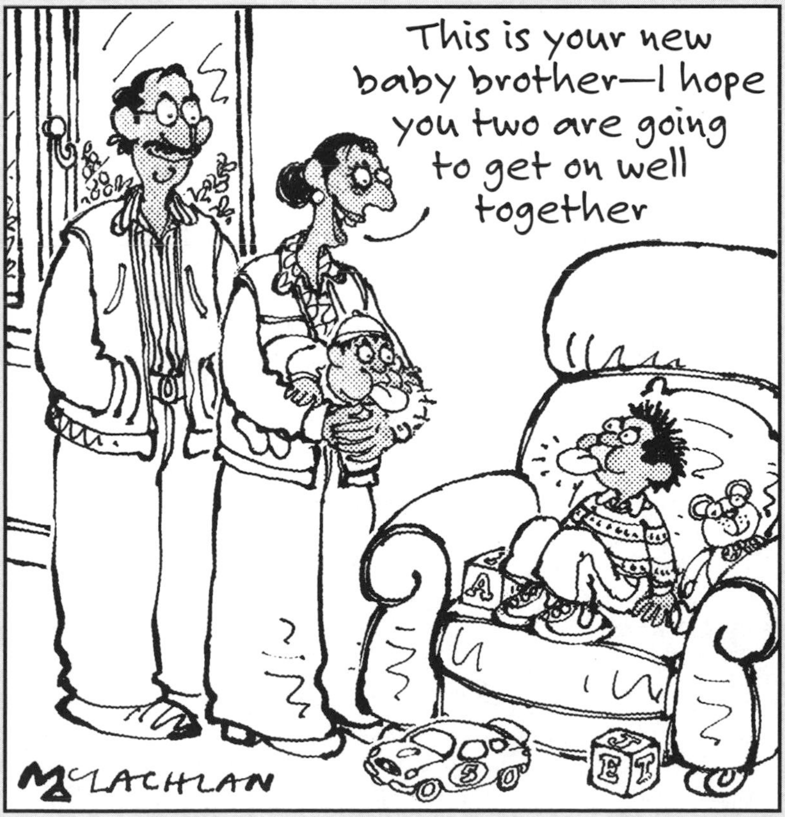

This is your new baby brother—I hope you two are going to get on well together
McLACHLAN

In this part . . .

You could actually go all the way through pregnancy without ever reading this part, especially if you're having your first child, you're not having twins (or more), and nothing – not even one tiny little thing – ever goes wrong or makes you uncomfortable. But very often, little things do come up. You get a cold and wonder how it affects your pregnancy. You develop an annoying rash. You're having twins or more. You have a significant medical problem or complication to deal with. No matter what your concern, we gather them all into this part. More than any other segment of the book, we design this part for you to read in pieces, depending on what particular situation you're in.

Chapter 15

Pregnancies with Special Considerations

In This Chapter

- Starting parenthood later
- Meeting the challenge of multiple births
- Having second babies – and third, fourth, fifth . . .
- Preparing older children for the new arrival

No two pregnancies are exactly alike. If you're like most women, you figure out pretty early in the game that your experience is different in some way from every friend and relative you talk to. You're not as queasy as your sister was during the first three months – or your morning sickness is 20 times worse than your best friend's. You feel comfortable exercising throughout your pregnancy, although your pregnant cousin was put on bed rest. Plenty of variation occurs within the boundaries of what is considered to be a normal, 'average' pregnancy. But some special kinds of pregnancies come with their own particular characteristics and challenges.

Figuring Out How Age Matters

Whether you're a prospective father or a prospective mother, age can make a difference – as many baby boomers are now finding out. Special problems and issues arise for men and women in their late 30s and older who are preparing to have children. Teenage mums also face unique challenges.

Over-35 (or older) mums

Long gone are the days when almost all pregnant women were in their early 20s or teens. Now, a greater number of women postpone having families until they've not only finished their education, but also have had at least a decade to become established in their careers. Divorce is also more common, and many women find themselves having children with a second husband – often when they're well into their 30s or 40s (and sometimes 50s).

How old is too old? The answer used to be when you reach the menopause – or even some years earlier, when your body no longer produces healthy eggs that can be fertilised to become embryos. But today, because of advances in assisted reproductive technologies – *in vitro fertilisation* (IVF), which may use eggs donated from another woman – even women who are past the age of the menopause can become pregnant.

Today, a more useful question is 'At what age do you need to watch out for special problems?' And here, the answer is more specific: Any woman who is at least 35 years old during her pregnancy falls into the medical definition of advanced maternal age, or AMA. (An impersonal term, to be sure, but perhaps less insulting than the alternatives that are also used: older gravida, mature gravida, and the particularly unfortunate elderly gravida.) The reason for singling out older mothers with any special term at all is that the incidence of certain chromosomal abnormalities increases with advancing maternal age. At age 35, the risks begin to increase significantly, as shown in Figure 15-1.

You should be offered a test to check for foetal abnormalities regardless of your age (you can find out the details in Chapter 9). The types of genetic tests available vary around the country and in most areas you'll initially be offered *non-invasive* tests such as blood testing or nuchal thickness scanning. If your *non-invasive* test shows a relatively high risk, you will then be offered an amniocentesis, which will give you a definite answer. You may also be offered an amniocentesis or chorionic villus sampling if you've had a previous baby with a chromosomal abnormality, if genetic problems run in your family, or if you're 37 or older.

The good news is that except for this increase in certain chromosomal abnormalities, babies born to women older than 35, or even older than 40, are as likely as any other babies to be healthy. The mums themselves do stand a higher than average risk of developing pre-eclampsia or gestational diabetes (see Chapters 16 and 17), and they stand an increased risk of needing a caesarean delivery. But these risks aren't terribly high, and in most cases, any problems that result are minor. Naturally, an older woman's experience with pregnancy depends to a large extent on her underlying health. If a woman is 48 years old or even 50, but she is in excellent health, she is likely to do extremely well.

Maternal Age and Chromosomal Abnormalities
(Live Births)

MATERNAL AGE	RISK FOR DOWN'S SYNDROME	TOTAL RISK FOR CHROMOSOME ABNORMALITIES*
20	1/1667	1/526*
21	1/1667	1/526*
22	1/1429	1/500*
23	1/1429	1/500*
24	1/1250	1/476*
25	1/1250	1/476*
26	1/1176	1/476*
27	1/1111	1/455*
28	1/1053	1/435*
29	1/1000	1/417*
30	1/952	1/384*
31	1/909	1/384*
32	1/769	1/322*
33	1/602	1/286
34	1/485	1/238
35	1/378	1/192
36	1/289	1/156
37	1/224	1/127
38	1/173	1/102
39	1/136	1/83
40	1/106	1/66
41	1/82	1/53
42	1/63	1/42
43	1/49	1/33
44	1/38	1/26
45	1/30	1/21
46	1/23	1/16
47	1/18	1/13
48	1/14	1/10
49	1/11	1/8

Figure 15-1: As maternal age rises, so do the risks of chromosomal abnormalities.

Data of Hook (1981) and Hook et al. (1983). Because sample size for some intervals is relatively small, confidence limits are sometimes relatively large. Nonetheless, these figures are suitable for genetic counselling.
**47.XXX excluded for ages 20–32 (data not available).*

Not-so-young dads

Pregnancies in older women call for some special scrutiny because of the increased risk of genetic complications and, to some extent, pregnancies involving older dads should likewise be singled out for observation. There is no absolute age cut-off for advanced paternal age, but many people use 45 or 50 (although some argue that it should be 35, just like for women).

Whereas for women the main genetic risk is having a foetus with a chromosomal abnormality (most commonly an extra chromosome), for men the risk is spontaneous gene mutations in the sperm that can lead to a child with an autosomal dominant disorder, such as *achondroplasia* (a type of dwarfism) or Huntington's disease. Only one copy of an abnormal gene can cause this kind of problem. (In so-called recessive genetic disorders – cystic fibrosis and sickle cell anaemia, for example – two copies of the abnormal gene are required for the problem to occur.) Autosomal dominant disorders are very rare, however, and many are impossible to test for, which is why no routine testing exists for advanced paternal age.

Very young mums

Pregnancy in teenage women raises a different set of concerns. Although this age group doesn't sustain any increase in chromosomal abnormalities, these women may experience a higher incidence of some birth defects. Because teenage mums tend to have less-than-ideal eating habits, they are also more likely to have low-birth-weight babies. Teenage mums are also at a higher risk of developing pre-eclampsia, are more likely to deliver by caesarean delivery, and are less likely to breast-feed. Due to their unique situation, these young mums need special guidance and counselling. If you're a teenage mum, we encourage you to receive adequate antenatal care, to follow a healthy diet, and to consider the benefits of breast-feeding.

Having Twins or More

Having twins may seem simple – to someone who's never faced the reality of it. Twins are either double the pleasure or a living nightmare (twice the work and only half the sleep). Twins are complicated, as any mother of twins can tell you – for hours and hours, if you're willing to listen. Indeed, you could fill an entire book with advice for parents of twins, triplets, and more. And if such a book were written, a sizable first part of it would have to be about the experience of pregnancy for women carrying twins or more.

If you're having triplets or more, what applies to twins generally applies to triplets (and more), only to a much greater extent.

Although the vast majority of twin pregnancies proceed smoothly and result in the birth of two beautiful, healthy babies, some risks are involved for both the foetuses and the mum. As a result, if you're pregnant with twins, you're more likely to have hospital-based rather than shared or midwife-led care (see Chapter 2). You'll probably have more antenatal appointments and more ultrasound scans. The number of twins that are conceived is much larger than the number of twins that are actually born. Many pregnancies that begin as twin pregnancies end as single births because one of the foetuses never develops. In many cases, one of the foetuses disappears before the pregnancy is even diagnosed (the so-called vanishing twin). The incidence of twin births is usually estimated to be about 1 per cent of all births. However, the incidence of twins is rising, mainly due to the increasing use of fertility techniques.

Ethnic background and family history can increase your chance of having twins; certain women are constitutionally more likely to ovulate more than one egg in a cycle. If twins occur in your family, let your practitioner know.

The incidence of spontaneous triplets is much more rare – about 1 in 7,000. Spontaneous quadruplets (or more) are exceedingly rare. However, with the increasing use of infertility treatments, the incidence of triplets has increased tenfold over the past few years.

Looking at types of multiples

Twins can be either identical or fraternal. These old-fashioned terms don't completely describe how twins occur. Identical twins look very much alike and are always the same sex. They come from a single embryo, meaning that they're a product of the same union of one egg and one sperm. In other words, they are *monozygotic* – they come from the same *zygote* (egg-sperm combination). Monozygotic twins have exactly the same genes as each other, which explains their resemblance. In the UK, roughly one-third of all twins are identical. An egg can split into three, leading to identical triplets, but it's very unusual.

A woman conceives fraternal twins when she ovulates more than one egg, and two different sperm fertilise the two eggs and then implant in her uterus at the same time. These *dizygotic* twins – which arise from two zygotes – don't share an identical set of genes. Instead, these twins' genetic make-up is as similar as that of any pair of children born of the same parents – they're just born at the same time. Dizygotic twins can be the same sex, or they can be of opposite sexes. Roughly two-thirds of all twins conceived spontaneously in the UK are dizygotic. If three eggs are fertilised, the result is fraternal triplets. A triplet pregnancy can also consist of two foetuses that are monozygotic and one that is from a second fertilised egg – leading to two babies that are identical and one that is fraternal.

The chance that a woman will have identical twins increases after she reaches the age of 35. The chance that a woman will have fraternal twins (because she ovulates more than one egg in any given month) rises until about the age of 35 and then drops off. Some families have more than their statistical share of fraternal twins. Fraternal twinning becomes more likely when a woman takes fertility drugs because these medications boost the chance that she ovulates more than one egg. Of course, a woman who takes fertility drugs can still produce an egg that gets fertilised and then splits in two to form identical twins.

Determining whether multiples are identical or fraternal

Many women who are pregnant with twins ask their doctor or ultrasonographer during an ultrasound examination if she can tell whether her twins are fraternal (they come from two different zygotes) or identical (they come from the same zygote). In some cases the technician or your doctor can tell – if you can see that the babies are two different sexes, you know they're fraternal; if they're the same sex, they may be either fraternal or identical.

REMEMBER

Because different types of twins are associated with different problems and risks, trying to figure out what type of twinning is present can be important. If the ultrasound signs are ambiguous and the medical situation suggests that determining the type of twinning is especially important, an amniocentesis can be performed for special studies to answer this question. These tests are called *zygosity* studies and require an invasive test, such as amniocentesis, chorionic villus sampling (CVS), or foetal blood sampling (see Chapter 9 for more on these).

Down's syndrome screening in pregnancies with twins or more

For many years, the most common way of screening pregnancies for Down's syndrome was by measuring different markers in the mother's blood at

16 weeks of pregnancy (see Chapter 9). The accuracy of this test with twins is still pretty good, but with triplets or more, it doesn't help at all. The newer method of Down's syndrome screening in the first trimester (*nuchal translucency*, see Chapter 9) appears particularly promising for mums with multiple gestations, because your doctor can obtain a nuchal translucency measurement for each foetus, thus giving each foetus its own specific risk of having Down's syndrome. The jury is still out, however, as to exactly what role the serum markers in mum's blood play in this situation. Serum markers may help with twins, but with triplets or more, probably the most helpful approach will be the nuchal translucency measurement alone.

Genetic testing in pregnancies with twins or more

Chorionic villus sampling and amniocentesis are a little trickier with twins or more. The two main challenges are to make sure that each foetus is sampled separately and that none of the tissue taken from one foetus contaminates the tissue taken from the other. In the case of identical twins, this issue isn't as critical, because the foetuses have the same genetic make-up. If you find a genetic abnormality (or lack of any genetic abnormalities) in one twin, the same is almost always true for the other. But with fraternal twins, triplets, or more, testing each foetus separately is critical.

Amniocentesis

Amniocentesis (see Chapter 9) is the most common way to genetic test in multi-foetal pregnancies. This method requires inserting a separate needle into the uterus for each foetus being tested. The amniocentesis is done under ultrasound guidance and the doctor should be able to check, using ultrasound, that the fluid taken for the two samples has come from the two different amniotic sacs. Occasionally, however, after the doctor removes some fluid from the first foetus, she may leave the needle in place to inject a harmless organic blue dye into that foetus's amniotic sac. (Don't worry – you won't give birth to a Smurf. This blue dye is absorbed over time.) Then, if the fluid from the second needle comes out clear (not blue), the doctor knows that she has sampled the second sac.

Chorionic villus sampling

Chorionic villus sampling, or CVS (see Chapter 9), can be somewhat complicated in multi-foetal pregnancies, but experienced doctors can usually handle the job. In some cases, the placentas are positioned in such a way that CVS is technically impossible. In these cases, the mother has the option of having an amniocentesis a little later in pregnancy (at about 15 to 18 weeks, rather than 12 weeks for CVS).

Our patients want to know . . .

Q: 'Is doing an amniocentesis or CVS for twin or triplet pregnancies riskier than for singleton pregnancies?'

A: Although scientists have conducted little research on this question, it appears that the chances of complications aren't substantially greater in multi-foetal pregnancies, if someone experienced in performing the procedure does it in mothers carrying twins or more.

Keeping track of which baby is which

Your doctor designates your babies before birth as Twin I and Twin II (or Triplets I, II, and III). These designations enable your doctor to communicate to you and others (nurses and other medical personnel) which baby is which and to follow the progress of each baby separately and consistently throughout the pregnancy. By convention, the foetus closest to the cervix (the opening to the womb) is designated as Twin I (or Triplet I). This baby is usually born first. In a triplet pregnancy, the highest triplet (closest to your chest) is designated as Triplet III. (Some patients come up with their own clever names. We had one patient with triplets who named her babies Itsy, Bitsy, and Ditsy before birth so she could keep track of them.)

Living day-to-day during a multiple pregnancy

If you're pregnant with multiples, don't ignore everything else we've written in this book. In many ways, your pregnancy proceeds like any other. The difference, as you may already know, is that your experience is more intense in various ways: You grow a larger belly, your nausea may be worse, your amniocentesis (if you have one) is a bit more complicated (as we describe earlier in this chapter), and the birth may take longer. With triplets or more, these physical changes and symptoms are even more exaggerated. Certain complications are also more frequent in multiples than in singletons. In the following list, we describe many of the ways that your experience may be somewhat different:

- **Activity:** In the old days, doctors recommended that women with twins be placed on bed rest beginning at 24 to 28 weeks. However, data shows that women placed on bed rest appear to be no less likely than others to experience preterm delivery or have babies of low birth-weight. Whether you need to reduce your activity depends upon your prior obstetric history as well as how smoothly your pregnancy goes week-to-week. If you develop preterm labour or have problems with foetal growth, your doctor may recommend that you take it easy. With triplets or more, the benefit is unclear, but many obstetricians routinely recommend bed rest starting in the second trimester.

- **Diet:** Many experts recommend that women carrying twins consume an extra 300 calories a day above what is required for a singleton (that is, an extra 600 calories per day above their pre-pregnancy intake). For triplets and more, no consensus exists, but obviously your food intake should be somewhat greater.
- **Iron and folic acid:** Women carrying twins, triplets, or more stand a greater chance of developing anaemia, which is due to dilutional anaemia (see Chapter 5), as well as greater demands for iron and folic acid. Doctors recommend supplemental iron and folic acid for women carrying two or more foetuses.
- **Nausea:** Most women carrying two or more foetuses definitely have more nausea and vomiting in early pregnancy than women with only one. This nausea may be related to higher levels of hCG (a pregnancy hormone) circulating through the bloodstream. The amount is greater with two or more foetuses. The good news is that nausea and vomiting for mothers of multiples, as for mothers of single babies, usually goes away by the end of the first trimester.
- **Antenatal visits:** Your practitioner is likely to follow pretty much the same routine she uses for mothers of single babies – you have your blood pressure, urine, and sometimes your weight, checked at each visit. But because you have more than one foetus, your practitioner may ask you to come in more frequently. Some practitioners perform routine pelvic examinations to make sure that your cervix isn't dilating prematurely; others may suggest that your cervix be checked with an ultrasound examination. If you don't have any preterm labour symptoms, your doctor may decide that you don't need these extra examinations.
- **Ultrasound examinations:** Most practitioners suggest that mothers of twins or more have ultrasound examinations periodically throughout their pregnancy in order to check foetal growth. If you have any problems, these examinations may need to be more frequent. With more than one foetus, your doctor can't use fundal height measurements to check the growth. And because women with twins, triplets, or more are at a higher risk of having problems with foetal growth (see 'Intrauterine growth restriction', later in this chapter), these ultrasounds are very important.

- **Weight gain:** The average weight gain for a twin pregnancy is 35 to 45 pounds (15 to 20 kg). But the exact amount that you gain depends on your pre-pregnancy weight. If you're pregnant with twins, the ideal weight gain is about one pound per week during the second and third trimesters. Recent studies show that you can achieve the optimal growth rates by taking into account your body mass index (see Chapter 5) prior to pregnancy and that weight gain in the first two trimesters may be especially important. Doctors recommend weight gains of 45 to 50 pounds (20 to 23 kg) by 34 weeks for triplets and more than 50 pounds (23 kg) for quadruplets.

Going through labour and delivery with twins

Almost always, women carrying triplets deliver by caesarean. Recently, however, some studies have suggested that in very specific situations and with very strict criteria, vaginal delivery of a triplet pregnancy may be possible. Because almost all triplets are delivered by caesarean, the following section on birth positions and delivery is addressed to women carrying twins.

Often, pregnancy goes smoothly for mothers of twins, but labour and delivery can still be complex. For this reason, we recommend that women carrying more than one foetus deliver in a hospital, where extra personnel are present to handle any complications that may arise.

Assuming that they are full term, your babies can be in different positions. The babies' positions fall into three possibilities:

- Both foetuses can be head-down (vertex), as they are in about 45 per cent of twin pregnancies (see Figure 15-2a). Vaginal delivery is successful 60 to 70 per cent of the time when the babies are in this position.
- The first foetus can be head-down and the second not, as is the case about 35 per cent of the time, making a caesarean delivery more likely, unless your practitioner can turn the second baby to a head-down position. Whether trying to manipulate the baby in this way makes sense is a matter of some debate among practitioners. Your doctor's choice of trying to turn the baby around, or delivering the baby breech, depends on her training, experience, and professional bias, and your views, too.
- The first foetus can be breech or transverse (lying horizontal across the uterus), and the second can be breech, head-down, or transverse, as they're about 20 per cent of the time (see Figures 15-2b and 15-2c).

With any of these combinations of positions, if the babies are preterm, the options may be different. Discuss the possibilities with your doctor before the time of delivery.

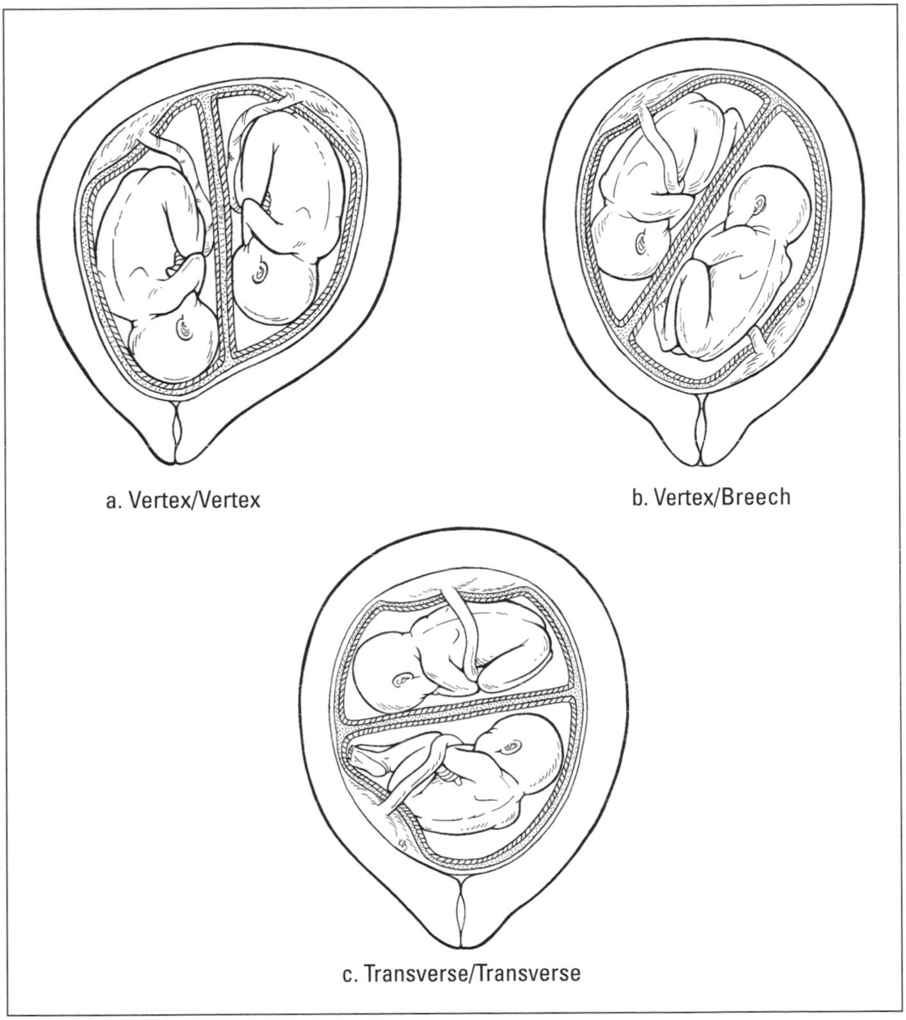

Figure 15-2: Three possible positions of twins before delivery.

Covering special issues for mums with multiples

If you're pregnant with twins or triplets (or more), your doctor puts you under closer surveillance, because the risk of certain complications is greater in multi-foetal pregnancies. The following topics are some of the things your doctor is watching out for.

Don't let this list scare you. The important thing is to be aware of potential problems so that if they develop, you and your practitioner can recognise them early and manage them appropriately to give you the best outcome possible.

Preterm delivery

The biggest risk you face in carrying more than one baby is that you may have preterm labour and delivery. The average length of pregnancy for a singleton is 40 weeks, but for a twin pregnancy it's only about 36 weeks; for triplets, 33–34 weeks; and for quadruplets, about 31 weeks. A pregnancy is full term if it lasts 37 weeks or more. Preterm delivery is technically between 24 and 37 weeks, but most babies born at 35 or 36 weeks are generally as healthy as babies delivered after 37 weeks.

Many women go into preterm labour without actually delivering their babies early. About 80 per cent of mothers carrying triplets and 40 per cent of those with twins experience preterm labour, but not all deliver early. (See details about preterm labour and delivery in Chapter 16.)

Chromosomal abnormalities

When you have more than one foetus and they aren't identical, the chance that either one of them has a genetic abnormality is somewhat higher. After all, each baby has its own individual risk of some abnormality, and the risks add up. Mothers of single babies are considered to be of advanced maternal age (AMA) at 35, as we describe earlier in the chapter, but in twin pregnancies derived from two separate eggs, AMA may be as early as 33, and for triplets, 31 or 32. This information all becomes relevant for women considering the genetic testing we mention earlier.

Diabetes

Because the incidence of gestational diabetes is higher with twins or more, many practitioners recommend that all women carrying more than one foetus be screened for this condition. (See Chapter 17.)

Hypertension and pre-eclampsia

Hypertension (high blood pressure) is more common in multi-foetal pregnancies. The risk is proportional to the number of foetuses present. Some women develop hypertension alone, without other symptoms or other physical signs. Other women develop a condition unique to pregnancy called *pre-eclampsia*, which involves high blood pressure in association with either oedema (swelling) or spilling protein in the urine (see the description of pre-eclampsia in Chapter 16). Forty per cent of mothers carrying twins and 60 per cent or more with triplets develop some form of hypertension during pregnancy. For this reason, your practitioner keeps a close eye on your blood pressure.

Intrauterine growth restriction

Problems with foetal growth occur in anywhere from 15 to 50 per cent of all twins. The problem is even more common in triplets and in foetuses that share the same placenta. In the case of a single placenta, the blood may not be distributed equally to both twins, which may cause one twin to get more nutrients than the other. In multiples that have different placentas, growth restriction can result when one placenta is implanted in a more favourable position within the uterus and therefore provides better nourishment than the other. Your doctor is likely to schedule periodic ultrasound examinations during your pregnancy to check that both (or all three) foetuses are growing properly.

Twin-twin transfusion syndrome

Twin-twin transfusion syndrome is specific to twins who share a single placenta (the technical name for this is monochorionic, and this condition only happens with identical twins). In some cases, the single placenta contains blood vessels that interconnect between the two foetuses. This connection enables the two foetuses to exchange blood – and allows the blood to become distributed unequally. The foetus that gets more blood grows bigger and produces extra amniotic fluid, while the one who gets less blood may suffer impaired growth and have significantly decreased amniotic fluid in its sac. This situation can be very serious, but fortunately, it affects only 10 to 15 per cent of monochorionic twins.

Multi-foetal pregnancy reduction

Some doctors perform the multi-foetal pregnancy reduction procedure to decrease the number of foetuses a woman is carrying in order to improve the chances that she delivers healthy babies. Doctors more commonly use the procedure in women who have at least three viable foetuses resulting from fertility treatments because of the high risk of preterm delivery if they try to carry all the foetuses. Also, some women carrying twins want to reduce their pregnancy to a singleton. Usually a maternal-foetal medicine specialist performs a multi-foetal pregnancy reduction during the last weeks of the first trimester, between 9 and 13 weeks, in a special centre. The risk involved is acceptably low when an experienced foetal-maternal specialist specifically trained in this procedure performs the reduction. Find out about all the multi-foetal pregnancy reduction options, so that you have as much information as possible to make the best decision for you.

Selective termination

A selective termination procedure can be used in a multi-foetal pregnancy to terminate one of the foetuses when that foetus has a significant abnormality. A maternal-foetal medicine specialist can perform this procedure if the foetuses have separate placentas, so that the medication used can't cross over and affect the normal foetus. In the case of identical twins that share a single amniotic sac, some other options are available (ask your doctor). Only a few specialist centres in the UK perform this procedure.

Getting Pregnant Again

Doctors and parents haven't come to a consensus on the optimal time to get pregnant again. Probably the most important consideration is your overall health. If you can get back to your pre-pregnancy or ideal body weight quickly after you deliver, and if you can replenish any lost nutrients and vitamins (particularly iron and calcium) from your last pregnancy, then you can probably consider getting pregnant again fairly soon – in about six months to a year. However, if you have had a complicated pregnancy, a difficult delivery, or excessive loss of blood, wait until you're in better shape before trying again.

REMEMBER

Many women are faced with getting pregnant within a few months of having their last baby – some are delighted, but many more are quite surprised! This situation frequently happens when getting pregnant took several months the last time round, and this time the woman thinks she should start trying several months before she actually wants to get pregnant. We do not recommend this technique. The time it takes to get pregnant one time has no bearing on the time it'll take to get pregnant another time. Before you start trying, ask yourself whether you're ready to be pregnant straight away.

TIP

Also ask yourself what you consider to be the ideal age difference between your children. Some people feel that having children close in age is better, so that the older child doesn't have so many years to settle into the role of only child and therefore may not feel so jealous when the new baby comes. Other people feel that spacing the children further apart, so that the older child is mature enough to handle the introduction of a new sibling, is better. Most important is how you and your partner feel and how ready you are to take on another child. The decision may involve emotional and financial issues as well as physical ones.

Realising how each pregnancy is different

Naturally, any mother compares her second pregnancy with her first, but every pregnancy is different. If your last pregnancy went smoothly, you may think that any little thing that happens out of the ordinary in the next pregnancy is a signal that things aren't going well; if your first pregnancy was difficult, you needn't assume that the same complications are going to happen again. And no matter what anybody tells you, remember that different symptoms don't mean the baby will be a different sex to your first child. See Chapter 20 for some old wives' tales about predicting your baby's sex.

These are some of the ways in which you may experience pregnancy differently the second (or third or fourth) time around:

- Many women feel that they're showing sooner or are at least more bloated and distended. This condition may be due to the fact that their abdominal muscles have been stretched by their previous pregnancy and are now more lax.
- Many women find that nausea isn't as severe as it was the first time around, and others find that it's worse.
- You can usually identify foetal movement earlier.
- Labour is usually shorter, and delivery is easier.
- Many women find that they feel Braxton-Hicks contractions earlier and more frequently than with their first child. (See Chapter 8 for more on Braxton-Hicks contractions.)
- Most women are less anxious the second time around.

One thing that remains the same: As hard as it is to believe, you will love your second child as much as your first.

DON'T WORRY

In their third pregnancy, many women commonly experience a special kind of worry: They feel that because their first two pregnancies were healthy and problem-free, the third one's bound to have complications. Many feel that they were lucky twice in a row, and that going for a third baby is pushing their luck. If you feel this way, believe us, you aren't alone. Keep in mind that the chances of trouble aren't inherently greater in a third pregnancy, even if the first two went smoothly.

Giving birth after a prior caesarean delivery

If you have had a caesarean delivery and you get pregnant again, you may wonder whether you can deliver vaginally this time or will need another caesarean.

The vast majority of caesarean sections in the UK are called lower segment caesarean sections (LCSC). In an LCSC, a transverse cut is made along your bikini line, and along the lower part of your uterus. With this kind of caesarean section, the chances are good that you'll be able to deliver a subsequent baby vaginally, as long as you don't have any complicating factors.

Recent studies show that 70 per cent of the time, women can successfully deliver a baby vaginally after they've had a caesarean. Of course, the likelihood of success depends to some extent on why a caesarean was performed in the first place. If it was because the baby was breech, the chance that the next baby can be delivered vaginally is nearly 90 per cent. If the caesarean was performed because the baby was too large to fit through the mother's pelvis, the chance of a future vaginal delivery falls to 50 to 60 per cent. Whatever the reason for your previous caesarean, you'll be closely monitored during your next labour, and if you have any problems, you'll probably have a caesarean again. Why would you want to deliver your next baby vaginally? The main benefit is that if you're successful, your recovery is much shorter. However, if you try labour and then end up with another caesarean, studies show that the complication rate is higher than if you went straight to a repeat caesarean without labour. Another potential benefit from a vaginal birth is that it's often associated with less postpartum pain. However, although most patients find the pain associated with vaginal birth to be less than that associated with caesarean delivery, some vaginal births have painful complications of their own. See Chapter 11 for more information.

Other benefits of a vaginal birth include the following:

- A lower risk of the kind of complications associated with abdominal surgery, including:
  - Anaesthetic problems
  - Inadvertent injury to adjacent organs
  - Infection
  - Possible blood clots from being immobile for a longer period of time
- For some women, a psychological benefit from experiencing a vaginal birth
- Shorter hospital stay
- The possibility, indicated by some studies, that the baby clears her secretions more efficiently if born vaginally

Preparing Your Child (or Children) for a New Arrival

Many parents look forward to having a second child specifically because they want to provide a sibling for the first one. But your first child may not easily understand this reasoning. She may feel completely content about being the only child, and it may take months or years before the first one appreciates the second one. For those of you who are having your second child – or third or fourth (or more!) – the following sections offer a few ideas about how to help prepare the older one(s) for the new arrival.

Explaining pregnancy

The ease or difficulty you may have introducing a new baby sister or brother depends quite a bit on how old the elder sibling is. Explaining a new baby to a 15-year-old is easy; getting the concept across to a 15-month-old can be tricky. And the challenge begins at the time you tell the first child that you're pregnant. A two-year-old has little concept of time and may not understand that mum is pregnant for months before the baby comes. She may be frustrated that the baby can't come immediately – so delay telling a very young child about your pregnancy until the second or third trimester unless you don't mind being hounded every day about when the new baby is coming.

TIP

Look out for children's books that cover the subject of a new baby or sibling rivalry. If you buy a couple of these books well in advance, you can give your child plenty of time to take on board the idea of a new brother or sister. Books can also be useful in introducing subjects you may never have thought of – such as the fact that you can't sell or return new siblings if your older child doesn't like them.

If your child is old enough – at least two or three years old – you may want to bring her along to antenatal doctor visits, ultrasound examinations, or when you're shopping for baby items. (While you're doing that shopping, consider getting a small present for your child so that she doesn't feel neglected.) A child who is old enough may also like to join in discussions about what to name the new baby.

TIP

If you anticipate moving your child to a new room or having her graduate from a cot to a bed, make the change before the baby is born. This change allows your older child to have a chance to acclimatise so that she doesn't associate the new situation directly with the new baby's arrival.

As you near the end of your pregnancy, don't be surprised if your child starts to act up or becomes unusually clingy and dependent. Many children get a sense that things are about to change when they see their mother getting physically bigger or when they overhear conversations about the impending arrival. During this time, be supportive and loving. Include your child in the preparations as much as possible. And remember that although having a new sibling affects almost all children in certain predictable ways, each child is unique, and how yours reacts depends in large part on her personality.

Making baby-sitting arrangements for your delivery

Obviously, you need to make arrangements for someone to take care of your child when you and your partner go to deliver the new baby. If your delivery is scheduled (if you're having a planned caesarean or an elective induction), arranging for a baby-sitter is relatively easy. But most women don't know exactly when the big moment will arrive – and you still need to be ready beforehand. If you go into labour spontaneously in the middle of the night, you want your child to be prepared in advance for what will happen and who will show up to take care of her while you're gone. Reassure your child that you will be okay and that she can come to see you and the new baby in the hospital very soon. If possible, phone your child at home while you're in the hospital to tell her that you're doing well, especially if your labour is unusually long. Many hospitals now have special sibling visiting hours, and you may want to check out the details ahead of time.

TIP

Pack a couple of gifts to take with you to the hospital – one for your child to give to the new baby and one for the baby to give to the child. Keeping your child waiting for a particularly precious treat, which the baby then gives them, can warm their feelings towards the baby very effectively. And don't forget – the present doesn't have to be expensive. Sarah made her son wait for months for a wooden pull-along train, and he was just as thrilled with the packaging as the present itself.

Coming home

During the first few days that the new siblings live together, you may be amazed at how well adjusted, happy, and excited your older child is. Part of this attitude is genuine enthusiasm. But keep in mind that part of it may also be your older child's attempt to share the limelight with the new baby. Some children have a short period of difficulty coping; others do fine at first but develop longer-lasting sibling rivalry. Don't be surprised if your child begins to regress in terms of some developmental milestones. A previously potty-trained child may resort to bedwetting, for example. Or a child may resume thumb-sucking or have difficulty sleeping. You may notice that your older child gets especially jealous while you're breast-feeding. During this period, understand that your child may need extra reassurance that you still love her and that the new baby hasn't replaced her in your heart at all.

Explain that your heart is big enough to love more than one child. If possible, allow your elder child to participate in helping to care for the baby. How much 'help' your child is capable of providing depends upon her age, but even small children can fetch a nappy if you need one or help give the baby a bath. Don't be surprised if at times your child expresses aggression toward you or the baby. Usually, these acts of aggression are harmless, but during this early stage of adjustment, don't leave your child alone with the baby unsupervised – she may not realise that certain ways of handling the baby may be harmful.

Several months may pass before your older child feels secure, but eventually most children do deal with the change successfully. Quite often friends, neighbours, and family shower the new baby with gifts. Again, having a stash of inexpensive new toys for your older child to prevent excessive jealousy may be a good idea. With extra love and understanding, you can help your child through what can be a difficult period.

Chapter 16

When Things Get Complicated

In This Chapter

- Going into labour too soon
- Understanding problems with blood pressure
- Monitoring placental conditions and amniotic fluid levels
- Keeping track of the baby's growth
- Examining blood issues
- Handling breech presentation
- Waiting for baby: When labour doesn't start on time

The vast majority of pregnancies are smooth, uncomplicated affairs – perfectly well managed by Mother Nature alone. Sometimes, though, your pregnancy can get a little complicated. Even when problems arise, ultimately both baby and mother are healthy in most cases. We have many patients who, after reading other books about pregnancy, call us frantically, assuming that they're going through every complication they read about. This chapter's information is meant to reassure you that your pregnancy is safe – or if you do have a particular problem, it's there to help you understand the problem better.

We're trying to avoid writing yet another textbook on maternal-foetal medicine – so we cover some conditions only briefly and omit some less common problems entirely. But our hope is that the following information gives you some idea of what can happen, so that if you develop any problem, you know how to proceed.

Dealing with Preterm Labour

Normally, during the second half of pregnancy, the uterus contracts intermittently. As the end approaches, these contractions grow more frequent and, finally, they become regular and cause the cervix to dilate. When contractions and dilation occur before 37 weeks gestation, labour is considered preterm. Some women notice periods of regular contractions prior to 37 weeks. If the cervix doesn't dilate or efface, however, the condition isn't considered preterm labour.

Of course, the earlier that preterm labour occurs, the more troublesome it can be. The problems that a premature baby has if he is born after about 34 weeks are usually much less to worry about than those he would face if born at only 24 weeks. Prior to about 32 weeks, the main problem is that the baby's lungs may still be immature, but you may have other complications as well. Nevertheless, the majority of babies born at 26 to 32 weeks can be fine and healthy, especially if they have access to modern neonatal intensive care. Premature babies stand a higher risk of contracting some infection, they may experience problems with the gastrointestinal tract (stomach and intestines), or they may have an *intraventricular haemorrhage,* which is bleeding into an area within the brain.

The following are signs and symptoms of preterm labour:

- Constant leakage of thin fluid from the vagina
- Increase in mucous-like vaginal discharge
- Intense and persistent pressure in the pelvis or vaginal area
- Menstrual-like cramps
- Persistent lower-back pain
- Regular contractions that don't stop with rest or decreased activity

Nobody knows for sure what causes premature labour, but clearly, some patients are at higher risk for developing it. If you fall into one of the high-risk categories, your practitioner probably wants to follow you more closely than usual. Your practitioner may ask you to come to the surgery or clinic more often, or to undergo certain tests. The following are some factors that put you at risk for preterm delivery:

- Abnormally shaped uterus
- Abuse of certain illicit drugs
- Bleeding during pregnancy, especially during the second half (*Note:* This doesn't include occasional spotting during the first trimester.)

- Prior preterm delivery
- Some infections, like bacterial vaginosis or a kidney infection
- Smoking
- Twins or more

Checking for signs of preterm labour

Practitioners have various ways to try to detect preterm labour, although the techniques aren't always effective. The most common way is for your practitioner to perform an internal examination to check the cervix and to monitor you for contractions.

Stopping preterm labour

Depending on how far along you are when you develop preterm labour, your doctor may attempt to stop your contractions (if he believes in this practice), and you may be admitted to hospital. Your doctor may use several medications (called *tocolytics*) to block preterm labour. Doctors have never come to widespread agreement that these medications are useful in the long run, though they have been shown to help for a few days to a week. Most tocolytics have side effects for the mother. Terbutaline, for example, may cause an increase in heart rate or a jittery feeling. Magnesium sulphate may cause nausea, flushing, or drowsiness. Indomethacin is well-tolerated, but can't be used for too long because of some effects on the foetus. If your doctor thinks that your preterm labour may lead to premature delivery prior to 34 weeks, he will probably recommend that you receive an injection of steroids, which have been shown to decrease the risk of breathing problems and other complications in the premature newborn. The risks to the mother of taking steroids are negligible, and large studies have shown that they offer benefits to the baby for about a week. Patients who continue to be at risk for preterm delivery and are more than seven days past the time that the steroids were given shouldn't repeat the course.

Preventing preterm labour

Several recent studies indicate that women who are at an increased risk for a preterm delivery (see the list in 'Dealing with Preterm Labour' earlier in this chapter) may have a reduced chance of delivering preterm if they take a specific type of progesterone during their pregnancies. The studies looked at both progesterone injections and progesterone vaginal suppositories. Researchers don't know yet which is best, but several studies currently underway are looking at administering progesterone to prevent preterm delivery.

Delivering the baby early

Sometimes delivering a baby early makes sense. If you go into preterm labour at 35 or 36 weeks, for example, just letting you go ahead and deliver is usually wise, because the outlook for the baby is so good and there's no reason to subject you to the side effects of medications to stop labour. If your baby has a condition that doctors can't treat inside the uterus, or if you have a condition that's getting worse, such as pre-eclampsia (see the next section, 'Handling Pre-eclampsia'), and continuing the pregnancy would be risky, early delivery is sometimes the best option.

Handling Pre-eclampsia

Also known as toxaemia, or pregnancy-induced hypertension (PIH), *pre-eclampsia* shows up as raised blood pressure along with fluid retention or protein spillage in the urine. About 1 in 12 pregnancies are complicated by pre-eclampsia, most commonly in first pregnancies. Pre-eclampsia usually occurs late in pregnancy but can develop in the late second or early third trimester. The condition goes away after delivery.

TECHNICAL STUFF

Doctors have different criteria for diagnosing pre-eclampsia, but, in general, blood pressure that stays above 140/90, or 20 millimetres of mercury above the first blood pressure you had taken after you became pregnant, is considered raised, if you have no history of blood pressure problems prior to pregnancy.

Following is a list of the signs and symptoms of pre-eclampsia:

- Abnormalities in certain blood tests (decreased platelets, important in clotting) and elevations in liver tests
- Blurry vision or seeing spots in front of your eyes
- Nausea, vomiting, and pain in the upper mid-abdominal area
- Onset of seizures
- Pain in the upper-right part of your abdomen, near your liver

- Severe headache that won't go away even if you take pain medication
- Sudden swelling of the hands, face, or legs
- Sudden weight gain

Most of the symptoms can occur harmlessly during any pregnancy. Unless these symptoms happen in combination with elevated blood pressure or protein spillage in the urine, they're quite normal. If one day you have a headache, or if for a second you see spots, don't jump to the conclusion that you have pre-eclampsia. If the symptoms persist, tell your doctor.

No one knows exactly what causes pre-eclampsia, but doctors do know that some women are at a higher risk for developing it than others. The following are risk factors for pre-eclampsia:

- Existing chronic hypertension
- First pregnancy
- History of pre-eclampsia in a prior pregnancy
- Long-standing diabetes
- Mother older than 40
- Significant obesity
- Some medical problems, such as serious kidney or liver disease, lupus, or other vascular diseases
- Triplets or more (twins, also, but to a much lesser extent)

Despite extensive ongoing medical research on pre-eclampsia, no one knows exactly how to prevent it. The only real treatment for pre-eclampsia is delivering the baby. When to deliver depends on how severe the condition is and how far along you are in your pregnancy. If you're close to your due date, induced delivery may be the wisest approach. If you're only 28 weeks along, your doctor may try bed rest and close observation, either at home or in hospital. Doctors weigh the risks to the mother's health against the risks to the baby of preterm delivery.

Understanding Placental Conditions

Two different problems with the baby's placenta can sometimes occur in the latter part of pregnancy: placenta praevia and placental abruption. In this section, we describe both these conditions.

Placenta praevia

Placenta praevia is when the placenta partially or completely covers the cervix, as shown in Figure 16-1. Doctors typically diagnose patients with placenta praevia during a routine ultrasound examination, but sometimes women find out about the problem only when they begin bleeding late in the second or early in the third trimester.

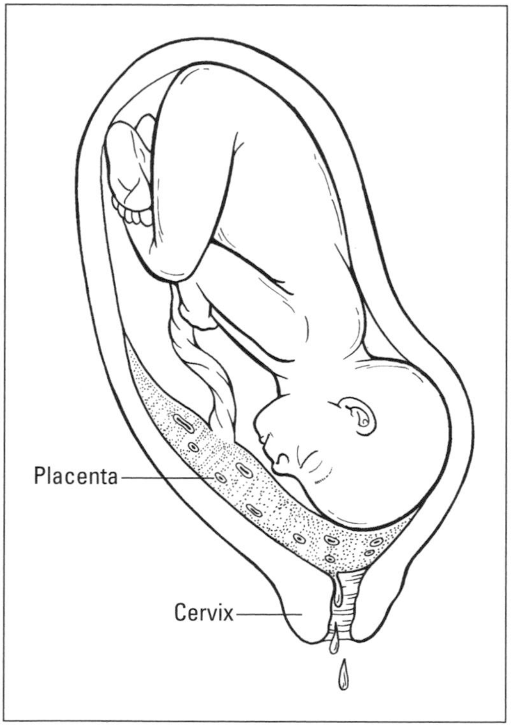

Figure 16-1: Placenta praevia.

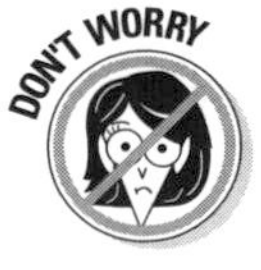

In early pregnancy, having the placenta near the cervix or even partially covering the cervix is common – this positioning can happen in as many as 1 in 5 pregnancies. In the vast majority of women (95 per cent), the placenta rises as the uterus enlarges with the growing baby, which is why you have no reason to worry about the placenta covering the cervix early in pregnancy. If placenta praevia is discovered during a routine ultrasound examination, the hospital doctor will arrange for you to have regular ultrasound scans to check progress throughout your pregnancy. Even if the situation persists through the late second trimester and into the third, it can still be harmless.

Although many women who have placenta praevia never bleed at all, the main concern is that heavy bleeding may occur. If bleeding is severe enough, the baby may have to be delivered just for this reason. Sometimes bleeding leads to preterm labour, so your practitioner attempts to stop the contractions, which often stops the bleeding.

If you're in your third trimester and you have placenta praevia, your practitioner may want you to have regular ultrasound scans to see whether the placenta will eventually move out of the way. He or she may tell you to avoid intercourse and internal examinations in order to lower the risk of any bleeding. If the praevia persists until 36 weeks, your doctor will usually recommend a caesarean delivery, because the baby can't come through the birth canal without disrupting the placenta, which can lead to heavy bleeding.

Placental abruption

In some women, the placenta separates from the uterine wall before pregnancy is over. This condition is called placental abruption (sometimes also called abruptio placentae or placental separation). Figure 16-2 shows you what placental abruption looks like.

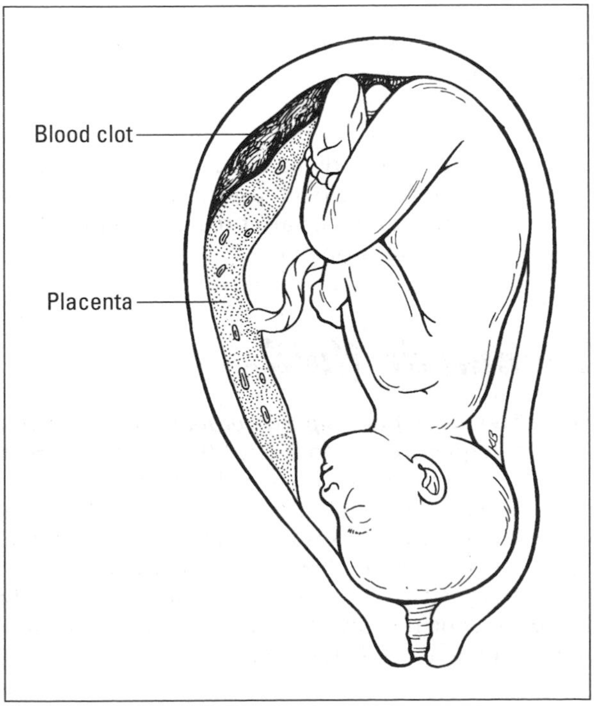

Figure 16-2: Placental abruption.

Placental abruption is a common cause of third-trimester bleeding. Because blood is an irritant to the uterine muscle, it can also cause premature labour and abdominal pain. An abruption is difficult to see on an ultrasound examination unless it is quite large. So in many cases, doctors can make the diagnosis of an abruption only after they rule out every other possible cause of bleeding. Rarely, a placental abruption occurs suddenly, and if the separation is large enough your baby may need to be delivered very quickly. See Chapter 8 for other causes of third-trimester bleeding.

If you experience a small placental abruption, your practitioner may recommend bed rest. He will also start to observe your pregnancy more closely to make sure that the problem has no harmful side effects on the foetus.

Recognising Problems with the Amniotic Fluid and Sac

The foetus grows within a bag of water – the amniotic sac, containing the amniotic fluid. This fluid increases in volume throughout the first part of pregnancy and reaches its maximum level at 34 weeks. After that, the volume gradually declines. During the second half of pregnancy, the amniotic fluid comprises mainly foetal urine. The foetus urinates into the sac and then also swallows the fluid. Don't worry, this won't cause any harm – the fluid circulating around the foetal lungs aids in lung development.

Sometimes, a practitioner may suspect that the amount of amniotic fluid is above or below average, and he may do an ultrasound examination to see what's happening. Minor increases or decreases in the amount of amniotic fluid usually aren't a problem. But large variations in amniotic fluid volume may be a symptom of some other problem.

Too much amniotic fluid

The medical term for too much fluid is *polyhydramnios* or *hydramnios*. This situation occurs quite frequently, in about 1 to 10 per cent of pregnancies. Often the increase in volume is small. Doctors don't always know what causes the increase of amniotic fluid, but they do know that a small increase usually isn't a problem. Larger increases in fluid may be associated with a medical condition in the mother – diabetes or certain viral illnesses, for example. In some rare cases, the excess fluid may be due to certain foetal problems – the foetus may be having difficulty swallowing the fluid, for example, so more of it accumulates inside the sac.

Expectant mothers ask . . .

Q: 'Is the amount of amniotic fluid determined to any extent by the amount of water I drink?'

A: No. The mother's fluid intake has little to do with it. Some recent studies suggest that a mother can cause small increases in the amount of amniotic fluid by drinking plenty of liquids, but the effect isn't that great. Nevertheless, stay well hydrated.

Too little amniotic fluid

A woman who has too little amniotic fluid has *oligohydramnios*. Amniotic fluid volume normally decreases after 34 to 36 weeks. If your fluid volume starts to fall below a specific range, however, your practitioner may want to observe the foetus more closely by performing certain tests. One common cause of low amniotic fluid is a rupture of the membranes, which allows fluid to leak out.

A fluid level that drops significantly prior to 34 weeks may indicate a problem with the mother or the baby. For example, some women with hypertension or lupus may have less blood flow to the uterus and, consequently, less blood flow to the placenta and the baby. When the baby receives less blood, his kidneys make less urine, and that results in lower levels of amniotic fluid.

If the reduction in fluid is mild or moderate, the baby is watched carefully and undergoes tests of foetal wellbeing. Sometimes, oligohydramnios is a sign that the baby's growth is restricted (see 'Describing Problems with Foetal Growth' later in this chapter) or, rarely, that there are abnormalities in the baby's urinary tract. Sometimes it's a sign that the placenta isn't functioning optimally.

If you have decreased amniotic fluid, your doctor may suggest that you get more rest and try to stay off your feet. By doing so, you may promote more blood flow to the uterus and placenta and thus increase the baby's urine output. (Just be glad you don't have to change all the nappies yet.)

Rupture of the amniotic sac

Premature rupture of the membranes or *amniotic sac*, sometimes called PROM, is when a woman's water breaks some time before labour starts. PROM can happen close to the due date (term PROM) or sometimes earlier than 37 weeks (preterm PROM).

- If you experience term PROM, your practitioner may simply wait until you go into labour on your own, or he may induce labour in order to avoid the risk that an infection may develop inside the uterus.
- If you experience preterm PROM, you may or may not go into labour, depending on how far along you are. If you're very far from your due date and don't appear to have an infection in your uterus, your doctor may use some medications (antibiotics, tocolytics, and steroids) to prolong the pregnancy as long as possible. Your doctor will probably arrange frequent ultrasound scans and monitor the foetal heart rate to ensure that the baby is managing okay.

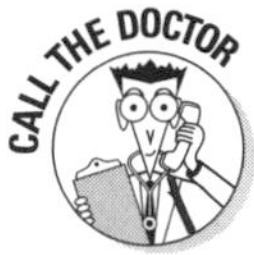

If you think your membranes may have ruptured and you're preterm, let your practitioner know immediately. He can perform tests to let you know for certain whether your membranes have actually ruptured.

Describing Problems with Foetal Growth

One of the main reasons to get antenatal care is to make sure that your baby is growing well. A practitioner typically gauges growth by measuring the fundal height (see Chapter 3). As a general rule (in a singleton pregnancy), the measurement in centimetres from the top of the pubic bone to the top of the uterus roughly equals the number of weeks' gestation. If your practitioner finds that this measurement is greater or less than expected, he may recommend that you have an ultrasound scan to assess the baby's growth more accurately. During the scan, the technician measures various foetal body parts to come up with an approximate foetal weight. That estimate is then compared with the average weight for foetuses at the same gestational age and assigned to a certain percentile. The 50th percentile is average. But because foetuses (like babies, toddlers, children, teenagers, and grown-ups) come in different sizes, there is a range of normal weights. Anything between the 10th and the 90th percentile is considered normal (see Chapter 8 for more information about foetal weight).

Expectant mothers ask . . .

Q: 'If I eat more, will my baby grow into the normal range?'

A: Unfortunately, the answer is no. Eating more doesn't correct the problem unless you're significantly malnourished.

These upper and lower limits are somewhat arbitrary and imply that 10 per cent of the population is larger than normal and that 10 per cent is smaller – but this statement isn't exactly true. Most foetuses below the 10th percentile or above the 90th percentile are completely normal. However, some of these foetuses may not be growing normally and may need extra surveillance.

Smaller-than-average babies

A foetus whose estimated weight falls below the 10th percentile may have *intrauterine growth restriction* (IUGR). IUGR can lead to the birth of a baby who is *small for dates* (SFD). IUGR has many possible causes, including the following:

- **The baby is measuring small, but is otherwise normal.** Just as healthy adults come in all sizes, so do foetuses.
- **Chromosomal abnormalities.** This cause is most common with early-onset IUGR, which occurs in the second trimester.
- **Environmental toxins.** Cigarette smoking causes a decrease in birth-weight between one-fourth and one-half of a pound, on average. Chronic alcohol consumption (of at least one to two drinks a day) and cocaine use also can cause low birth-weight.
- **Genetic factors.** Some genetic factors cause the foetus to grow less than average.
- **Heart and circulatory abnormalities in the foetus.** Examples include a congenital heart defect or umbilical cord abnormalities.
- **Inadequate nutrition for the mother.** Proper nutrition is especially important in the third trimester.
- **Infection such as rubella, and toxoplasmosis.** Chapters 5 and 17 provide more information.
- **Multiple gestation.** Fifteen to 25 per cent of twins have IUGR, and even more triplets. Twins grow at the same rate as singletons until 28 to 32 weeks, when the twin growth curve drops off.
- **Placenta factors and uterine-placental problems.** Because the placenta provides nutrition and oxygen to the foetus, if it's functioning poorly or if the blood isn't flowing smoothly from the uterus to the placenta, the foetus may not grow properly. Women with antiphospholipid antibody syndrome (a blood-clotting problem), recurrent bleeding, vascular diseases, or chronic hypertension are at risk for IUGR because those conditions cause poor placental function. Pre-eclampsia may also impair placental function and lead to IUGR.

The way your practitioner responds to IUGR depends on your individual situation. Foetuses with mild IUGR, normal chromosomes, and no evidence of infection are likely to be fine. Sometimes early delivery is warranted, however, because the foetus may grow better in the nursery than inside the uterus. The way your practitioner responds to signs of IUGR depends on both the cause of the problem and the gestational age at which it is diagnosed. In many cases, *small for dates* (SFD) babies turn out to be perfectly normal. Unfortunately, though, severe cases have been associated with learning difficulties later in life and even foetal death, which is why a mother and baby with this condition are closely monitored.

Larger-than-average babies

A baby whose estimated weight is above the 90th percentile may have *macrosomia* (big body). Many different reasons can explain why a woman may have an exceptionally large baby, including the following:

- Delivery of a previous large baby.
- Excessive maternal weight gain during pregnancy.
- Obesity in the mother.
- One parent was born very large – or both were.
- The pregnancy lasts longer than 40 weeks.
- Poorly controlled diabetes in the mother.

The mother's main risk is that the delivery is more difficult. If she delivers vaginally, she may suffer increased trauma to the birth canal, and she has an increased chance of needing a caesarean delivery. The main risk to the baby is injury during delivery. Birth injury is more likely when a large baby is delivered vaginally, but it can also occur during a caesarean delivery. Most commonly, birth injury involves excessive stretching of the nerves in the baby's upper arm and neck resulting from a shoulder dystocia during delivery (see Chapter 11).

DON'T WORRY

If your practitioner thinks that your baby may be exceptionally large, based on either an ultrasound estimate of foetal weight or an abdominal examination, and it appears that your pelvic bones may make for a tight fit, he will discuss your delivery options with you.

Looking at Blood Incompatibilities

If a baby's parents have two different blood types, the baby's blood type can be different from the mother's. Usually this situation creates absolutely no problem for the mother or the baby. In some rare cases, these blood-type mismatches warrant special consideration – even then, however, there is hardly ever a significant problem.

All women are routinely checked in early pregnancy for their blood's Rhesus status, which can be positive or negative. The *Rhesus antigen* is part of your body's immune system. If you are *Rhesus negative*, you don't have this Rhesus antigen. If your baby is *Rhesus positive* (your baby can inherit the Rhesus antigen from his father, even if you don't have it), he does have this Rhesus antigen. During pregnancy, there's a small risk of your Rhesus negative blood coming into contact with your baby's Rhesus positive blood, priming your immune system to fight off future contact with Rhesus antigens. This situation won't harm your present baby, but does mean that if you have another Rhesus positive pregnancy, your body's immune system might see the foetus as an intruder, and try to fight it off. This can cause the baby to be stillborn, or give rise to *haemolytic disease of the newborn* (HDN). HDN can give your baby jaundice or anaemia, and in a few cases may be fatal. Fortunately, this risk can be prevented very effectively by giving you an injection of a substance called Anti-D at certain points in your pregnancy. Your doctor may recommend Anti-D at the following times, if you are Rhesus negative:

- Within 72 hours of delivery. A midwife gives the injection after delivery in order to prevent problems in future pregnancies.
- Routinely at 28 and 34 weeks gestation (as a precaution, just in case any passage of blood across the placenta has already occurred).
- After amniocentesis, CVS (chorionic villus sampling), or any invasive procedure (see Chapter 9).
- After a miscarriage, abortion, or ectopic pregnancy (see Chapter 6 for more on ectopic pregnancy).
- After significant trauma to your abdomen during pregnancy, if your doctor thinks that some of the baby's blood may have leaked into your circulation.
- After significant bleeding during pregnancy.

Dealing with Breech Presentation

A baby is in a so-called *breech* position when its buttocks or legs are down, closest to the cervix. Breech presentation happens in 3 to 4 per cent of all singleton deliveries. A woman's risk of having a breech baby decreases the further along she goes in her pregnancy. The foetus is more likely to assume a breech position for one of the following reasons:

- The foetus is preterm or especially small.
- An increased amount of amniotic fluid exists (all the more room to turn around in).

- A congenital malformation of the uterus is present (for example, a bicornuate, or T-shaped, uterus).
- Fibroids that impinge on the uterine cavity are present.
- You have placenta praevia (see Chapter 16).
- You're having twins – or more.
- Your uterus is relaxed from having had several babies already.

If your baby is in a breech position, your doctor will talk with you about the potential risks and benefits of a vaginal breech delivery. Special concerns about a breech delivery include the following:

- Trapping the baby's head (which comes out last in a breech delivery) in a cervix that has been incompletely dilated by the passage of the baby's body, which is smaller than the head. (This situation is especially troublesome if the baby is very small or premature.)
- Trauma resulting from an *extended foetal head* (meaning the head is tilted back).
- Difficulty delivering the arms, which can lead to potential arm injuries.

Because of these potential problems, many practitioners recommend that all breech babies be delivered by caesarean section. However, some foetuses in breech position are actually good candidates for vaginal delivery. Conditions that should be present for you and your doctor to consider a vaginal breech delivery include the following:

- Estimated foetal weight is between 1.8 and 3.6 kilograms (4 to 8 pounds).
- The baby is in a *frank* breech position, which means that the buttocks, not the feet, are in position to come out first.
- The buttocks are engaged in the pelvis.
- Your doctor doesn't detect (by physical examination or by X-ray) any problem with the baby's head fitting through the birth canal.
- Ultrasound shows that the foetal head is either flexed or in the *military* position (looking straight ahead, not tilted back).
- Immediate anaesthetic is available so that caesarean delivery can be done in an emergency.
- The doctor is experienced in vaginal breech deliveries.

A few recent large studies have shown that breech babies delivered vaginally are at a higher risk for certain complications. The information is so compelling that many obstetricians have stopped performing vaginal breech deliveries. If you and your practitioner decide that a vaginal breech delivery isn't right for you, another option is *external cephalic version,* a procedure in which the doctor tries to turn the baby into normal delivery position by externally manipulating the mother's abdomen, which is a common and usually safe procedure. Sometimes this manipulation is fairly uncomfortable, but it works in about 50 to 70 per cent of cases. There are certain conditions in which external cephalic version isn't advisable, such as bleeding, low amniotic fluid level, or in multiple births.

Pondering Post-Date Pregnancy

The average pregnancy lasts about 40 weeks (or 280 days) after the last menstrual period, but only about 5 per cent of women deliver on their due date. Some women deliver a couple of weeks earlier and some a couple of weeks later, and all are considered to be at term. You don't have a post-date pregnancy, according to the medical definition, until you go beyond 42 weeks. Only a small number of pregnancies last longer than 42 weeks, and no one knows why they do.

Why should you or your practitioner care whether you go past your due date? Because the chance of certain complications rises as time goes on – from 40 to 42 weeks, the increases are small, but after 42 weeks, they climb into a range that is more worrying. The worst complication is perinatal death (also called perinatal mortality). The chances of perinatal death start to increase after 41 to 42 weeks and double by 43 weeks.

DON'T WORRY

Perinatal death isn't as scary as it may sound, because the actual number of deaths is very low. The vast majority of late babies are born healthy. The increase in mortality rates in post-date pregnancies involves several factors, including:

- The placenta, which supports and feeds your baby, can function efficiently for only a finite length of time – about 40 weeks. Fortunately, most placentas have some amount of 'reserve', and they still work beyond 40 weeks.
- In a post-date pregnancy, the volume of amniotic fluid may decrease. Most of the time, adequate fluid is left after 40 weeks. Sometimes, however, the fluid level drops into a range that doctors consider too low. In this situation, the umbilical cord has a chance of becoming compressed, and doctors may recommend that labour be induced.
- Babies can sometimes pass their first bowel movement while they're still inside the uterus, and the longer a pregnancy lasts, the more likely it is that this happens. In rare instances, the baby may breathe in this thick *meconium*, either before or during birth, which can cause problems with breathing in the first few days or weeks after birth (for more information, see Chapter 10).

- In a post-date pregnancy in which the placenta continues to function normally, the baby keeps growing. Therefore, late babies are more likely to be very large (known as *macrosomic*; see 'Describing Problems with Foetal Growth' earlier in this chapter), or large for gestational age. So these babies may be at risk for all the problems that come with being extra large.

The National Institute of Clinical Excellence (NICE) has issued guidance on options for post-date pregnancy, and Chapter 10 gives more details.

Chapter 17

Pregnancy in Sickness and in Health

In This Chapter

- Treating infections from the common cold to cystitis
- Handling asthma, diabetes, and other pre-existing health problems during pregnancy

Pregnancy may give you a maternal glow and make you feel as if something magical is happening to your body. But let's face it: Pregnancy doesn't make you superhuman. You're still susceptible to all the illnesses and other health problems that can affect anyone who's not expecting a baby. When illnesses arise during pregnancy, they can have special consequences. In this chapter, we talk about how a variety of medical conditions affect pregnant women.

Getting an Infection during Pregnancy

Try as you may, avoiding every person who's carrying an infection during your pregnancy may be impossible. Keep in mind that most infections don't hurt the baby at all; they just make life more uncomfortable for you for a while. In this section, we cover the most common infections and some of the more unusual ones.

Bladder and kidney infections

Bladder infections come in two basic types: women who have symptoms and women who don't. The silent (symptom-free) ones are common, occurring in about 6 per cent of pregnant women. The other kind, called *cystitis*, comes with symptoms that include:

- Constantly feeling that you need to urinate
- Discomfort above your pubic bone (where the bladder is)

- More frequent urination
- Pain with urination

If you develop either type of bladder infection, your doctor treats it with antibiotics.

If left untreated, a bladder infection can progress into a kidney infection, also known as *pyelonephritis*. A kidney infection produces the same symptoms described for cystitis, plus high fevers and flank pain – pain over one or both kidneys (see Figure 17-1). Flank pain also can occur in someone who has kidney stones. The difference: A kidney infection causes a constant pain, whereas kidney stones produce more severe, but intermittent, pain. Also, kidney stones are more often accompanied by small quantities of blood in the urine.

If your practitioner diagnoses you with pyelonephritis, she may want to admit you to hospital for a few days so that you can get intravenous antibiotics. Because kidney infections tend to recur during pregnancy, your practitioner may also want to keep you on a daily antibiotic for the remainder of your pregnancy.

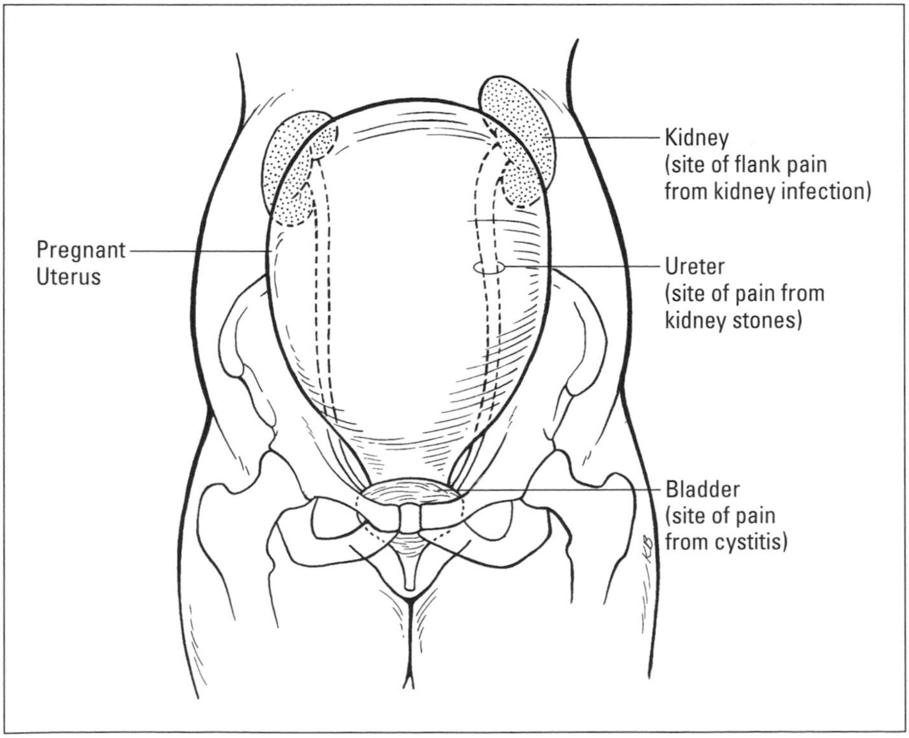

Figure 17-1: Bladder infections, kidney infections, and kidney stones have their own unique symptoms.

Chickenpox

The varicella zoster virus causes chickenpox. The first time someone comes down with an infection caused by this virus, usually in childhood, she gets chickenpox. Chickenpox is pretty rare in adults, and pregnant women stand no greater risk of contracting this virus than non-pregnant people do. Even better, if you've already had chickenpox, you're not likely to get it again (but never say never).

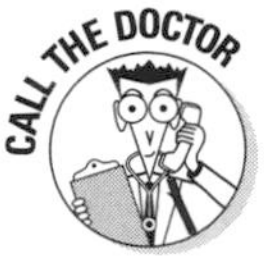

If you don't know whether you've ever had chickenpox and you're exposed to someone with the infection, let your GP or midwife know immediately. Your practitioner will arrange for a blood test to determine whether you're immune, and if you're not immune, you'll receive an injection known as VZIG (*varicella zoster immune globulin*), which may reduce the risk of infection to you and the baby. Get this injection within three days of exposure, if possible. If you contract chickenpox within several days of giving birth (before or after), your baby should receive VZIG.

Chickenpox can cause three potential problems during pregnancy:

- It can make the mother ill with flu-like symptoms, plus the famous skin rash (lots of little red blemishes). In rare circumstances, pneumonia develops two to six days after the rash appears. If you have chickenpox, and you develop symptoms like shortness of breath or a dry cough, let your doctor know immediately.
- If you contract chickenpox during the first four months of pregnancy, the foetus has a small chance of developing the infection, too, leading to congenital varicella syndrome. With this syndrome, the foetus can have scarring (the same kinds of scars that little kids get on their bodies from chickenpox), some abnormal development of the limbs, problems with growth, and developmental delays.

  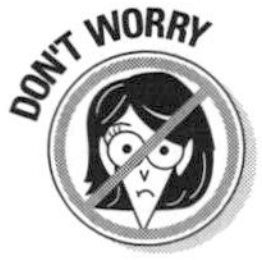

  Fortunately, congenital varicella syndrome is very rare. (It happens in less than 1 per cent of cases in which the infection occurs in the first trimester, 2 per cent if in the early second trimester.)
- If you contract chickenpox within the interval from five days before to five days after giving birth, the baby is at risk for developing a serious varicella infection in the newborn period. You can greatly reduce this chance by giving the baby VZIG.

The same varicella zoster virus that causes chickenpox can also produce a recurrent form of the infection called shingles or herpes zoster. Most babies born to pregnant women who develop shingles are completely normal. Because shingles is much less common than chickenpox in pregnancy, doctors don't really know how common birth defects are after a pregnant woman develops this condition, although the incidence is thought to be less than the 1 to 2 per cent seen with chickenpox.

If you know that you're susceptible to chickenpox, avoid direct contact with anyone who has shingles or herpes zoster, because their lesions contain the varicella zoster virus and can cause a chickenpox infection in susceptible women.

The common cold

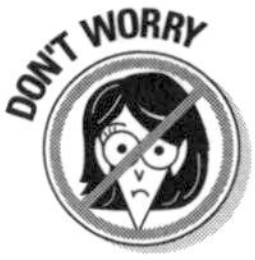

Most people get a cold about once a year, so the fact that most women get one during pregnancy isn't surprising. Nothing about pregnancy makes you more vulnerable to a cold virus, but the fatigue and congestion that go along with pregnancy can make a cold seem worse. The common cold is perfectly harmless to the developing foetus. Because there's no cure for the common cold, the only option is to treat the symptoms. Although some medications (you can find out more in Chapter 3) are perfectly safe in pregnancy, many women want to avoid taking them unless doing so is absolutely essential – so with that in mind, here are a few suggestions for dealing with cold symptoms:

- **Drink fluids, fluids, and more fluids.** All viral illnesses promote dehydration, and being pregnant makes the problem more extreme. Drink plenty of water, juice, or fizzy drinks when you have a cold or the flu, but stay away from milk.
- **Give yourself a steam inhalation.** Inhaling steam for colds and coughs may be the oldest remedy in the book, but it works. Fill a bowl with boiling water, and add a few drops of decongestant oil. Then sit down in front of the bowl with a towel covering your head and the bowl, for about fifteen minutes. Not only is steam an incredibly effective way of helping you to cough up mucus, but it'll give you a facial at the same time!
- **Go citrus-fruit crazy.** Citrus fruit is very high in vitamin C, which has been found in some studies to reduce the duration of colds. By taking your vitamin C in whole fruit form, you get all the other benefits that fruit and vegetables bring (see Chapter 5 for more on the wonders of diet).
- **Take paracetamol.** Paracetamol, in the recommended doses, will bring your fever down as well as help with the aches and pains that accompany a cold. Paracetamol is also perfectly safe at the standard adult dose, so don't be scared to take it.

- **Eat some comfort food.** Last, but certainly not least, have some soup. Scientific studies have shown that soup has properties that help cold sufferers feel better, even though no one knows exactly what those properties are.

TIP

You can use the same treatments for the common cold and for influenza infections. If you get the flu while you're pregnant, you're likely to have the same experience as when you're not pregnant.

German measles (rubella)

The rubella virus causes German measles, which are the only kind that have any significant impact on pregnancy. If you contract rubella within the first trimester, the baby has about a 20 per cent chance of developing congenital rubella syndrome. The chance of developing this syndrome, however, varies even within the first trimester from the first month to the third month. Fortunately, acute rubella infection during pregnancy is extremely uncommon.

Herpes infections

Herpes is a common virus that infects the mouth, throat, skin, and genital tract. If you have a history of herpes, rest assured that the infection poses no risk to the developing foetus. The main concern is that you may have an active genital herpes lesion when you go into labour or when your water breaks. If you do have a lesion there is a small risk that you transmit the infection to the baby as she passes through the birth canal. If it's your first herpes infection, the chance that the foetus contracts the virus is greater, because you have no antibodies to the virus. Studies show that women with a history of recurrent herpes may lower the chance of having an active herpes infection at delivery by taking a medication called *aciclovir* in the last month of pregnancy.

REMEMBER

If you have a history of genital herpes, tell your practitioner at your booking appointment (see Chapter 6 for more on this meeting). If you have active genital herpes lesions at the time of labour or ruptured membranes, let your practitioner know. She is likely to perform a caesarean delivery to avoid infecting the baby. If you see no lesions, but you feel as if you may be developing them, also tell your doctor – having a caesarean may also be advisable.

Human immunodeficiency virus (HIV)

Over the past few years, studies have shown that some of the medications used to treat HIV infection can dramatically reduce the chance that the virus is transmitted from a mother to her baby. Many doctors now recommend that women undergo HIV testing early in pregnancy, and that if a woman is HIV-positive she receives these medications during pregnancy as well as during labour. In order to decrease the chance that a baby becomes infected with HIV, avoid any invasive procedures that can cause bleeding, such as amniocentesis or CVS (refer to Chapter 9), unless they're absolutely required. If your doctor performs these procedures, it is recommended that you receive intravenous doses of antiviral medications immediately beforehand to minimise the chance of infecting the foetus.

Don't breast-feed if you're infected with HIV because you may transmit the virus to your baby. Whatever form of birth control you choose, the use of condoms, in addition, is absolutely necessary.

If you're HIV-positive, maintain close contact with HIV specialists so that you can benefit from the ever-improving treatments.

Tummy bugs (gastroenteritis)

A tummy bug can occur at any time, whether or not you're pregnant. Symptoms of gastroenteritis include stomach cramps, fever, diarrhoea, and nausea, with or without vomiting, and they last anywhere from 24 to 72 hours. The viruses that cause gastroenteritis usually don't harm your baby.

Don't worry that your baby won't get adequate nutrition if you can't eat for a few days. Foetuses do just fine even when their mothers miss a few meals.

If you get a tummy bug, make sure that you drink plenty of liquids. Dehydration can lead to premature contractions and can contribute to fatigue and dizziness. Try soup, as well as other liquids – water, ginger beer, tea, or broth. Take care of yourself in the same way you would if you weren't pregnant. If your symptoms persist for more than 72 hours, call your doctor.

Vaginal infections

Bacteria and other organisms, when given half a chance, readily make themselves at home in a vagina, where the conditions – warm and moist – are perfect for them to grow and reproduce. A woman can get an infection at any time, even when she's pregnant. Some vaginal infections, such as thrush (see the following section on 'Yeast infections'), actually become more common when you're pregnant.

Yeast infections

Yeast infections, known as *thrush*, are very common in pregnancy. The large amounts of oestrogen that circulate in the bloodstream during pregnancy promote the growth of yeast in the vagina. Symptoms of an infection are vaginal itching and a thick, whitish-yellow discharge. However, many women get infections without any symptoms. The only treatment usually needed is a short course of vaginal suppositories or creams – talk to your GP or pharmacist for more advice.

DON'T WORRY

Yeast infections usually don't cause problems for the foetus or newborn.

Chlamydia

Chlamydia is one of the more common sexually transmitted diseases. This infection often comes with no symptoms, meaning you may be affected for years without knowing it. This lack of short-term symptoms makes chlamydia dangerous – not only do people pass the infection on without knowing it, but chlamydia can also cause long-term problems with fertility, or increase your risk of having an ectopic pregnancy (see Chapter 6). Although no national chlamydia screening programme exists, some areas offer routine checks at a well-woman clinic or during a cervical smear test.

If you're found to have chlamydia, whether or not you're pregnant, your doctor will prescribe a medication to treat the infection. Chlamydia can be passed to your newborn during vaginal delivery, increasing the chance that the baby will develop conjunctivitis (an eye infection) or, less likely, pneumonia.

Handling Pre-Pregnancy Conditions

The following sections detail conditions that you may have before you get pregnant and how those conditions may affect your pregnancy and vice versa.

Asthma

Predicting how pregnancy can affect a woman's asthma is difficult. Some women find that their condition improves when they're expecting, some find it gets worse, and about half notice no difference at all.

The main concern that women with asthma have is whether they can safely continue taking their medications during pregnancy. Remember, the biggest problem with asthma isn't the medications but the possibility that pregnant women with asthma under-treat themselves. If you're having trouble breathing, you may not be getting enough oxygen to the baby.

The guidelines of the British Thoracic Society (an organisation for people with respiratory disorders) contain a whole section on pregnant women with asthma, and the importance of making sure optimum treatment is given. The Society recommends that the benefits of all inhaled medicines for asthma (and some oral ones) outweigh the risks during pregnancy, so pregnant women with asthma should take exactly the same medication as when not pregnant. You can find out more about the British Thoracic Society's work by contacting them: The British Thoracic Society, 17 Doughty Street, London WC1N 2PL; phone 020 7831 8778; Web site www.brit-thoracic.org.uk.

Your doctor will tell you which oral asthma medications are safe during pregnancy. If you have asthma, make sure you talk to your GP before you get pregnant, or as soon as possible after finding out.

Chronic hypertension

Chronic hypertension refers to high blood pressure that occurs independently from pregnancy. Although many women who have this condition are aware that they have it before they conceive, doctors occasionally diagnose it during pregnancy. If you have mild or moderate chronic hypertension, chances are good that you'll have an uneventful pregnancy. However, your doctor will be on the lookout for certain conditions that can affect you or the baby.

Women with chronic hypertension stand an increased risk of developing pre-eclampsia, so your doctor looks for any signs that you're developing this condition. The main risk for the baby is intrauterine growth restriction (IUGR) or placental abruption (see Chapter 16). Your doctor may use repeated ultrasound scans to check on the baby's growth and to make sure that you have adequate amniotic fluid; she may also suggest that you undergo some tests later during your pregnancy for foetal wellbeing, such as non-stress tests (see Chapter 9). The overall management of your pregnancy depends on how well controlled your blood pressure is, your overall health, and how the baby grows.

Deep-vein thrombosis and pulmonary embolus

A deep-vein thrombosis (DVT) is a blood clot that develops within a deep vein, most commonly in the leg. A pulmonary embolus is a blood clot within the lung, which is often a clot that has dislodged from a deep-vein thrombosis in the leg and made its way to the lung. Both of these conditions are rare, affecting far less than 1 per cent of pregnant women, but both are also more common during pregnancy than outside of pregnancy.

Symptoms of a DVT include pain, swelling, redness, and tenderness, usually in the calf, and a rope-like hardness running down the back of the lower leg. Symptoms of a pulmonary embolus include sudden onset of shortness of breath, sharp chest pain, which is worse when you breathe, and coughing up blood.

Keep in mind that muscle pain, cramping, and swelling are common symptoms of a normal pregnancy, and a DVT is quite unusual. Likewise, getting more easily out-of-breath as your pregnancy progresses is almost inevitable, but a pulmonary embolus is highly unlikely. Tell your doctor when you're experiencing the sudden onset of these symptoms, but don't panic about them.

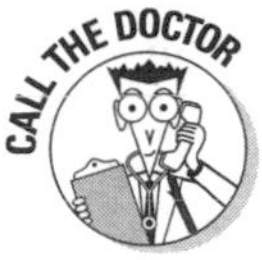

If you get a sudden onset of shortness of breath that gets rapidly worse, especially if it's accompanied by sharp chest pain and/or coughing up blood, call your doctor immediately.

Diabetes

You can find out much more about diabetes in pregnancy by reading *Diabetes For Dummies* by Sarah Jarvis and Alan L. Rubin (Wiley). Diabetes comes up as a problem in pregnancy in two ways:

- You already have the condition before you become pregnant.
- You develop gestational diabetes, which is unique to pregnancy and which usually goes away after pregnancy.

Our patients want to know . . .

Q: 'Are blood pressure medications safe?'

A: Most medications are safe, but many haven't been well studied during pregnancy. Discuss this important question with your doctor. Certain medications, however, should be avoided. Angiotensin-converting enzyme inhibitors (known as ACE inhibitors) pose some risk for kidney problems in the foetus. Beta-blockers, although considered quite safe, pose a very small risk of IUGR (intrauterine growth restriction). Also, diuretics (often called water tablets) are better avoided, unless this is the only way of treating the high blood pressure.

Diabetes before pregnancy

If you have a history of diabetes, talk to your doctor about it before you get pregnant. If you have your blood sugar level under good control before you conceive, your pregnancy is more likely to proceed smoothly. Women with pre-gestational diabetes stand a higher-than-average risk of having a foetus with certain birth defects, but you can reduce this risk down to the normal range if you achieve excellent glucose control.

If you take an oral medication to control your blood sugar, your practitioner will probably suggest you switch to insulin injections for better control. Some women with diabetes suffer kidney complications, but this isn't likely to worsen during pregnancy. If you have eye problems related to diabetes (proliferative retinopathy), get your doctor to monitor closely and possibly treat your eyes during pregnancy.

The vast majority of diabetic women proceed through pregnancy without a hitch. However, your doctor may need to adjust your insulin dose. Your doctor also follows the baby's growth with periodic ultrasound scans and is on the lookout to see that you don't develop high blood pressure. When you're in labour, your doctor keeps a close eye on your glucose level and may give you insulin. With optimal glucose control and close monitoring of the baby and mother-to-be, most women with diabetes have an excellent outlook for pregnancy.

Gestational diabetes

Gestational diabetes is one of the most common medical complications in pregnancy, occurring in 2 to 3 per cent of all pregnant women. Your practitioner can diagnose gestational diabetes by giving you a special blood test. (Refer to Chapter 9 for more information about this test.)

If you have gestational diabetes and you don't control your glucose levels, your baby may be at higher risk for certain problems. If your blood sugar levels are high, the foetus's are too. And high blood sugar levels cause the foetus to produce certain hormones that stimulate foetal growth, which may cause her to grow too large (refer to Chapter 16). Furthermore, if the foetus has high blood sugar levels while still in the uterus, she may have temporary problems with sugar regulation after birth. If the mother's (and foetus's) glucose levels are controlled during pregnancy, the risk of these complications drops dramatically.

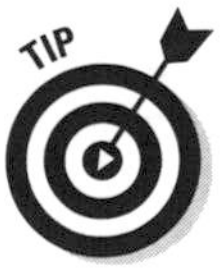

You need to control your sugar levels if you have gestational diabetes. Usually, altering your diet is enough. (Most women have a consultation with a nurse and/or a dietician to come up with a specific diet plan.) Exercise also helps. Only in rare cases do women need to resort to taking medication to keep their sugar level under control. If you do need to take medication, you'll probably be referred to a specialist clinic at the hospital. If you develop gestational diabetes, your doctor may ask you to check your sugar level several times during the day or on a weekly basis. You check your sugar level by pricking your finger (called a fingerstick) and placing the drop of blood onto a strip, or into a little machine, giving almost immediate results.

Fibroids

Fibroids are benign growths of the muscle cells that make up the uterus – they're extremely common, and your practitioner often diagnoses them during routine ultrasound scans. The high levels of oestrogen in a pregnant woman's bloodstream can encourage fibroids to grow larger. Yet predicting whether any woman's fibroids grow, stay the same, or shrink during pregnancy is difficult. Generally, fibroids cause no problems for a pregnancy and shrink in size after delivery.

In extreme cases, fibroids can cause difficulties, such as:

- Fibroids may grow so fast that they outgrow their blood supply and begin to degenerate, which sometimes causes pain, uterine contractions, and even preterm labour. Symptoms of degeneration include pain and tenderness directly over the fibroid (in the lower abdomen). Short-term treatment with anti-inflammatory painkilling medications may help.
- Very large fibroids in the lower portion of the uterus or near the cervix may interfere with the baby's ability to make its way through the birth canal. Fibroids may thus increase the risk for caesarean delivery, although this situation is quite unusual.
- Large fibroids within the uterus can sometimes increase the likelihood that the baby will be in the breech or transverse position. But this possibility, too, is rare.

Seizure disorders (epilepsy)

Most women who have epilepsy can have an uneventful pregnancy and give birth to a perfectly healthy baby. However, epilepsy does require that a woman's obstetrician and her neurologist work together to come up with the right strategy for controlling seizures. If you have epilepsy, work with your GP or hospital consultant before you get pregnant to control your seizures with the lowest possible dose, and the smallest number, of medications. Studies show that women whose seizures are well controlled on a minimal dose of a single medication before they get pregnant have the best pregnancy outcomes. So consult your neurologist before you get pregnant, and don't stop taking your medications unless your doctor advises you to.

All medications used to treat seizures pose some risk of birth defects. The problems they can cause vary, depending on the particular medication, but they include facial abnormalities, cleft lip and cleft palate, congenital heart defects, and neural tube defects. Women who take seizure medications therefore need to have an ultrasound to evaluate foetal anatomy and a foetal echocardiogram (see Chapter 9) to look for abnormalities in the baby's heart.

Women with seizure disorders should begin taking extra folic acid about three months before trying to conceive, because some seizure medications can affect folic acid levels.

Don't adjust your medications on your own, especially after you become pregnant. Your seizure activity could increase, which would probably be worse for the developing baby than the medications themselves.

Thyroid problems

Problems with thyroid function are relatively common in women of reproductive age; we see many women with overactive or underactive thyroids during pregnancy. Although these conditions require extra testing, they usually don't cause significant problems for pregnancy.

Hyperthyroidism (overactive thyroid)

There are many different causes of hyperthyroidism, but the most common by far is Grave's disease, which is associated with its own special set of antibodies (thyroid stimulating immunoglobulins, or TSIs) in the blood. These antibodies cause the thyroid to make too much hormone. Women with an overactive thyroid must receive adequate treatment during pregnancy (ideally, beginning before conception) in order to reduce their risk of such complications as miscarriage, preterm delivery, and low birth-weight.

If you have an overactive thyroid, unless your condition is extremely mild, your doctor will probably recommend that you take certain medications to lower the amount of thyroid hormone circulating in your blood. Some of these medications may cross the placenta, so your doctor will watch the foetus closely, usually by performing regular ultrasound scans, to look for any evidence that the medications are lowering the baby's thyroid levels too much. Specifically, your doctor will monitor the baby's growth and heart rate to see that they're normal and check for any evidence that the foetus has developed a *goitre* (an enlarged thyroid).

Your doctor will probably also monitor the levels of thyroid-stimulating antibodies in your blood because these antibodies may, in some rare cases, cross the placenta and stimulate the baby's thyroid as well. After delivery, your baby's paediatrician will monitor the baby carefully for any evidence of thyroid problems.

Hypothyroidism (underactive thyroid)

A woman with an underactive thyroid (hypothyroidism) can have a healthy pregnancy as long as her condition is adequately treated – if it's not, she stands a higher risk of developing certain complications, such as a low birth-weight baby. The condition is treated with a thyroid replacement hormone called thyroxine. Thyroxine is safe for the baby, because very little of it crosses the placenta. If you have an underactive thyroid, your doctor will want to check your hormone levels every so often to see if your medication needs to be adjusted.

Chapter 18

Coping with the Unexpected

In This Chapter

- Dealing with multiple miscarriages
- Suffering a loss late in pregnancy
- Making a decision when the baby develops an abnormality
- Finding help: Where to turn for support
- Healing – and getting ready to try again

We wish we had no reason to include this chapter. We wish every pregnant couple could end up delivering a healthy baby. Most couples do, but not everyone is so fortunate. And so there are times when couples need to know what happens and how to respond when things go wrong. If you're experiencing any of the problems we cover in this chapter, we hope that you find some of this information helpful.

Perhaps you're drawn to this chapter because you have had an unsuccessful pregnancy in the past. If so, you may be anxious about your current pregnancy – that's entirely normal. We take care of many women who have had poor outcomes in the past, and we realise that the only thing that can truly alleviate their anxiety is to hold a healthy baby.

TIP

One way to at least minimise your worry is to sit down with your doctor and discuss the situation. Ask him to map out a plan for your current pregnancy that maximises your chances for a favourable outcome. When you feel certain that you're doing everything you possibly can do to avoid a recurring problem, you may rest a little easier. Your worry probably won't entirely disappear, but remember that although a certain part of the process is in Mother Nature's hands, you can take medical steps to maximise your chances of having a healthy baby.

Surviving Recurrent Miscarriages

Unfortunately, a first-trimester miscarriage is a fairly common occurence. Doctors estimate that about 15 to 20 per cent of recognised pregnancies – those that have yielded a positive pregnancy test – end up in miscarriage. Still more early embryos are lost before they're actually known to exist – that is, before a woman takes a pregnancy test. About half the time, the cause of first-trimester miscarriage is the presence of some chromosomal abnormality in the embryo or foetus. Another 20 per cent of early miscarriages are due to structural abnormalities in the embryo.

REMEMBER

Fortunately, 80 to 90 per cent of women who experience a single early miscarriage subsequently deliver a normal baby.

Recurrent miscarriage – technically, the loss of three consecutive pregnancies – is far less common. This problem occurs in only ½ to 1 per cent of women. A variety of causes contribute to recurrent miscarriage, including the following:

- Genetic causes
- Uterine abnormalities
- Immunologic causes (though not all doctors agree that this is a factor)
- Inadequate progesterone secretion
- Certain infections (though this cause is also controversial)
- Antiphospholipid antibody syndrome (see Chapter 17)
- Certain environmental toxins or drugs (such as anti-malarials and some anaesthetic agents)

Most doctors suggest that women undergo certain tests after having three miscarriages; some begin testing even sooner. Because chromosomal abnormalities are the most common cause of miscarriage, an important first diagnostic step is to run tests on the chromosomes of the foetal tissue.

Various strategies for treating recurrent miscarriage are available, but doctors may disagree about which one, if any, is best. Choosing a strategy is easier if you know what the problem is. For example, your doctor may be able to repair an abnormally-shaped uterus surgically. If doctors can't find a cause for recurrent miscarriage, knowing which treatment is best may be difficult. Note, however, that even if no treatment is attempted, women who have had three consecutive miscarriages still have a 50 per cent or higher chance of having a normal, successful pregnancy.

Coping with Late-Pregnancy Loss

Late-pregnancy loss refers to a foetal death, stillbirth, or death of an infant in the immediate newborn period. Fortunately, these losses are infrequent and rarely occur more than once. Some causes of late losses include

- Chromosomal abnormalities
- Other genetic syndromes
- Structural defects
- A massive placental abruption (refer to Chapter 16)
- Antiphospholipid antibodies (refer to Chapter 17)
- Umbilical cord compression
- Unexplained reason, which is, unfortunately, very common

Women who suffer a loss of pregnancy often ask, 'Did I do something to cause this?' The answer is almost always no. So you have no reason to add to your grief by mixing in guilt. Many patients find it helpful, after the initial hurt has begun to subside, to gather all their pregnancy records, including any pathology reports, and consult with their doctor or a specialist. Sometimes your doctor can identify a cause, and sometimes not. Either way, most patients benefit from sitting down with their doctor and mapping out a strategy for preventing a loss in future pregnancies. Having a plan to focus on makes many patients feel less helpless. Support groups are also very helpful (see 'Finding Help' later in this chapter).

In subsequent pregnancies, your doctor may recommend that you undergo blood tests to check for certain abnormalities that have been associated with foetal loss. Often, if you have experienced a prior late-pregnancy loss, doctors follow your progress with regular ultrasound examinations and tests of foetal wellbeing. Your doctor may recommend that you deliver somewhat early, before you go into labour. You're likely to feel anxious during subsequent pregnancies, which is completely normal. But keep in mind, suffering a pregnancy loss a second time is quite unlikely.

Dealing with Foetal Abnormalities

All prospective parents wonder whether their baby will be 'normal' – and most are. Still, 2 to 3 per cent of babies end up having a significant abnormality. Some of these abnormalities can be repaired and have very little impact on the baby's overall quality of life. Occasionally, however, the condition can be significant, whether it is a structural, chromosomal, or genetic abnormality.

When an abnormality occurs, the first question many women ask us is, 'Is this my fault?' And the answer, most often, is no. From what is known about foetal abnormalities, most are what are called sporadic, meaning that they occur randomly and have no identifiable cause. If your doctor can't identify a cause, it's unlikely that the same kind of abnormality will recur in a subsequent pregnancy. (If the cause is genetic, there may be some chance that the abnormality could occur again.)

If your foetus is diagnosed with an abnormality, by ultrasound or some other test, your doctor may recommend that you have additional tests to look for other factors that have been associated with that particular abnormality. He may recommend that you see a genetic counsellor to discuss the implications of the abnormality. If the abnormality is a defect that can be surgically repaired or treated, you doctor may recommend that you meet with the specialist who can treat the baby after he is born. These discussions help you prepare for what lies ahead during the newborn period and also later on in the child's life.

Nobody wants to get the news that they have a foetus with an abnormality, but having this information is helpful for several reasons:

- If you're aware of some disorders, such as foetal anaemia or obstructions in the urinary tract, doctors can treat them.
- The knowledge helps to prepare you for what happens after the baby is born.
- This information helps you manage your pregnancy and consider all possible options.
- The information can give you important insights into the management of future pregnancies.

Finding Help

If your pregnancy didn't turn out as you had hoped, the first and most obvious place to look for support is from your partner. Family members, friends, and clergy can also be very helpful. Professional advice or treatment from a psychotherapist or social worker may be useful for many couples. Most hospitals have counsellors, who can help you to come to terms with your loss. Support groups also can provide understanding and expert insight into your problem. These groups include:

- The Stillbirth and Neonatal Death Society (SANDS): Tel: 020 7436 5881 (Mon–Thurs 10 a.m. to 4 p.m.); `www.uk-sands.org`
- Compassionate Friends: Tel: 0117 9539639 (Mon–Fri 9.30 a.m. to 5 p.m.); `www.tcf.org.uk`

- Foundation for the Study of Infant Deaths: Tel: 020 7235 1721 (24-hour helpline, or in Northern Ireland: 028 9077 2215 6–10 p.m.); www.sids.org.uk
- The Miscarriage Association: Helpline: 01924 200 799; Scottish helpline: 0131 334 8883; www.miscarriageassociation.org.uk

Beginning to Heal

Couples naturally feel a strong emotional attachment to their unborn child, beginning as early as the first trimester. As a result, many couples experience the same grief after the loss of a foetus as they would after the loss of a family member or close friend. The loss of a foetus is no less significant than the loss of a child. Parents who decide to terminate a pregnancy because of an abnormality also go through tremendous grief.

Both parents should acknowledge their need – and their right – to grieve after a pregnancy loss. The emotional response takes time and typically goes through a number of stages, beginning with shock and denial, progressing to anger, and eventually reaching acceptance and the ability to carry on with life.

After you have gone through the stages of grief and feel that you're physically and emotionally strong, you're probably ready to start trying again. In some couples, one person progresses through the grieving process faster than the other. Make sure that both of you are ready before you begin trying to get pregnant again. And remember that a successful pregnancy, while joyful, doesn't replace a lost one – so the grieving process is necessary. From a medical perspective, make sure that you finish looking into possible causes for the loss and have a plan of action for the next pregnancy. Realise that your next pregnancy will be somewhat stressful and that you will need extra attention and compassion from your family, friends, and health care professionals.

Part V
The Part of Tens

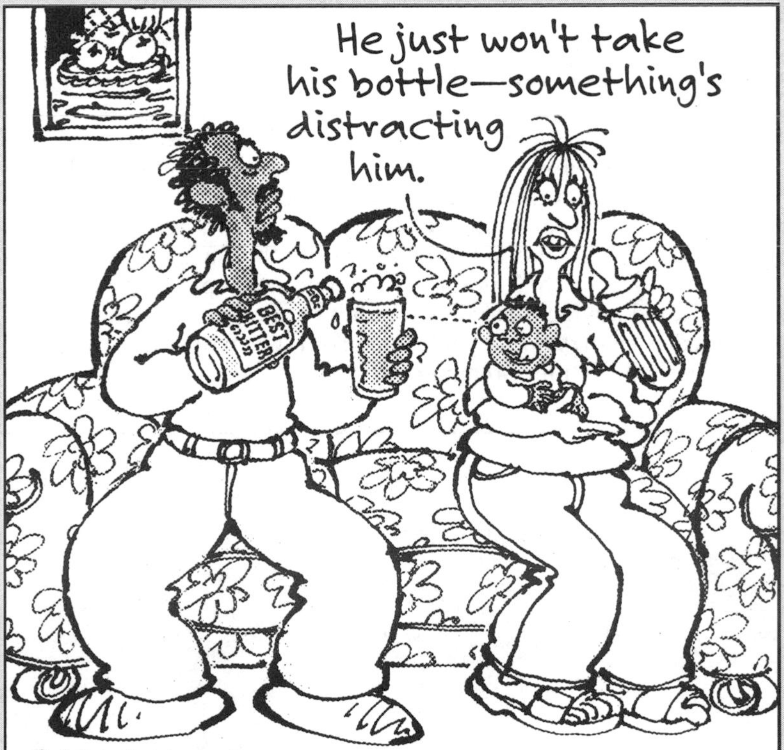

In this part . . .

In this part, we put things in a nutshell. We describe how the baby grows over the course of pregnancy and how your practitioner can observe that growth and development via ultrasound. We also tell you ten things that pregnant women don't often hear from their friends and family or even their practitioners. And in keeping with our repeated advice that you shouldn't get bogged down with needless worry while you're pregnant, we expose old wives' tales about pregnancy.

Chapter 19

Ten Things Nobody Tells You

In This Chapter

- Fighting fatigue and other discomforts of pregnancy
- Finding out that your belly has become public property
- Being prepared for the aftermath of delivery

Don't worry. We don't know of any conspiracy to keep you from knowing all there is to know about pregnancy. But your friends, sisters, cousins – whoever tells you what to expect with your pregnancy – often forget the little details, especially the more unpleasant ones. Furthermore, other books often gloss over this stuff, perhaps in the interest of decorum. Well, at the risk of being indecorous, we're going to give it to you straight.

Pregnancy Lasts Longer than Nine Months

Patients always ask, 'How many months pregnant am I?' and we have trouble giving them a precise answer. Pregnancy is said to last nine months, but that number isn't exactly accurate. The average pregnancy lasts 280 days, or 40 weeks, starting from the date of the mother's last menstrual period. (You think 40 weeks lasts a long time? Just be glad you're not an elephant, which has a gestation period of 22 months!) If a month is four weeks, then that calculation comes out to ten months. On the calendar, however, most months contain four weeks plus two or three days, so nine calendar months often do contain close to 40 weeks. Practitioners speak in terms of weeks when measuring gestational age because it's more accurate and less confusing.

Other People Can Drive You Crazy

Friends, relatives, acquaintances, strangers, and even your partner give you unsolicited opinions and advice and want to share with you every pregnancy horror story they've ever heard. These people may tell you that your bottom looks big, that you're too fat (or too thin), that your bump is too big or too small, or that you shouldn't be eating whatever you're putting in your mouth.

We realise that these people usually have only good intentions when they tell you how their sister's pregnancy ended badly, or about the trouble a friend of a friend had. They don't realise that they're increasing your anxiety. Don't pay attention. Try to politely smile and ignore them. Tell them you really don't want to hear this story right now. If you have any real problems or concerns, talk them over with your practitioner.

You Feel Exhausted in the First Trimester

You may already have heard that you're going to feel tired during the first trimester, but until you go through it, you really have no idea how overwhelming the fatigue can be. You may find yourself looking for every possible opportunity to catch a few winks – on the bus, on the train, at work, or even in the waiting room before your antenatal appointment. Rest assured that this fatigue does go away, usually by the end of the first trimester (at about 13 weeks), and you do get your usual energy back. Look out, though. Around 30 to 34 weeks, the physical stress of pregnancy may overwhelm you again, and you may go back to feeling pretty washed out for several weeks.

Round Ligament Pain Really Hurts

The round ligaments run from the top of the uterus down into the labia. As the uterus grows, these ligaments stretch, and many women feel discomfort or pain on one or both sides of the groin area, especially at about 16 to 22 weeks. Practitioners tell you that this symptom is only round ligament pain and that it's nothing to worry about. And they're right – don't worry. But you deserve some sympathy (you have ours), because this pain can be fairly intense.

You can probably ease round ligament pain a bit by getting off your feet, thereby taking the pressure off the ligaments. The good news is that round ligament pain usually diminishes by about 24 weeks.

Your Belly Becomes a Hand Magnet

After your stomach protrudes noticeably with pregnancy, you're likely to find that suddenly everyone presumes touching it is okay – not only your friends, family members, and the people you work with, but also the postman, the cashier at the supermarket, and other people you've never even met. Although some women appreciate the extra attention, many find it an invasion of privacy. You can either grin and bear it or practise your icy stare and withering 'Do you mind?'

Piles Are a Royal Pain in the . . .

Your best friend may say that she's told you everything about her own pregnancy. But has she remembered her piles? Believe us, piles happen pretty often, and when they do, you're in for some very noticeable pain and discomfort.

Piles are dilated veins near the rectum that become engorged because of the pressure on that part of the body or because of pushing during delivery. Some women notice piles during pregnancy, others don't have any problem with them until after delivery, and some very lucky women never have piles at all.

If your piles are significant, be prepared for some discomfort after vaginal delivery (see Chapter 13). Most piles go away within a few weeks. If you're fortunate enough not to have them, realise how lucky you are – and have sympathy for all the other new mothers who do have them.

Sometimes Women Poo While Pushing

Our patients frequently ask us about having a bowel movement during labour, so although it may not be the most genteel subject to bring up, we're going to anyway. Pooing while pushing doesn't happen every time, but it isn't that uncommon. In all likelihood, you and your partner aren't even aware of it happening, because your midwife quickly wipes away any mess and keeps you clean throughout the pushing process. If it does happen, don't give it a thought. No one – neither your doctor nor your partner – is going to be revolted.

The Weight Stays On after the Baby Comes Out

Most women can't wait to weigh themselves after delivering 10 pounds or so of baby, placenta, and fluid. But contain yourself. Wait at least a week. After delivery, many women swell up like dumplings, especially their hands and feet. This extra water retention adds pounds. If you step on the scales straight away, you may be very disappointed at the number that comes up. The swelling generally takes about a week or two to go away.

Hospital Towels Are Relics from Your Mother's Era

Most hospitals don't provide sanitary towels routinely. If you forget to take any with you, the hospital staff provide you with a couple to tide you over – but they're likely to be great cumbersome affairs straight out of the 1920s, with nothing to stick them to your knickers. You can usually stock up at the hospital shop during your stay – but that's no consolation if you deliver in the middle of the night! So don't forget to pack your own box of large-size towels with wings, as well as some sturdy underwear. Think old-fashioned school knickers rather than thongs – you'll be much more concerned with comfort than glamour in the first few days after you deliver!

Breast Engorgement Really Sucks

Of course you know that your breasts fill up with milk after you deliver your baby. But what you may not have heard is how painful and cumbersome this engorgement can be if you aren't breast-feeding, or when you decide to stop breast-feeding. Your breasts may become rock hard, tender, and warm, and they sometimes seem to grow to the size of melons. Fortunately, the discomfort is temporary; this intense period of engorgement lasts only a couple of days.

Chapter 20

Ten (Or So) Old Wives' Tales

In This Chapter

- Facing non-problems you don't have to worry about
- Pondering weird notions you don't even have to think about
- Looking at strange beliefs you can only shake your head in wonder about

Pregnancy has a certain mystique. Millions of women have been through it, yet predicting in detail what any one woman's experience is going to be like is difficult. Perhaps that's why so many myths have formed (and survived) over the centuries, most of which are designed to foresee the unknowable future. Here are ten (or so) tales that, thankfully, are really nothing but nonsense.

The Old Heartburn Myth

If a pregnant woman frequently experiences heartburn, her baby will have a full head of hair. Simply not true. Some babies have hair; some don't. Most lose it all within a few weeks, anyway.

The Mysterious Umbilical Cord Movement Myth

If a pregnant woman lifts her hands above her head, she will choke the baby. Give us a break. People used to think (and, alas, some *still* believe) that the mother's movement could cause the baby to become tangled in the umbilical cord, but that's just not true.

The Curse Myth

Anyone who denies a pregnant woman the food that she craves will get a sty in his eye. Nope. This myth doesn't mean that someone who stands between a pregnant woman and her craving is in the clear, though: He will most certainly be subjected to threats, name-calling, or icy glares, but no sties.

The Heart Rate Myth

If the foetal heart rate is fast, the baby is a girl, and if the heart rate is slow, the baby is a boy. Medical researchers actually looked into this myth. They did find a very slight difference between the average heart rate of boys and that of girls, but it wasn't significant enough to make heart rate an accurate predictor of sex.

The Ugly Stick Myth

If a pregnant woman sees something ugly or horrible, she will have an ugly baby. How could this possibly be true? There's no such thing as an ugly baby!

The Coffee Myth

If a baby is born with cafe au lait spots (light-brown birthmarks), the mother drank too much coffee or had unfulfilled cravings during her pregnancy. Nope.

The Myth of International Cuisine

Many people still believe that eating spicy food brings on labour. It doesn't, but it may be an effective marketing tool: We know of an Indian restaurant that advertises its Chicken Vindaloo as a surefire labour inducer. The dish may be delicious (hot, but delicious), but it simply can't bring on labour.

The Great Sex Myth

Interestingly, this may be one of the few myths with a grain of truth in it. Love-making can stimulate your body to produce the hormone oxytocin, which can help your cervix ripen in readiness for labour. Your partner's semen also contains hormones called prostaglandins, which can cause contractions.

I (Sarah) have been recommending a 'patent method' of induction to my patients for years (with the proviso that it's not a sure-fire guarantee). Take a long walk (which might allow gravity to bring your baby's head down lower into your pelvis), followed by making love, and then eating Belgian chocolates and drinking a glass of champagne. The chocolates and champagne have no scientific significance whatsoever, but they should stop you being quite so disappointed if it doesn't work.

The Round Face Myth

If a pregnant woman gains weight in her face, the baby is a girl. And the corollary myth says that if a woman gains weight on her backside, the baby is a boy. Neither statement is true, obviously enough. The baby's sex has no influence whatsoever on the way the mother stores fat.

Another seemingly related myth is that if the mother's nose begins to grow and widen, the baby is a girl. The so-called reasoning here is that a daughter always steals her mother's beauty. Strange concept – and quite untrue.

The Ring Myth

Hang a gold wedding ring on a thread above the mother's stomach. If the ring swings back and forth the baby is a girl; if the ring moves in circles, the baby is a boy. I (Sarah) humoured a friend during her pregnancy by letting her try this, then repeated the test on the bedside chest of drawers and proved that it, too, was going to have a girl. Enough said.

The Moon Maid Myth

This one holds that more women go into labour during a full moon. Although many labour and delivery personnel insist that the labour floor is busier during a full moon (police say their cells are livelier then, too), the scientific data just doesn't support the idea.

The Belly Shape Myth

If a pregnant woman's belly is round, the baby is a girl, and if the woman's belly is more bullet-like, it's a boy. Forget about it. Belly shape differs from woman to woman, but the child's sex has nothing to do with it.

The Ultrasound Tells All Myth

Ultrasound can always tell the baby's sex, right? Nope, not always. Often, by about 18–20 weeks gestation, seeing a foetus's genitalia on ultrasound is possible. But being able to determine the baby's sex depends on whether the baby is in position to give you a good view. Sometimes the ultrasonographer can't see between the unco-operative baby's legs and therefore can't determine the sex. Sometimes, too, the ultrasonographer may be wrong, especially if the ultrasound is done very early in the pregnancy. So even though you can technically find out the baby's sex through ultrasound in most cases, it's not 100 per cent guaranteed. That's one of the reasons you're not routinely told at your 20-week scan what sex your baby is.

Chapter 21

Ten Landmarks in Foetal Development

In This Chapter

- Finding out how pregnancy begins
- Knowing when the baby takes shape
- Recognising when the baby starts calling attention to herself

Pregnant women are naturally curious to know how their babies grow. On any given day during pregnancy, they want to know which body parts have developed, which organs are working, and, later on in pregnancy, whether the baby has matured to the point where she can survive outside the uterus. In this chapter, we describe ten major landmarks in foetal development.

The Baby Is Conceived

The essential first moment of pregnancy occurs when the sperm penetrates or fertilises the egg. Conception occurs, on average, about 14 days after the first day of the mother's last menstrual period. The average pregnancy lasts 40 weeks after the last menstrual period (38 weeks after conception).

The Embryo Implants Itself

Implantation usually occurs about seven days after conception. The embryo (or zygote, as it's known in the very early stages) spends the first week travelling down the fallopian tube. The embryo reaches the inside of the uterus on about day 5 and begins to implant on about day 6 or 7. The zygote takes several days to implant in the uterus's lining.

The Heart Begins Beating

The first organ system to start operating in a developing foetus is the cardiovascular system. The embryonic heart starts beating only three weeks after conception. The motion of the beating heart is often one of the first signs of a viable pregnancy that practitioners can detect on ultrasound – in fact, you can sometimes see the beating heart before you can see the embryo itself.

The Neural Tube Closes

The neural tube is the beginning of the central nervous system – the brain and spinal cord. The neural tube starts as a flat plate of cells that rolls up into a tube during development. After the ends of this tube close, the primitive nervous system begins the long process of maturing, which continues after the baby is born. The neural tube is normally closed on both ends by day 28 after conception.

The Face Develops

Although foetal facial features mature throughout gestation, the critical period for face development is from five to eight weeks after conception.

The Embryonic Period Ends

The rudiments of all the organs and structures of a normal baby are formed during the so-called embryonic period, the first eight weeks of gestation. The foetal period that follows is characterised by further maturation of these primitive organs until a happy, healthy, crying baby is born.

The Sexual Organs Appear

Although your baby's sex was determined at the time of conception, the very early embryo appears the same whether it's a male or female. Only after about 12 weeks gestation do either the penis and scrotum or the clitoris and vagina become apparent.

Quickening Occurs

Quickening refers to the mother's first perception of foetal movement. Quickening typically occurs at about 18–20 weeks gestation. Although you can see foetal movements on ultrasound much earlier than this, quickening is the first sign of life that the expectant mother can feel.

The Lungs Reach Maturity

The foundations of the foetal respiratory system are present and functioning by 26–28 weeks gestation. Some babies born at this time can breathe by themselves, but many need the help of a mechanical ventilator. Some babies' lungs mature earlier than others do, but the overwhelming majority of babies have well-developed lungs by 36–37 weeks gestation.

A Baby Is Born

This one needs no (further) explanation.

Chapter 22

Ten Key Things You Can See on Ultrasound

In This Chapter

- Seeing what the ultrasonographer sees
- Checking your baby's health from ultrasound
- Working out what's what

If you've ever had a parent-to-be show you an ultrasound picture of their baby, you know determining what you're looking at, let alone detecting a family resemblance, isn't always easy. But ultrasound pictures can be amazingly clear and useful if you know what you're looking for. In this chapter, we show you what doctors and ultrasonographers try to pick out on ultrasound to find out whether the baby is growing and developing well.

Measurement of Crown-Rump Length

The crown-rump length is also referred to by its acronym, CRL. This measurement (see Figure 22-1) is made from the top of the foetus's head (crown) to the buttocks (rump) during the first trimester. It is the most precise sonographic measurement that your practitioner can use to estimate gestational age.

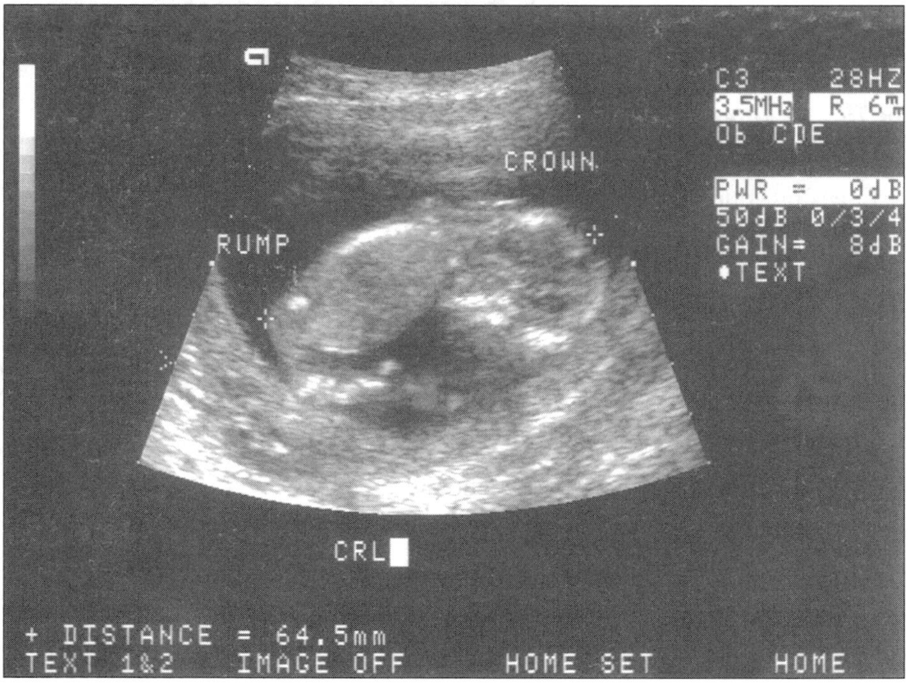

Figure 22-1: The crown-rump length is a first-trimester measurement used to determine how far along your pregnancy is.

The Face

Many people think that the view of the foetus in Figure 22-2, taken during the second trimester, is sort of ghoulish. Some say that the baby looks like E.T. But remember that it's not a traditional photograph of the baby's face. The ultrasound beam passes through the foetus wherever it's directed and renders a picture of a 'section' of the inside of the baby, not the surface.

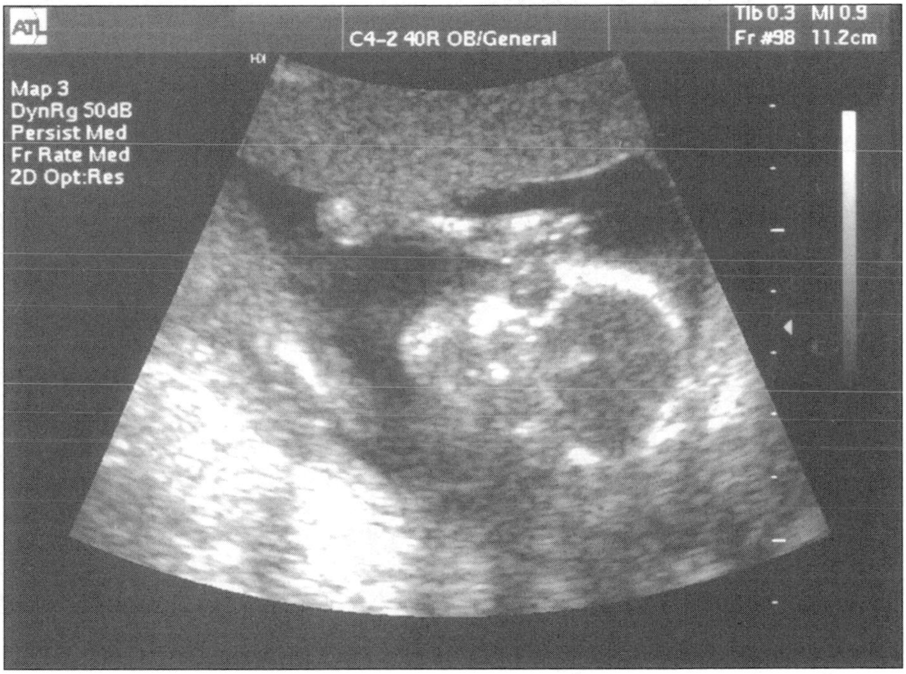

Figure 22-2: Smile for the camera!

The Spine

The spine is one thing that even most novices at ultrasound can easily find. Take a look at it in Figure 22-3. In the second trimester, imaging the entire spine is important in order to rule out neural tube defects (see Chapter 9).

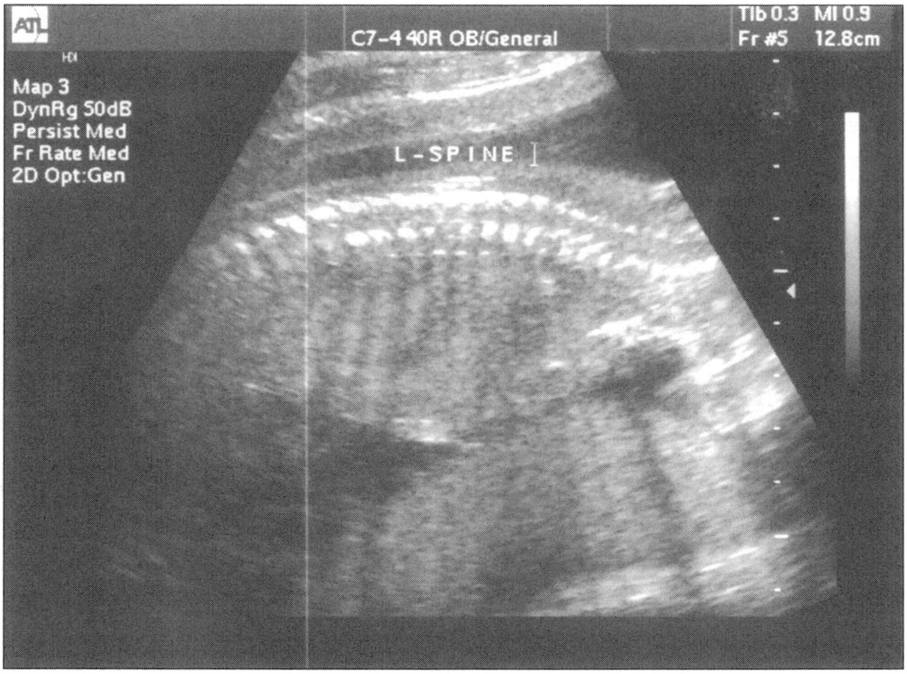

Figure 22-3: You can easily see the foetal spine on ultrasound in the second trimester.

The Heart

Your baby's heart, like yours, is made up of four chambers – two atria and two ventricles. (The connections between the chambers in the foetus's heart are different from yours, as they change around the time your baby's born.) The image in Figure 22-4 is the classic four-chamber view of the foetal heart that your practitioner looks for on ultrasound in the second trimester. You can clearly see two atria and two ventricles. A normal four-chamber view rules out the most major heart abnormalities. During an actual ultrasound, you can see the heart beating and the valves moving.

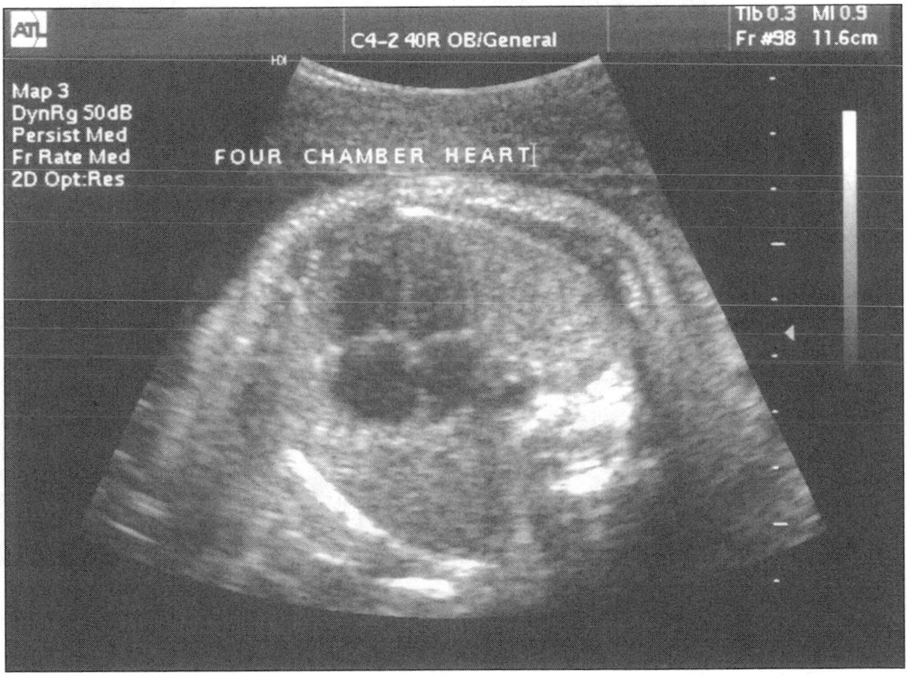

Figure 22-4: In this picture, you can see the heart's four chambers. During the actual examination, you can also see the heart beating.

The Hands

In the second trimester, counting foetal fingers and toes is a challenge because the foetus moves constantly. But Figure 22-5 captures them all in the picture. You can see five fingers in the lower hand and five in the upper (that's just the tip of the upper hand's thumb you see).

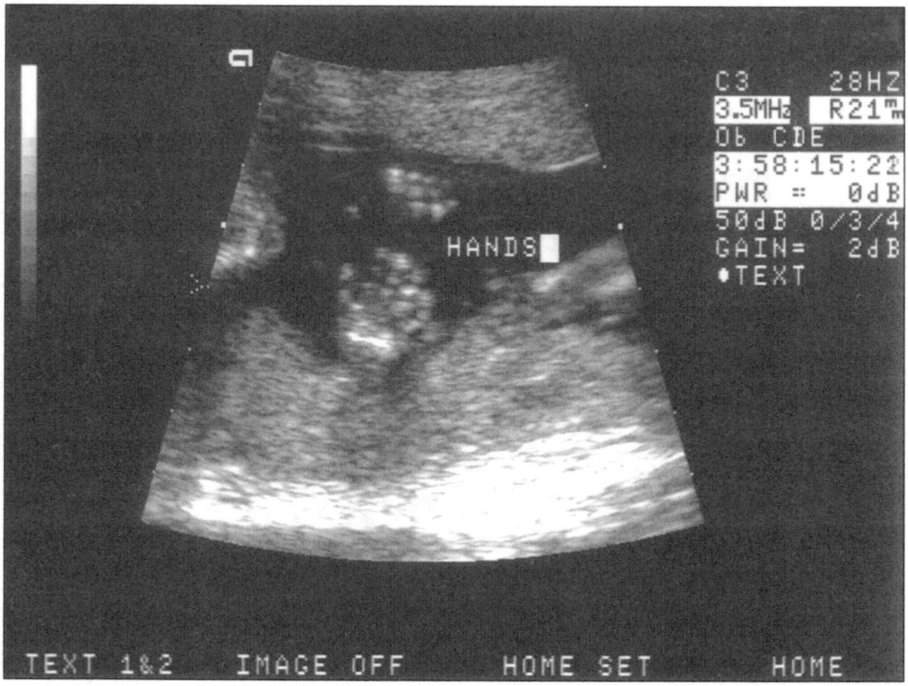

Figure 22-5: All five fingers . . .

The Foot

Although you can't predict shoe size yet, you can see five toes on the foot in Figure 22-6, caught on ultrasound in the second trimester.

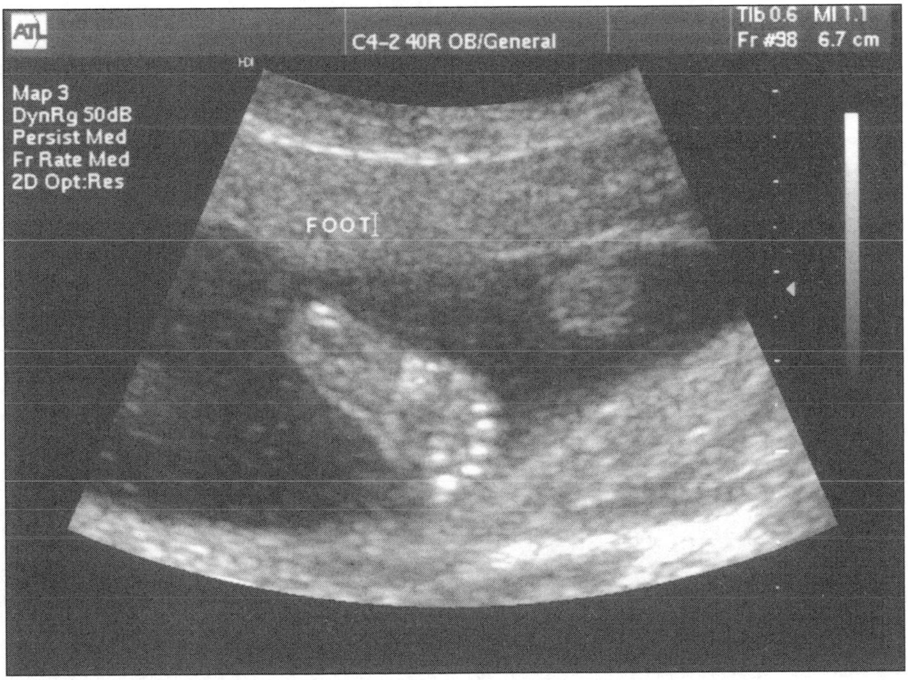

Figure 22-6: . . .and all five toes.

The Foetal Profile

In Figure 22-7, you can see a foetus in the second trimester taking a rest from his busy play schedule.

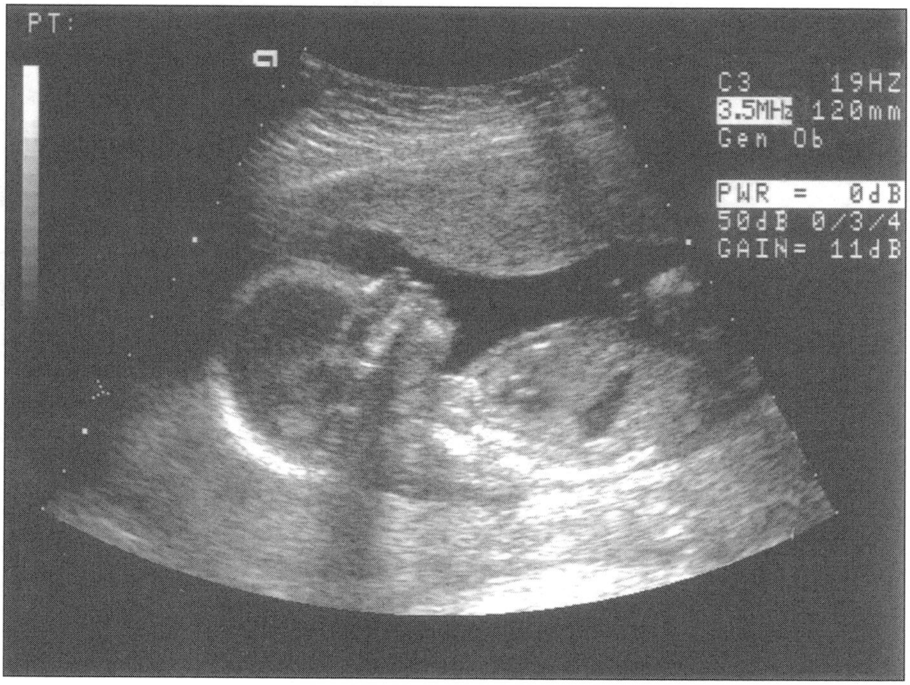

Figure 22-7: In this ultrasound image, you can see the foetus resting in clear profile.

The Stomach

Anything that is fluid-filled shows up dark on ultrasound. Because the baby is constantly swallowing amniotic fluid, the stomach shows up as a dark bubble. (The foetus in Figure 22-8 is also second trimester.)

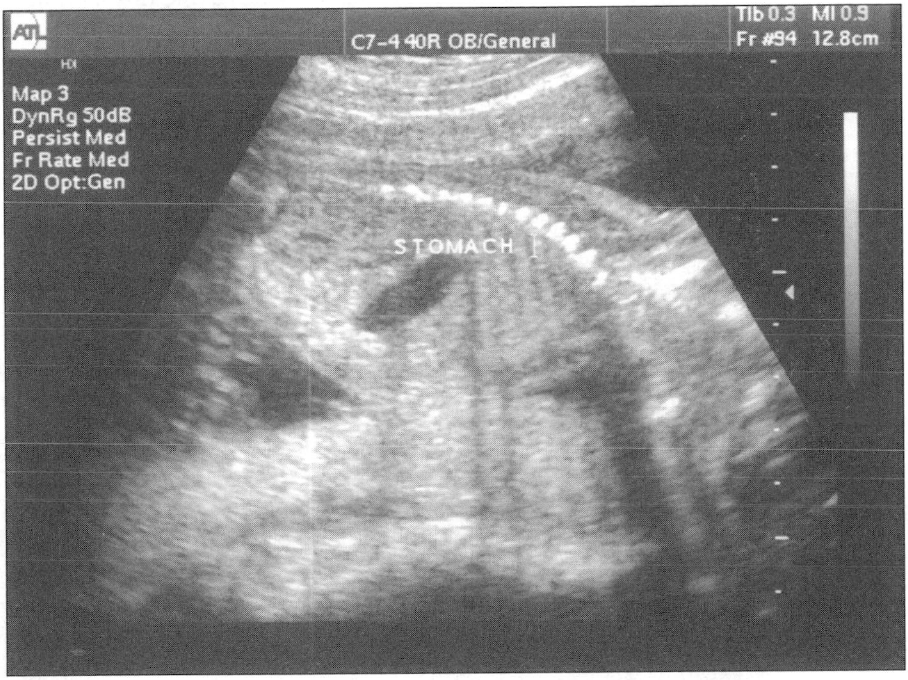

Figure 22-8: The foetus's stomach shows up as a dark bubble on ultrasound.

It's a Boy!

As you can see in Figure 22-9, getting a very clear view of the developing penis is often possible. (Isn't daddy proud!)

REMEMBER

Even though these scans give a very clear picture of the foetus's sex, the sex isn't always so obvious. Many women only have one ultrasound scan, which may be carried out too soon to give a reliable indication of the baby's sex. Of course, this doesn't matter if you don't want to know what sex your baby is – and many women like to save the excitement of finding out until delivery. However, you do need to be aware that if you do ask, you still have a small chance that 'Janet' may turn out to be 'John'!

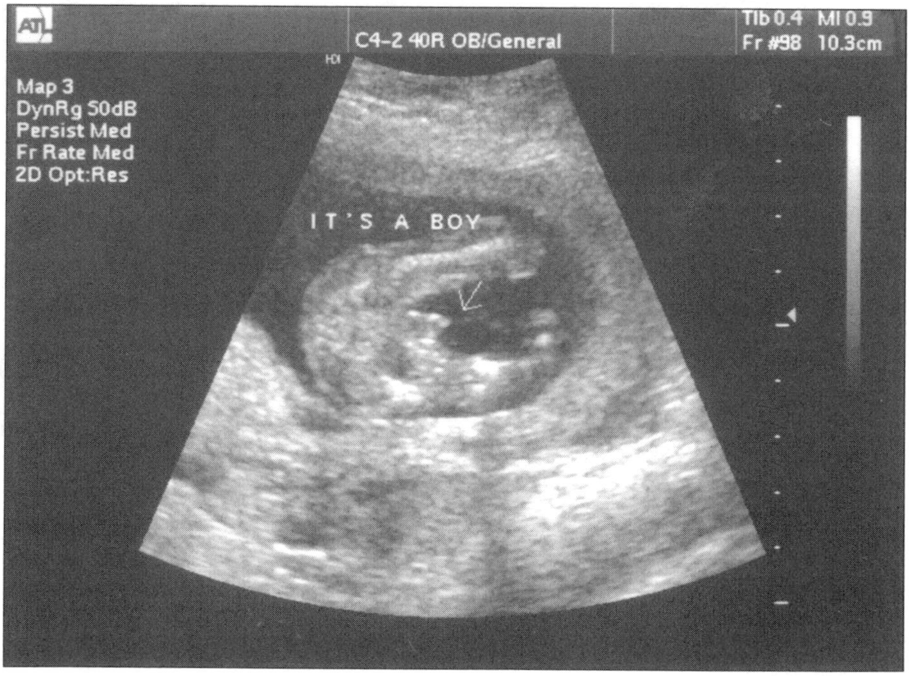

Figure 22-9: One look at this ultrasound image is enough to tell that the baby is a boy.

It's a Girl!

Figure 22-10 shows an easily recognisable image of the labia. As explained in the preceding section, 'It's a Boy!', differentiating boys from girls isn't always so easy. In the case of girls, you often can't see the labia, and deciding it's a girl may simply be based on not seeing a penis.

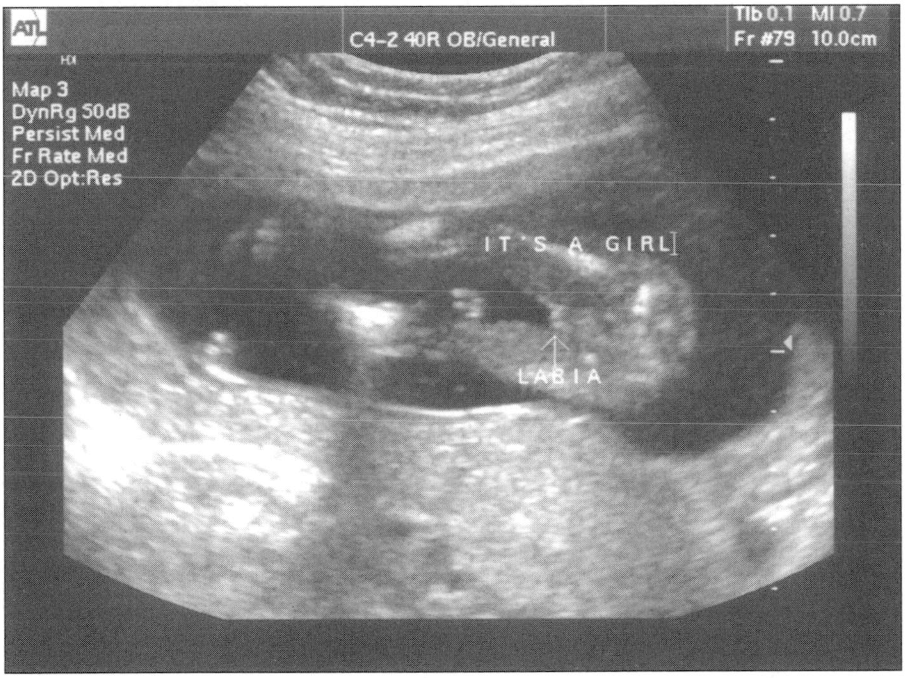

Figure 22-10: The ultrasound image clearly shows that this baby is a girl.

Appendix

The Pregnant Man: Having a Baby from a Dad's Perspective

A woman's role in pregnancy is undoubtedly pivotal, but, biologically speaking, she can't do it alone. Your part is vital, too, right from the start. Your sperm's DNA provides half the baby's total DNA. And your share of DNA determines the baby's sex. If you donate an X chromosome, it's a girl; if you hand in a Y, it's a boy. (A woman's egg always contains an X chromosome.)

Sperm, of course, is only the first contribution you make to the project. The support you provide the mother during pregnancy is at least as important. Just as pregnancy is a time of tremendous change in a woman's body, so is it a time of tremendous emotional change for both the father and mother, and it's a time of transition for you as a couple – a transition to parenthood. Recognising this fact can make it easier for you to become comfortable with the whole process and play your role as well as possible. You can make life easier for both of you. Studies clearly show that pregnancy, labour, and delivery are associated with fewer complications when the father is involved and supportive.

Reacting to the News

'I think I'm pregnant!' You hear the words that millions of other men before you have heard – and you feel pure joy and excitement. Well, not really. You probably also feel some concern, even fear for the future. Rest assured that these feelings are completely normal. You may be concerned about how parenthood may change your relationship with your partner. You may be concerned about how parenthood could change your life in general. You may worry that you and your partner won't be able to support a family financially, or that you won't be a good father. Just remember that your partner's feelings about having a baby probably aren't all that different – she's probably having a few worries herself. So talk to your partner about what you're both feeling.

Everything every dad wants to know about sex

One of the most common questions that dads ask is about sex during pregnancy. Your desire for sex – like that of your partner – may increase or decrease. Many men worry that inserting the penis into the vagina, next to the cervix, may injure the baby or lead to preterm delivery. In an uncomplicated pregnancy, you have nothing to worry about at all in this regard. Another common worry is that you may crush the baby by lying on top of your partner. Again, if the pregnancy is normal (especially during the first months), being on top isn't a problem. A cushion of amniotic fluid surrounds the baby. Later on in pregnancy, the size of the mother's abdomen may make the missionary position awkward, or your partner may find it uncomfortable. If your partner is willing, take the time to find alternative positions that are comfortable for her.

Remember that libido can wax and wane during pregnancy, or it may wane only (refer to Chapter 3). For some women, pregnancy is just a sexual turnoff. So try to be understanding if your part-ner isn't interested in sex. Keep in mind that intercourse isn't the only way that you and your partner can express your sexual feelings for each other. Often, embracing, cuddling, or fondling can be satisfying alternatives. Remember, pregnancy (and the possible interruption in your sex life) won't last forever, even though you may sometimes feel like it will.

In a somewhat stressful (even if very joyful) situation such as having a new baby, sex may not be a huge priority. Give yourself and your partner the time you both need to adjust your sex drives. Even after your partner's practitioner gives her the go-ahead to resume sex (usually about six weeks after delivery) and you're both ready, take things slow and easy at first. If your partner is breast-feeding, her body will be low in oestrogen, which means that, among other things, she's more likely to be experiencing vaginal dryness. So take things gently when you first have sex – remember, without adequate lubrication, sex may be uncomfortable enough for her to put her off for some time. Many couples find it useful to use a water-based lubricant for the first few times.

Knowing What to Expect from the First Trimester

After both of you get over the initial surprise, you're faced with the realities of pregnancy during the first trimester. To find out more about the first trimester, take a peek at Chapter 6.

Your partner is likely to feel exceptionally tired and may need to urinate with remarkable frequency. Chances are she also has morning sickness. You can help by assuming more of the day-to-day responsibilities of running the household. And be aware of what a drag it can be to be nauseated all the time. Be as supportive as you can. If your partner asks you to run out for more pickled gherkins and ketchup at midnight, just smile and ask, 'Whole or slices?'

Try to make room in your schedule to accompany your partner to her first antenatal visit to her practitioner. Your participation is important not only because it telegraphs your support, but also because you may need to answer questions about your family medical history. In addition, you probably have questions to ask the practitioner.

Watching Mum Grow – the Second Trimester

'Darling, do you think I'm fat and ugly now?' You may start to hear this question during the second trimester when the mother's body really begins to change. Here's a tip: It's not a multiple-choice question. You only have one answer, and you may as well commit it to memory so that you can answer without hesitation: 'Absolutely not, darling. You're the most beautiful woman I've ever laid eyes on.' If you want a few more potentially Dad-saving tips, read through Chapter 7 to find out more about the second trimester.

Enjoy the second trimester – often, it's the most fun part of pregnancy for both parents. Morning sickness fades away, fatigue subsides, and your partner begins to feel the baby move around inside her. Often, you, too, can feel the baby move by placing your hand on the mum's abdomen. During this trimester, many mothers get an ultrasound examination to check the baby's anatomy.

Try to go along to see the ultrasound examination (see Chapter 22); it's one of the most enjoyable antenatal tests. You get to see the baby's hands, feet, and face, and you get to watch the baby move around. For the first time, you see the living, moving, growing little human inside, and suddenly the whole enterprise seems so much more real.

By the end of the second trimester, you may begin antenatal classes. Don't make excuses! Go with your partner! The classes are designed for both father and mother. During this time, you can find out how to be useful during labour and delivery. And you can also ask questions about what to anticipate – to relieve some of your own anxiety.

Under Starter's Orders – the Third Trimester

'I can't sleep.' 'I look like a beached whale.' 'I've lost my ankles.' The third trimester has arrived. Your partner may begin to feel uncomfortable because of all the changes in her body – and because of her sheer size. Check out Chapter 8 to find out plenty more about the third trimester.

Many women do have trouble sleeping late in pregnancy, which only makes it harder for them to tolerate their discomfort. As you did during the first trimester, take on more of the day-to-day household duties and give your partner the time she needs to rest. Consider treating her to a 'day of beauty' at her favourite salon, or send her out for a massage or something else that makes her feel special – she deserves to feel good about herself and the changes her body is going through. And things will go easier for both of you if you can find a way to help her accept her pregnant body, relax, and take things a little easier.

Later in the third trimester, naturally, both of you start to focus on labour and delivery. You may have a million questions: Will the baby be okay? Do I really want to be in the delivery room? How will my partner tolerate labour? How will I tolerate labour? Will I get queasy during the delivery? Psychologically, childbirth can be a real challenge for the father. You care about the course of events very much, but you're clearly not in the driver's seat, and this situation may make you feel anxious.

TIP

Many women write a birth plan (you can find out more about doing so in Chapter 8), so have a look at mum's birth plan before the big day. Maybe you could write it together. The advantages of doing so include:

- You can discuss how best you can help her
- You'll feel more included in the whole birth process
- You'll have a better idea of her needs, so you can make sure her wishes are made clear to the practitioner
- You'll avoid any nasty surprises ('What do you mean, my wife has written that she wants me to deliver the baby and cut the cord while she sits on my lap?')

At the same time, imminent fatherhood faces you head-on. And the onset of this new responsibility may cause still more anxiety and more questions: Will I be able to provide for my family? Will I be a good father? Can I work out how to change a nappy? How will I know how to handle a fragile newborn? These questions are all normal. Again, they're probably very similar to the questions running through your partner's head. Communication is everything. Most couples find that they can talk each other through their respective panic attacks.

Dad in the Delivery Room

If you plan to join your partner in the delivery room (and we wholeheartedly encourage you to do so), remember that after you arrive on the labour floor, all attention is focused on mum. Your primary role is to support your partner. Play that role to the hilt. If she occasionally snaps at you, don't be surprised, and don't think it means that she wishes you weren't there. After it's all over, she will appreciate your presence. If your partner needs to make decisions about pain management – about whether to have an epidural, for example – help her make them, without being judgemental. She has to make the final decision; after all, it's her body, her pain.

REMEMBER

The middle of labour is not the best time to be debating your differences of opinion on natural childbirth, your new child's name, or anything else.

Some fathers may prefer not to watch the actual delivery. Some mothers prefer that their partner not see them in this less-than-sexy light. Chapter 11 tells you about the weird and wonderful things that happen during labour. We won't rehash it here, but be warned – more will come out of your partner than a baby (as if that weren't enough).

If you choose to join your partner in the delivery room, make yourself useful however you can. Above all, be patient and understanding. The mother-to-be, out of anxiety, fear, or pain, may become somewhat angry or short-tempered – this reaction is completely normal during labour. You can help her use her breathing exercises and relaxation techniques (see Chapter 8 for a crash course). You can also help by

- Reassuring her that everything is going well
- Understanding when she gets frustrated or short-tempered
- Empathising with her
- Distracting her (with games, humour, and so on, at least in the first stage of labour . . . although a game of chess is probably out of the question)
- Helping to communicate her needs to the professional staff at the hospital or birthing centre

When labour reaches the final stage, you can do a lot to help your partner through it:

- Help her count to ten during pushes.
- If necessary, let her know when a contraction is starting. (You can tell by watching the monitor.)
- Lift up her legs or hold her head forward, chin to chest. This position makes the pushes more efficient.
- Do whatever she asks to make her more comfortable. Offer to dab her forehead with a moist cloth if that makes her feel better.
- Be supportive and encouraging.
- Hold her hand. Watch it because she'll squeeze hard. Actually, make that very hard.
- Massage her when she asks you.
- Do whatever she says, even (or *especially*) if she tells you to shut up.

After the baby is born, make sure you congratulate your partner on a job well done.

Home at Last – with the New Family

If pregnancy, labour, and delivery weren't enough to jolt you into the realisation that your life is changing forever, getting home from the hospital with your new family certainly does. You and your partner now have a new set of responsibilities. You can help change nappies (they even have changing tables in men's loos these days), feed the baby, shop, and do household chores. Even if the mother is breast-feeding, you can sometimes feed the baby breast milk she has pumped and put into a bottle. In fact, you may want to ask her to prepare bottles this way for you regularly, because feeding the baby is an important and highly satisfying way to bond.

Your partner is going to need at least six weeks to get back to pre-pregnancy shape, and probably longer. During the first couple of months, she may be exhausted – she's recovering from labour and delivery, after all. And chances are good that both you and she are somewhat sleep deprived. Conditions like these make it easy for anyone to lose his patience from time to time or to lose her temper more often than usual. Simply being aware of the fact that you're operating under special circumstances for a while is helpful. See that your partner has time for rest – and try to take naps yourself.

Finally, don't be surprised if you feel unprepared for parenthood, lacking in the skills and understanding of what it takes to do a good job. Unlike cats, dogs, or jungle animals, humans aren't born with sure-fire instincts about how to be perfect parents. Both you and your partner need time to develop the skills it takes to handle babies – and children, and teenagers. Along the way, you often work by trial and error. Just realise and accept this situation. Talk about it with each other – often. And fasten your seat belts. You're in for an incredible adventure.

Index

• A •

• B •

• C •

• D •

• E •

• F •

• G •

• H •

• I •

• J •

• N •

• O •

• P •

• T •

Notes

Notes

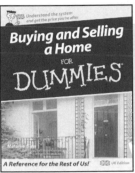

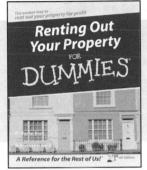

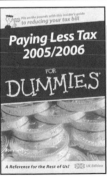

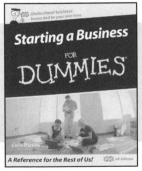

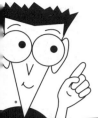

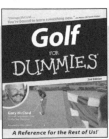

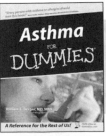

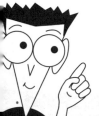

FOR DUMMIES®

Helping you expand your horizons and realize your potenti

INTERNET

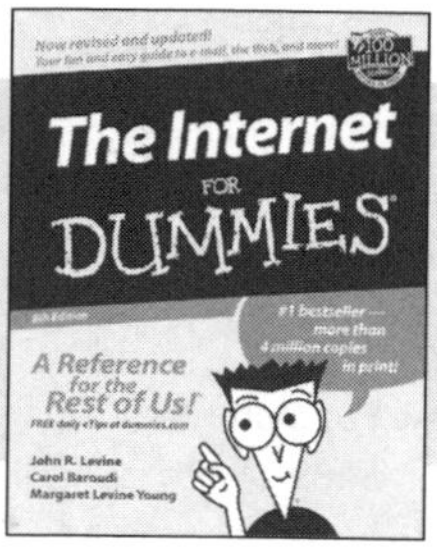

0-7645-4173-0

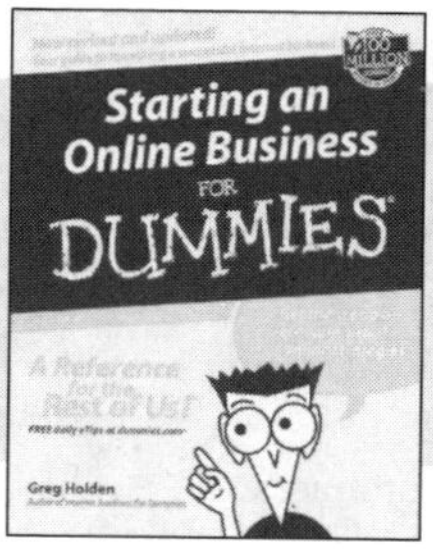

0-7645-1655-8

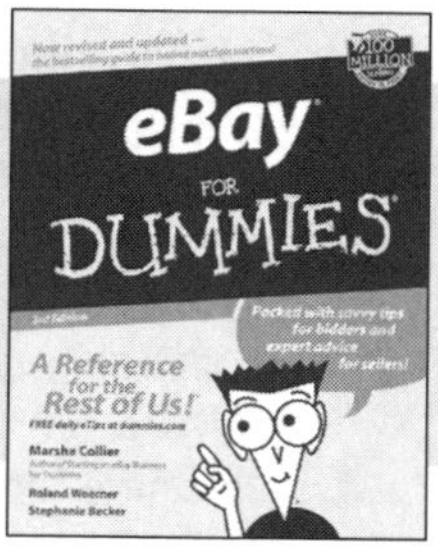

0-7645-5654-1

Also available:

America Online 7.0 For Dummies (0-7645-1624-8)

The Internet All-in-One Desk Reference For Dummies (0-7645-1659-0)

Internet Explorer 6 For Dummies (0-7645-1344-3)

Internet Privacy For Dummies (0-7645-0846-6)

Researching Online For Dummies (0-7645-0546-7)

eBay Bargain Shoppin For Dummies (0-7645-4080-7)

Google For Dummies (0-7645-4420-9)

2005 Online Shop Dire for Dummies (0-7645-7495-7)

DIGITAL MEDIA

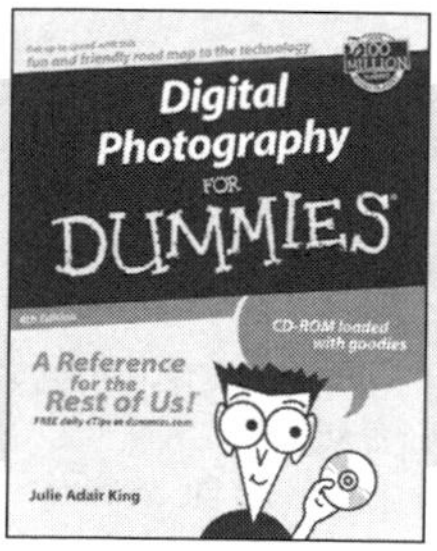

0-7645-1664-7

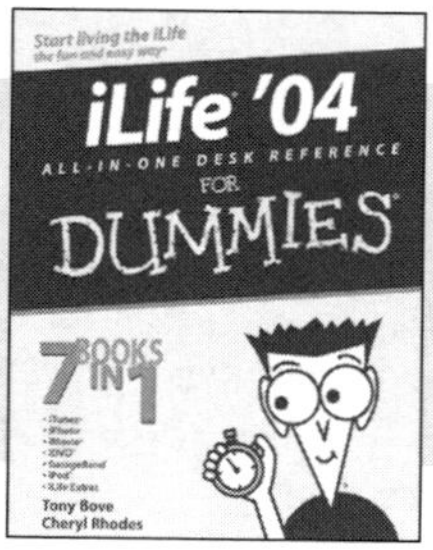

0-7645-7347-0

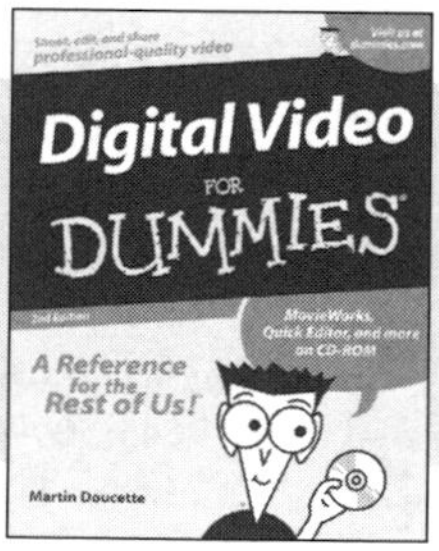

0-7645-4114-5

Also available:

CD and DVD Recording For Dummies (0-7645-5956-7)

Digital Photography All-in-One Desk Reference For Dummies (0-7645-7328-4)

Home Recording for Musicians For Dummies (0-7645-1634-5)

MP3 For Dummies (0-7645-0858-X)

Paint Shop Pro 8 For Du (0-7645-2440-2)

Photo Retouching & Restoration For Dumm (0-7645-1662-0)

Scanners For Dummies (0-7645-6790-X)

Photoshop Elements 2 For Dummies (0-7645-1675-2)

Digital Photos, Movies Music Gigabook For Dummies (0-7645-7414-0)

COMPUTER BASICS

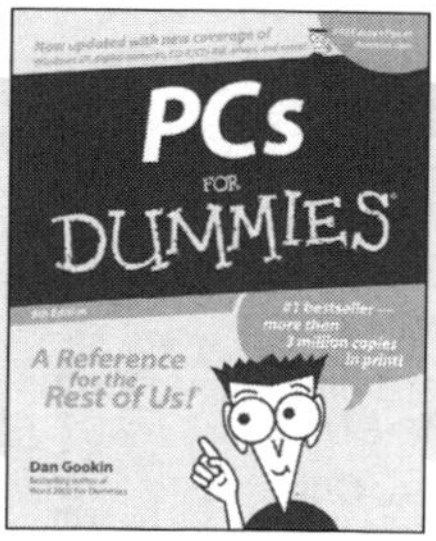

0-7645-4074-2

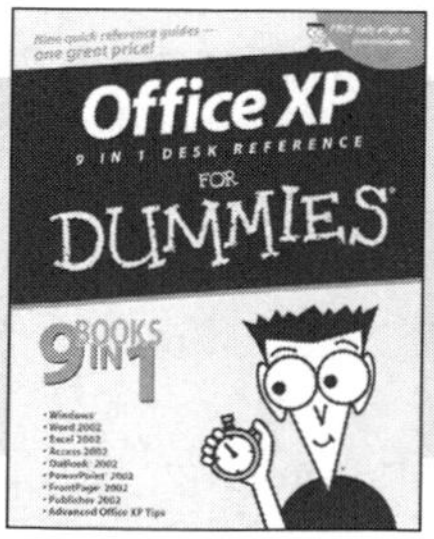

0-7645-0819-9

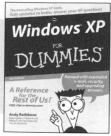

0-7645-7326-8

Also available:

PCs All-in-One Desk Reference For Dummies (0-7645-3941-8)

Pocket PC For Dummies (0-7645-1640-X)

Troubleshooting Your PC For Dummies (0-7645-1669-8)

Upgrading & Fixing PCs For Dummies (0-7645-1665-5)

Buying a Computer For Dummies (0-7645-7653-4)

Windows XP All-in-One Reference For Dummie (0-7645-7463-9)

Macs For Dummies (0-7645-5656-8)

Available wherever books are sold. For more information or to order direct go to www.wileyeurope.com or call 0800 243407 (Non UK call +44 1243 84